Functional Cognition and Occupational Therapy

A Practical Approach to Treating Individuals With Cognitive Loss

Edited by
Timothy J. Wolf, OTD, PhD, OTR/L, FAOTA; **Dorothy Farrar Edwards,** PhD;
and **Gordon Muir Giles,** PhD, OTR/L, FAOTA

AOTA PRESS

AOTA Vision 2025

Occupational therapy maximizes health, well-being, and quality of life for all people, populations, and communities through effective solutions that facilitate participation in everyday living.

Mission Statement

The American Occupational Therapy Association advances occupational therapy practice, education, and research through standard-setting and advocacy on behalf of its members, the profession, and the public.

AOTA Staff

Sherry Keramidas, *Executive Director*
Christopher M. Bluhm, *Chief Operating Officer*

Chris Davis, *Associate Chief Officer for AOTA Press and Content Strategy*
Caroline Polk, *Digital Manager and AJOT Managing Editor*
Ashley Hofmann, *Development/Acquisitions Editor*
Barbara Dickson, *Production Editor*

Rebecca Rutberg, *Director, Marketing*
Amanda Goldman, *Marketing Manager*
Jennifer Folden, *Marketing Specialist*

American Occupational Therapy Association, Inc.
4720 Montgomery Lane
Bethesda, MD 20814
Phone: 301-652-AOTA (2682)
Fax: 301-652-7711
www.aota.org
To order: 1-877-404-AOTA or store.aota.org

Disclaimers

This publication is designed to provide accurate and authoritative information in regard to the subject matter covered. It is sold or distributed with the understanding that the publisher is not engaged in rendering legal, accounting, or other professional service. If legal advice or other expert assistance is required, the services of a competent professional person should be sought.
—*From the Declaration of Principles jointly adopted by the American Bar Association and a Committee of Publishers and Associations*

It is the objective of the American Occupational Therapy Association to be a forum for free expression and interchange of ideas. The opinions expressed by the contributors to this work are their own and not necessarily those of the American Occupational Therapy Association.

ISBN: 978-1-56900-601-6
Ebook ISBN: 978-1-56900-477-7
Library of Congress Control Number: 2019937109

Cover design by Debra Naylor, Naylor Design, Inc., Washington, DC
Composition by Manila Typesetting Company, Manila, the Philippines
Printed by Automated Graphics, White Plains, MD

Contents

Boxes, Case Examples, Exhibits, Figures, Tables, Appendices, and Videos

Appendices

Videos

Videos are available online; see note on the inside front cover.

Acknowledgments

First, I want to acknowledge those who have worked in the area of functional cognition for many years, who made a book like this possible in the first place. I have had the great pleasure to count many of them as mentors, colleagues, and friends, and they have helped shape who I am as an occupational therapist. I specifically want to thank Carolyn Baum, Glen Gillen, Joan Toglia, Gordon Muir Giles, Dorothy Farrar Edwards, Leonard Matheson, Tracy Morrison, and Helene Polatajko. Second, I want to thank the faculty, staff, and students at the University of Missouri. Having your support while I worked on this project was vital, and I thank you all.

Last, but not least, I want to thank my family: my wife, Angie; my three boys, William, Henry, and Benjamin; and my extended family. I know it sounds cliché to say "I couldn't have done this without you," but I couldn't have done this without you. Thank you for always supporting me no matter what I jump into. I love you all.

—TIMOTHY J. WOLF

I have had the great pleasure to work with many extraordinary occupational therapy scholars over the course of my career. They generously supported my work and guided my research. In particular, I want to thank my colleague and research partner Carolyn Baum, who made it possible for me to join the community of occupational therapy scholars. I also want to thank Joan Rogers, Florence Clark, Winnie Dunn, Helene Polatajko, Elizabeth Skidmore, Noomi Katz, and Gordon Muir Giles for their guidance as I worked to bridge the gap between traditional neuropsychological and occupational science perspectives.

Also, my research has been brought to life by my students and now colleagues Tracy Morrison, Michelle Hahn, and Hui Chun Chen. My master's in occupational therapy and doctoral students at the University of Wisconsin–Madison, particularly Muhammad Al-Heizan and Timothy Marks, have made my contributions to this text possible. I also want to thank my partner, Jan Greenberg, who asked me to join him here at the University of Wisconsin in 2006. He has enriched my work and personal life in so many ways.

—DOROTHY FARRAR EDWARDS

I would like to thank the clients I have worked with for the education and inspiration with which they have provided me. I would also like to thank my colleagues at Crestwood Treatment Center and Idylwood Care Center, especially Lillian Fong and Karen Scott, and the faculty at Samuel Merritt University for making my working conditions endlessly fascinating and fun. Jo Clark-Wilson was my collaborator in developing the Neurofunctional Approach and has been my friend and a research partner for 30 years.

Working with my coeditors, Professors Dorothy Farrar Edwards and Timothy J. Wolf, has been a joy. The chapter authors, many of whom are leaders in the profession, have made the job of editing painless, and I thank them all. To my friends and loved ones, I would like to blame the demands of writing for not keeping my office tidy and not keeping up with my chores, but you all know better.

—GORDON MUIR GILES

Contributors

Muhammad O. Al-Heizan, MS, OT
Assistant Professor, Department of Rehabilitation Sciences
King Saud University
Riyadh, Saudi Arabia

Caroline Thompson Fellow
Department of Kinesiology–Occupational Therapy
University of Wisconsin–Madison
Madison

Peggy P. Barco, OTD, OTR/L, SCDCM, CDRS, FAOTA
Assistant Professor
Program in Occupational Therapy
Washington University School of Medicine in St. Louis
St. Louis

Carolyn M. Baum, PhD, OTR/L, FAOTA
Elias Michael Director, Program in Occupational Therapy
Professor of Occupational Therapy, Neurology, and Social Work
Washington University in St. Louis
St. Louis

Anna E. Boone, MSOT, PhD, OTR/L
Assistant Professor
Department of Occupational Therapy
University of Missouri
Columbia

Kari C. Burch, OTD, OTR/L
Occupational Therapist
Memory Care Home Solutions
St. Louis

Theressa Burns, OTR
Clinical Occupational Therapist Specialist
Geriatric Research, Education, and Clinical Center
Minneapolis Veterans Affairs Medical Center
Minneapolis

Denise Chisholm, PhD, OTR/L, FAOTA
Professor
University of Pittsburgh
Pittsburgh

John DeLuca, PhD
Senior Vice President for Research
Kessler Foundation
West Orange, NJ

Katherine Dittmann, BSc, MKin, MPT
Physiotherapist
St. John's Rehab
Sunnybrook Health Sciences Centre
Toronto

Physiotherapist
Princess Margaret Hospital
Toronto

Physiotherapist
The Ottawa Hospital
Ottawa

Meghan Doherty, OTD, OTR/L
Assistant Professor
Saint Louis University
St. Louis

Dorothy Farrar Edwards, PhD
Professor of Kinesiology–Occupational Therapy
University of Wisconsin–Madison
Madison

Jeremy Furniss, OTD, MS, OTR/L, BCG
Director of Quality
American Occupational Therapy Association
Bethesda, MD

Gordon Muir Giles, PhD, OTR/L, FAOTA
Professor
Samuel Merritt University
Oakland, CA

Director of Neurobehavioral Services
Crestwood Behavioral Health, Inc.
Sacramento, CA

Glen Gillen, EdD, OTR, FAOTA
Professor and Program Director
Columbia University Programs in Occupational Therapy
New York

Hortensia Gimeno, Dip (OT), MSc, PhD
Clinical Research Fellow
King's College London
London

Clinical Research Fellow
Evelina London Children's Hospital
London

Yael Goverover, PhD, OTR/L
Associate Professor
New York University
New York

Lou Ann Griswold, PhD, OTR/L, FAOTA
Associate Professor and Department Chair
Department of Occupational Therapy
University of New Hampshire
Durham

Margo B. Holm, PhD, OTR/L, FAOTA, ABDA
Professor Emerita
University of Pittsburgh
Pittsburgh

Alexis Lussier, MS, OTR/L
Mercy College
Dobbs Ferry, NY

Adina Maeir, PhD, OT
School Chair and Director of Graduate Studies
School of Occupational Therapy
The Hebrew University
Jerusalem

Sara McEwen, BSc (PT), MSc, PhD
Affiliate Scientist
St. John's Rehab Research Program
Sunnybrook Research Institute
Toronto

Assistant Professor
Department of Physical Therapy and Rehabilitation Science Institute
University of Toronto
Toronto

M. Tracy Morrison, OTD, OTR/L
President
Engage Health and Wellness Center, PLLC

Research Faculty
Occupational Therapy Program
University of Minnesota
Minneapolis

Helene Polatajko, BOT, MED, PhD, OT Reg. (Ont.), OT(C), FCAOT, FCAHS
Professor
Department of Occupational Science and Occupational Therapy
University of Toronto
Toronto

Joan C. Rogers, PhD, OTR, FAOTA
Professor Emerita
University of Pittsburgh
Pittsburgh

Shlomit Rotenberg, PhD, OT
Postdoctoral Fellow
Rotman Research Institute
Baycrest Health Sciences
Toronto

Sharmila Sandhu, JD
Counsel and Director of Regulatory Affairs
American Occupational Therapy Association
Bethesda, MD

Chelsea J. Steinberg, MS, OTR/L
Occupational Therapist
New York–Presbyterian/Weill Cornell
New York

Joan Toglia, PhD, OTR/L, FAOTA
Dean and Professor
Mercy College
Dobbs Ferry, NY

Jacqueline Wesson, BAppSc (OT), MA, PhD
Dementia Specialist and Research Coordinator
Montefiore Residential Care
Randwick, New South Wales, Australia

Honorary Postdoctoral Research Fellow
Ageing Work and Health Research Unit
Faculty of Health Sciences
University of Sydney
Sydney, Australia

Timothy J. Wolf, OTD, PhD, OTR/L, FAOTA
Associate Professor and Chair
Department of Occupational Therapy
University of Missouri
Columbia

Sharon Zlotnik, PhD, OTR/L
Occupational Therapist
University of Haifa
Haifa, Israel

Introduction

TIMOTHY J. WOLF, OTD, PhD, OTR/L, FAOTA; DOROTHY FARRAR EDWARDS, PhD; AND GORDON MUIR GILES, PhD, OTR/L, FAOTA

Cognitive rehabilitation has always been a broad tent without a clearly defined content area (American Occupational Therapy Association [AOTA], 2019). However, with its foundation in clinical neuropsychology, cognitive rehabilitation has been heavily dominated by impairment-based approaches. Such approaches seek to identify deficits in isolated cognitive functions and then address these deficits using remediation-based approaches.

Remediation-based approaches view cognitive functions as hierarchically organized, and within this hierarchy, cognitive abilities are treated like mental muscles that, when exercised with activities of gradually increasing difficulty, should improve. The goal of these approaches is that as clients' isolated cognitive functions improve, a broad translation will occur in which their ability to participate in everyday life activities that rely on these cognitive abilities will also improve (Giles, 2010).

Although remediation-based approaches have been popularized in the media for the general public and have seen years of use in clinical practice across diagnostic groups (e.g., traumatic brain injury, stroke, schizophrenia), their limitations are increasingly apparent to those in health care and in science (das Nair, Cogger, et al., 2016; das Nair, Martin, & Lincoln, 2016). Although they are conceptually appealing, cognitive remediation treatment programs have not been shown to improve performance of everyday life activities (Kumar et al., 2017). However, there is an emerging appreciation of alternative cognitive rehabilitation methods, such as strategy training, training in habits and routines, and environmental modification (Giles & Clark-Wilson, 1993), and different intervention methods, most of which can have a significant impact on occupational performance (AOTA, 2019).

In tandem with changes in how researchers and clinicians are thinking about intervention has been a change in how assessment of the skills that are requisite for occupational performance can be approached. Rather than isolating specific cognitive functions and trying to predict ADL and IADL capacity, clinicians are using more broad-based approaches to evaluate clients' abilities and to identify the competencies necessary for occupational performance. In particular, performance-based testing of the construct of *functional cognition* (defined in Chapter 1) has been identified as superior to other approaches, such as self-report or proxy report.

In general, functional cognition is thought of as how people integrate their cognitive abilities in the context of completing a real-world activity. As this text highlights, the concept of *functional cognition* is not new and has a long history in occupational therapy. Occupational therapists have been assessing and addressing functional cognition since the creation of the profession more than a hundred years ago.

The field has, however, lacked the standardization of measures to assess functional cognition, and a coordinated attempt is needed to integrate the multiple frameworks, assessments, and interventions that have been developed in this area in an effort to help disseminate knowledge to the profession in a way that will promote implementation into practice. Achievement of this goal is essential not only to best help the clients with cognitive challenges whom we serve but also to establish occupational therapy's primary role in the health care system in addressing functional cognition. This text was developed specifically to address this goal.

As the title *Functional Cognition and Occupational Therapy: A Practical Approach to Treating Individuals With Cognitive Loss* implies, this text is intended to serve as a practical guide for how to use a functional–cognitive approach with individuals with cognitive loss. Section I (Chapters 1 and 2) introduces the concept of functional cognition as it relates to other widely known theories and concepts of cognitive function. This section also includes a discussion of issues related to health care policy and how functional cognition fits within the rapidly evolving U.S. health care system. Most important, Section I uses existing evidence to establish why it is essential for occupational therapy practitioners to adopt a functional–cognitive approach in practice.

Section II (Chapters 3–16) is focused on assessment. Section II.A (Chapters 3–6) introduces principles central to functional–cognitive assessment and a framework for functional–cognitive assessment. These chapters provide context for the different forms of screening tools (both cognitive screening tools [e.g., the Montreal Cognitive Assessment, or MoCA; Nasreddine et al., 2005] and tools for screening functional cognition) and assessments used to evaluate cognitive function, how they fit together, and how to use them to inform treatment planning using a functional–cognitive approach.

Sections II.B and II.C review specific assessment tools that occupational therapists can use in practice. Section II.B (Chapters 7–12) focuses on the community and IADLs, and Section II.C (Chapters 13–16) focuses on the home and ADLs. All of these chapters focus on practical application of an assessment tool—where it came from, how it is used, how it is scored, how it is interpreted, how it fits in the framework of cognitive assessment, how to obtain the tool or more information about it, and how to use the information it provides to inform next steps. Almost all of these chapters have associated video content to help provide guidance on the use of the assessment in practice.

Section III (Chapters 17–21) is focused on intervention. Chapter 17 provides a framework for how to use the results of a functional–cognitive assessment to inform treatment planning. Key concepts that guide intervention are introduced and discussed, including concepts related to awareness, Learning Theory, and transfer. Chapters 18–21 review specific intervention approaches. Again, these chapters have a specific focus on practical application—where the assessment came from, whom it is appropriate for, how to use it, how to get trained or obtain more information, and so forth. These chapters also have associated video content to help demonstrate the approach for the reader.

Finally, the text ends with an appendix that includes 2 case examples, based on real clients, that apply the frameworks, processes, assessment tools, and intervention approaches discussed in the text.

To maximize their benefit from using this text, readers need to be aware of several points. First, a functional–cognitive approach requires occupational therapists to focus their efforts at the activity performance level. When the therapist is focused at this level, there is a continuity in the process of assessments and intervention that is grounded in an evidence-based approach to help individuals use their retained functional–cognitive ability to engage in activity, regardless of their condition.

As a result, the assessments and interventions discussed are not diagnosis specific, and this is reflected in the structure of this text. For example, readers will note there is no chapter titled "Treatment for Individuals With Traumatic Brain Injury." Disease etiology and prognosis, comorbid conditions, concurrent conditions, and the like are important in this approach inasmuch as they inform what a client's residual cognitive function may be and how their functional cognition may improve or deteriorate over time.

Second, we have attempted to maintain consistent language across chapters. One of the barriers to implementing knowledge into practice is the frequently inconsistent use of language within and between disciplines. A term such as *awareness*, for example, is used differently in occupational therapy than it is in neuropsychology. Therefore, when authors use this term to describe an assessment, the behavior to which they are referring can at times be unclear. As the editors of this text, we worked with the authors to use common terms to describe behaviors and also with the production team at AOTA Press to use common definitions for key terms in the chapters as much as possible. There may still be some instances in which the language is inconsistent, but we encourage the readers to evaluate how the terms are used in context and to tie a specific definition back to the common key terms.

Third, this text is focused mostly on adults. This is in large part because the majority of assessments and interventions that have been developed in the relatively new area of standardized functional cognition are intended for use in adult populations. This does not reflect that pediatric populations would not also benefit from a functional–cognitive approach, and in many ways functional–cognitive approaches are already more widely used and appreciated with the pediatric population. The frameworks, concepts, and general functional–cognitive approach used in this text still apply to children; however, some of the specific assessments may not. The intervention approaches discussed have been or are currently used in practice with pediatric populations.

Finally, as the editors, we worked with the publisher to select the specific assessments and intervention approaches discussed in this text. We took many considerations into account when making these selections, including evidence to support use, accessibility to practitioners, and preference given for tools and approaches developed by occupational therapists. We acknowledge that this text does not represent a comprehensive review of all the assessments and intervention approaches that are available for use in practice. Our goal was to make sure the text covered a broad spectrum and to include a framework that the readers could then use to fit other assessments and interventions into.

Like all of occupational therapy practice, the area of functional cognition is constantly evolving. We hope this text helps ignite a passion for this area of practice and continues the conversation and development of the science to help inform future versions of this text.

References

American Occupational Therapy Association. (2019). Cognition, cognitive rehabilitation, and occupational performance. *American Journal of Occupational Therapy*.

das Nair, R., Cogger, H., Worthington, E., & Lincoln, N. B. (2016). Cognitive rehabilitation for memory deficits after stroke. *Cochrane Database of Systematic Reviews, 9*, CD002293. https://doi.org/10.1002/14651858.CD002293.pub3

das Nair, R., Martin, K. J., & Lincoln, N. B. (2016). Memory rehabilitation for people with multiple sclerosis. *Cochrane Database of Systematic Reviews, 23*, CD008754. https://doi.org/10.1002/14651858.CD008754.pub3

Giles, G. M. (2010). Cognitive versus functional approaches to rehabilitation after traumatic brain injury: Commentary on a randomized controlled trial. *American Journal of Occupational Therapy, 64,* 182–185. https://doi.org/10.5014/ajot.64.1.182

Giles, G. M., & Clark-Wilson, J. (Eds.). (1993). *Brain injury rehabilitation: A neurofunctional approach.* San Diego: Singular.

Kumar, K. S., Samuelkamaleshkumar, S., Viswanathan, A., & Macaden, A. S. (2017). Cognitive rehabilitation for adults with traumatic brain injury to improve occupational outcomes. *Cochrane Database of Systematic Reviews, 20,* CD007935. https://doi.org/10.1002/14651858.CD007935.pub2

Nasreddine, Z. S., Phillips, N. A., Bédirian, V., Charbonneau, S., Whitehead, V., Collin, I., . . . Chertkow, H. (2005). The Montreal Cognitive Assessment, MoCA: A brief screening tool for mild cognitive impairment. *Journal of the American Geriatrics Society, 53,* 695–699. https://doi.org/10.1111/j.1532-5415.2005.53221.x

SECTION

Foundations

1

Understanding Functional Cognition

JACQUELINE WESSON, BAppSc (OT), MA, PhD,
AND GORDON MUIR GILES, PhD, OTR/L, FAOTA

LEARNING OBJECTIVES

After completing this chapter, readers should be able to

- Describe *functional cognition* as a construct and its importance to occupational therapy practitioners,
- Describe how *functional cognition* differs from *cognition* as typically defined and how assessment of functional cognition differs from other types of cognitive assessment,
- Identify why standardized performance-based testing is central to evaluation of functional cognition,
- Identify characteristics of performance-based tests of functional cognition,
- Describe common patterns of performance that indicate impaired functional cognition, and
- Describe how evidence from performance-based testing influences intervention selection.

KEY TERMS AND CONCEPTS

- Cognitive impairment • Cognitive load • Complexity • Dynamic–interactive assessment
- Ecological validity • Functional cognition • Intellectual self-awareness • Life roles • Metacognition
- Naturalistic observation • Occupational performance • Online self-awareness • Performance-based testing
- Performance efficiency • Top-down measures • Universal cognitive access

Exploring Functional Cognition and Its Advantages

Functional cognition combines the constructs of *function* and *cognition* and refers to the use of cognitive processes in the widest sense—in the context of performing everyday activities and occupations. Traditionally, cognition and function have been studied separately because of the way various disciplines have developed their theories, conceptualizations, and measurement techniques (Streiner et al., 2015).

Furthermore, occupational therapy practitioners historically have quantified an individual's function in terms of skill level in distinct, specifically defined activities, such as managing money or taking medication, rather than focusing on estimating the integration of cognitive abilities used to perform ADLs and IADLs. Bringing the constructs of function and cognition together is a timely and natural progression for occupational

therapy practitioners who believe that "cognitive functioning can only be understood and facilitated fully within the context of occupational performance" (American Occupational Therapy Association [AOTA], 2019). The term *functional cognition* refines the concept of ability, returning the attribute back to the person in the environmental context rather than describing it in relation to discrete tasks. It follows that assessing functional cognition is central to the concerns of practitioners and the profession's client-centered assessment practices.

The occupational therapy assessment of functional cognition is not intended to replace the assessment of distinct cognitive functions conducted by other disciplines, such as neuropsychology or speech–language therapy. An occupational therapy assessment of functional cognition differs from these assessments in that it takes place at the level of ***occupational performance*** and, as such, allows therapists to estimate the amount and type of support individuals need to manage the activity demands of their daily life.

Functional cognition is relevant to all life roles. It is a global, "top-down" construct that is not task limited. Functional cognition is conceptualized as incorporating

- Metacognition,

- Executive function (EF),

- Other cognitive domains,

- Performance skills (e.g., motor skills), and

- Performance patterns (e.g., habits, routines).

Rather than assess specific cognitive skills in isolation, the goal of functional–cognitive evaluation is to assess individuals' capacity to perform essential tasks given the totality of their abilities (including their use of strategies, habits and routines, and environmental resources). Accordingly, assessments are not constructed to quantify specific cognitive skills. Instead, individuals' ability to function despite the presence of particular cognitive deficits is the issue of interest. Functional cognition is more than the sum of its parts. It incorporates a conceptualization of both abilities and strengths simultaneously with impairment.

Assessing functional cognition can identify individuals who are having difficulty performing real-life tasks; as a result, the approach is generally applicable across patient populations (i.e., not to be limited to any 1 diagnostic group; Chaytor & Schmitter-Edgecombe, 2003; Chaytor et al., 2006).

The first use of the term *functional cognition* that approximated the current meaning was in teaching children with intellectual disability. The term described the use of realistic tasks in children's education, as opposed to more theoretical educational approaches (Turnure, 1985). Early researchers of functional cognition recognized the ability of individuals to perform tasks in the presence of **cognitive impairment** (i.e., functioning below expected normative levels, or loss of ability in any area of cognitive functioning), viewing this ability as "residual 'functional' cognition" (Labi et al., 1998, p. 46). Others have described a similar construct as *applied cognition* (Coster et al., 2004).

Pollard and Olin (2005) used the term in the context of Allen's (1985) Cognitive Disabilities Model, which proposes that functional cognition is the central construct evaluated by the model and its assessment tools (Allen et al., 2007). Allen and subsequent authors (e.g., Earhart, 2006) included discussions of the construct but did not provide a concise definition.

Donovan and colleagues (2008) defined *functional cognition* as "the ability to accomplish everyday activities that rely on cognitive abilities, such as locating keys, conveying information, or planning activities" (p. 122). However, this conceptualization retained a focus on the tasks to define ability and did not adequately incorporate the integration of performance components, such as motor and cognitive skills, or additional factors influencing ability, such as task complexity and the nature of the task environment. The earlier discussions therefore failed to fully capture the current conceptualization of functional cognition.

Recent definitions in the literature have highlighted the dynamic relationship between cognitive processes and occupational performance. *Functional cognition* has been defined simply as "the ability to use and integrate thinking and performance skills to accomplish complex everyday activities" (Giles et al., 2017, p. 1).

An extended conceptualization from Wesson et al. (2016) incorporated additional influences on occupational performance, with *functional cognition* defined as the "observable performance of everyday activities resulting from a dynamic interaction between motor abilities, activity demands and the task environment, which is guided by cognitive abilities" (p. 336). Wesson et al.'s definition includes how the activity and the environment contextualize performance. It offers an expanded framework that allows practitioners to consider opportunities to provide therapeutic interventions that are broader than targeting the individual alone.

Evaluating functional cognition prepares practitioners to consider the multifaceted nature of occupational performance (Bottari, Iliopoulos, et al., 2014; Giles et al., 2017). These elements include

- The individual's ability to use multiple cognitive processes during task performance,

- The environmental demands,

- Task complexity,

- The dynamic nature of naturalistic environments, and

- Whether the individual can adapt as 1 or more of these elements change during the enactment of a dynamic activity.

Individuals vary in their ability to synthesize and respond to all of these factors. Individuals with limited functional–cognitive ability may be unable to successfully perform novel activities that require on-the-spot decision making. In contrast, others with greater functional–cognitive resources are able to respond appropriately to more complex task demands involving novel problem solving, reasoning, and other EFs (Gold, 2012; McAlister et al., 2016; Willis, 1996).

Understanding functional–cognitive ability also helps to determine whether individuals' estimates of their own abilities (i.e., metacognition) either serves or hinders task performance. Adequate self-assessment influences individuals' use of strategies and whether they

- Recognize and correct errors,

- Perform activities based on concrete or abstract goals, and

- Apply skills consistently during task performance.

The practitioner can use such information to direct intervention. For example, some individuals may need approaches that compensate for their impaired cognitive processes directly, such as self-awareness training, or approaches that rely on strategy development and implementation. Others may need therapies that focus on specific activities—modifying or supporting performance through adaptive technologies, such as pill organizers to manage medications or checklists and cueing systems. Some individuals receive minimal direct intervention, and the focus of intervention with them is improving the support skills of the care provider. (Chapter 17, "Intervention Selection," discusses how assessment informs the process of selecting the mode of intervention.)

In occupational therapy, occupation is both the means and the end of therapy. Using occupation as the mediator of the evaluation process also has some distinct advantages. Individuals may be better motivated by and more likely to attempt tests that have better face validity. This approach to assessment also maximizes clinical utility by allowing a direct translation of assessment results to the types of intervention needed to support occupational performance (Schutz & Wanlass, 2009). In addition, the term *functional cognition* is neutral and avoids a focus on impairment or deficits.

Functional cognition is not an all-or-none phenomenon; it is a quality that all individuals possess to varying degrees— even in the presence of cognitive loss. It allows for a transition toward **universal cognitive access** (i.e., providing cognitive supports as a natural and intrinsic part of the lived environment) in communities for people who have impaired functional cognition—an extension of the concept of *universal physical access* that was advocated in the late 1980s. These advantages in terms of the acceptability of the assessment process, intervention selection, and neutral language give practitioners strong theoretical reasons for adopting functional cognition into their scope of practice and adjusting their clinical practice to ensure the construct is addressed in the occupational therapy evaluation process.

Approaches to Evaluating Functional Cognition

Occupational therapy practice centers on occupational performance and the client's engagement in culturally sanctioned and self-selected **life roles** (i.e., "behaviors expected by society and shaped by culture and context that may be further conceptualized and defined by the client"; AOTA, 2014, p. S27). Occupational therapists seek to understand the relationship between how individuals *attempt* an activity and their *actual* task performance.

Customarily, occupational therapists use **naturalistic observation** (i.e., watching what people do in context) of everyday activities or occupations that are meaningful to the client to assess abilities, using a sampling of behavior in context to infer general capacity. Therapists typically set up scenarios that are relevant to an individual and the individual's specific challenges, then make ad hoc performance-based observations to assess specific competencies, understanding that "function is what people do" (Allen et al., 1992, p. 4).

Part of occupational therapists' skill set is the ability to construct assessments that are highly relevant to individuals using everyday activities, so that the assessments have both face validity (i.e., an activity that the client is likely to recognize as relevant to their problem) and the appearance of predictive relevance (i.e., the client is likely to recognize the applicability of test results to real-life performance; Brown & Finlayson, 2013; Chaytor & Schmitter-Edgecombe, 2003; Douglas et al., 2013). Both the client and practitioner can believe in the integration between cognition and function through occupation-based assessment.

However, because these ad hoc scenarios are developed for a specific individual, the assessment procedures are not standardized, and there are no outside parameters against which to judge performance. There is no way to measure or compare competencies between clients to help establish performance norms, and occupational therapists must be aware of several potential biases when interpreting results. For example, therapists may rely on their own subjective opinion regarding what constitutes impairment (Douglas et al., 2007), and their individual ability to link performance specifically to cognitive processes may vary (Belchior, Korner-Bitensky, et al., 2015). Therapists are not always able to interpret performance accurately, especially with clients who have milder cognitive impairment (Belchior, Korner-Bitensky, et al., 2015; Bottari & Dawson, 2011; Bottari, Iliopoulos, et al., 2014). This limits the conclusions that can be drawn from nonstandardized assessment results about clients' competencies. Additionally, the absence of established psychometrics for these ad hoc assessments limits their currency outside of the profession.

A common situation practitioners encounter during discharge planning is being asked to determine whether individuals with cognitive impairment will be "safe" at home (Douglas et al., 2013). The therapist is really being asked to predict the risk that patients will engage in unsafe behaviors and their ability to avoid hazards. Historically, this question was often addressed with nonstandardized observations. The assumption made in these situations was that such assessments were able to predict individuals' future performance, but nonstandardized approaches do not have any established predictive validity (Giles et al., 2017). Moreover, such a dichotomous classification (i.e., safe or unsafe) is too simplistic, because it does not represent the scope of occupational performance.

Practitioners may often use familiar (overlearned and simple), nonstandardized measures in a "mechanical" process that provides limited information regarding functional–cognitive skills, especially the client's ability to adapt to new situations. Because "safe or unsafe" assessments are based on the often highly educated and experienced but nonetheless subjective view of practitioners, they may have little currency outside of the profession.

Many standardized measures to assess everyday activities are available, but there is no gold-standard instrument (Desai et al., 2004; Royall et al., 2007; Sikkes et al., 2009). Most measures assess basic ADLs, IADLs, or both, using either performance-based or questionnaire-based methods (Gold, 2012). Many combine both basic ADLs and IADLs, which makes it difficult to establish the nature of the discrete relationship between complex everyday activities and cognition (Loewenstein & Acevedo, 2010). Additionally, the number of functional domains that are assessed varies among measures, and the extent of in-depth examination within domains is also highly variable. There is little consensus regarding exactly what should be assessed (Gold, 2012).

Practitioners most commonly use questionnaires because they take less time to administer, can cover many functional areas, are less expensive, and can be completed as a self-report or by a proxy (Gold, 2012; Sikkes et al., 2009). However, self-report does not account for lack of insight or for various forms of reporter bias, with both under- and overreporting abilities observed (Doble et al., 1999; Farias et al., 2005; Jonas et al., 2011; Martyr & Clare, 2018).

Occupational therapy practitioners may use the results of neuropsychological testing to infer clients' ability to perform everyday activities, but the relationship between cognition and function has been described as modest, at best (Marcotte et al., 2010; McAlister et al., 2016; Royall et al., 2007). The strength of the relationship between neuropsychological measures and ADL–IADL function also varies according to the method used in the comparator assessment, such that use of different methods (e.g., questionnaires vs. performance-based measures) can result in markedly different degrees of association (Burton et al., 2009; Martyr & Clare, 2018; Schmitter-Edgecombe & Parsey, 2014).

Finally, many neuropsychological tests have limited face validity and so do not seem to meaningfully relate to individuals' everyday life. Such tests accordingly may have increased risk of being rejected by the test taker. Nevertheless, neuropsychological testing is important in providing specific information about cognition and may provide essential diagnostic information. It can help occupational therapists understand clients' capacities and develop occupational therapy interventions, but it has more limited utility in predicting functional performance.

Assessment of functional cognition is, by definition, performance based, because it involves test administrators directly observing individuals "executing a task in a real-world environment" (Belchior, Holmes, et al., 2015, p. 2) and provides "an objective behavioral evaluation of functional skills" (Loewenstein & Acevedo, 2010, p. 98). There is a growing consensus that subtle cognitive impairment is best evaluated with standardized, performance-based measures (Jekel et al., 2015; Puente et al., 2014; Wesson et al., 2016). Additionally, such measures have been shown to detect "preclinical disability" that is not identified with questionnaires (Puente et al., 2014; Rodakowski et al., 2014). Although there is a trend for newly developed measures to include everyday activities to improve *ecological validity* (i.e., the prediction or simulation of everyday life functions) across all disciplines (Marcotte et al., 2010), occupational therapists are particularly concerned with the refinement and validation of performance-based assessment of functional cognition.

Historical Development of Performance-Based Testing of Functional Cognition

The performance-based measures of functional cognition described in this text are the result of a gradual evolution of assessment practice, influenced by multiple factors. As noted, occupational therapists have a tradition of naturalistic observation, and Claudia Allen (1985) was 1 of the first therapists to address the need to standardize observational cognitive assessment. She worked with colleagues at the Eastern Pennsylvania Psychiatric Institute in the late 1960s, focusing on clients with severe and chronic mental illness who did not respond to the therapeutic approaches in use at the time (Allen et al., 2007; McCraith et al., 2011).

Allen (1982) hypothesized that individuals' cognitive abilities could be inferred through the observation of their voluntary motor actions and their use of objects in the context of performing meaningful activities. On the basis of systematic behavioral observations and analyses of patterns of behavior, Allen established a hierarchy for classifying different levels of cognitive ability, known as the *Allen Cognitive Level Scale* (Allen, 1985; Allen & Allen, 1987; Allen et al., 1992).

Together with her colleagues, Allen developed and tested a standardized screening tool of functional cognition—the Allen Cognitive Level Screen (ACLS; Allen et al., 2007). This instrument assesses functional cognition using leather lacing, an activity that is not mediated by language, to screen functional cognition. Information from the ACLS is interpreted with Allen's Cognitive Level Scale (Allen et al., 2007), and ACLS scores are validated against other assessments on the basis of Allen's (1985) Cognitive Disabilities Model or against observations of performance of everyday activities.

The ACLS and the Cognitive Disabilities Model have continued to develop, and therapists have used them internationally since their introduction in the late 1970s and 1980s (Burns et al., 2004; Gitlin et al., 2008; Mayer, 1988; Penny et al., 1995; Rojo-Mota et al., 2017; Scanlan & Still, 2013; Secrest et al., 2000). Other assessment tools include the Allen Diagnostic Module (Earhart, 2006) and the Routine Task Inventory-Expanded (Katz, 2006). Information from these assessments helps occupational therapists understand clients' "best ability to function" (Allen, 1985, p. 8) and thereby guides intervention and the functional cognition support needed to facilitate occupational performance.

A decade later, neuropsychologists Tim Shallice and Paul Burgess (1991) were encountering challenges with patients at the National Hospital for Neurological Diseases in the United Kingdom. The patients they described demonstrated no or only minor impairment on neuropsychological testing but were failing to manage their daily life in spectacular ways (Shallice & Burgess, 1991). Together, Shallice and Burgess developed the Multiple Errands Test (MET) to elicit the types of deficits that their clients were manifesting in their daily life.

The MET was based on ecological psychology theories focusing on behavioral assessment of people doing activities in unrestricted environments. This approach was very different from the theories guiding traditional neuropsychological assessment at the time. The MET requires test takers to navigate a shopping area, performing what seem to be simple tasks, and to develop their own solutions to task performance while under the constraint of unfamiliar rules (Shallice & Burgess, 1991).

It is assumed that adequate performance on the MET draws on the EFs of planning, problem solving, and response inhibition in a naturalistic social environment. However, occupational therapists have developed modified scoring systems that focus on behavioral performance. These rely on task completion and performance efficiency and are more consistent with a functional cognition framework (see Chapter 7, "The Executive Function Performance Test").

The MET was effective in identifying behavioral deficits not captured by standard neuropsychological measures. From a scientific perspective, however, it sacrificed the standardized control of the testing environment that is typical of neuropsychological tests, in favor of ecological validity. That is, as a consequence of using more real-world tasks in the assessment (for greater accuracy in predicting real-world performance), the test offered less clarity regarding environmental influences on test performance and therefore less clarity about what was being assessed (Marcotte et al., 2010; Rabin et al., 2007). Work continued on developing the MET (Alderman et al., 2003; Dawson et al., 2009), but this type of assessment was too far removed from the natural-science and laboratory-based traditional approach of neuropsychology to gain wide currency among most clinical psychologists or neuropsychologists (Rabin et al., 2007).

In response, Barbara Wilson et al. (1987, 1991, 2003), Paul Burgess (e.g., Wilson et al., 1996), and others (e.g., Robertson et al., 1994) developed tests that were intended to retain an ecologically valid approach but were more acceptable to psychologists, in that they continued to be both standardized and office based. These measures used simulated real-world scenarios to assess discrete cognitive functions and may be considered a hybrid approach between traditional neuropsychology testing and ***performance-based testing*** of functional cognition (an approach that "requires the patient to perform the particular activity under the observation of the examiner"; Loewenstein & Acevedo, 2010, p. 98). For example, the Behavioral Assessment of the Dysexecutive Syndrome (Wilson et al., 1996) presents several "practical scenarios" that are assessed with pencil-and-paper tasks (e.g., plotting how a person would search for a lost key in a field by drawing the search strategy on a sheet of paper).

Occupational therapists have refined and used the original MET (Clark et al., 2017; Dawson et al., 2009; Morrison et al., 2013), and, despite limitations in clinical utility due to lack of normative data, it continues to be used by therapists. It is probably the most sensitive performance-based test for the assessment of subtle impairments in functional cognition (Dawson et al., 2009; Morrison et al., 2015).

Other occupational therapists were aware of the limitations of pencil-and-paper-based tests taken in the office and moved toward using real-life practical activities to assess general competency in ADLs and IADLs. The 1990s were marked by an increased focus on cognition by therapists, who typically adopted assessments that were developed by other disciplines (Gillen, 2013). However, over time, several therapists have developed and tested occupation-based functional–cognitive assessments. These therapists started shifting the focus away from a neuropsychology lens, which pinpointed specific cognitive deficits, and onto performance skills: the "goal-directed actions that are observable as small units of engagement in daily life occupations" (AOTA, 2014, p. S7). Assessments were developed, such as

- The Performance Assessment of Self-Care Skills (PASS; Rogers & Holm, 1989; Rogers et al., 2016),

- The ADL-focused Occupation-Based Neurobehavioral Evaluation (Arnadottir, 1990, 2011),

- The Kitchen Task Assessment (Baum & Edwards, 1993), and, later,

- The Executive Function Performance Test (EFPT; Baum et al., 2003).

The work of these researchers and that of Joan Toglia (1998; Dynamic Interactional Model of Cognition) and Anne Fisher (Fisher & Jones, 2010a, 2010b; Assessment of Motor and Process Skills [AMPS]) in this period was influential in shifting how occupational therapists thought about occupational performance and cognition in context. The subsequent examination of the degree and types of support individuals needed to function in their environment was based on understanding how people use residual cognitive processes together to allow participation in everyday activities.

Both psychologists and occupational therapists continue to refine and develop performance-based tests. Examples from neuropsychology colleagues include

- The Day-Out Task (Schmitter-Edgecombe et al., 2012), and

- The Naturalistic Action Test (Giovannetti et al., 2008; Schwartz et al., 2003; Seidel et al., 2013).

More recent performance-based occupational therapy measures include

- The Kettle Test (Hartman-Maeir, Harel, & Katz, 2009);

- The IADL Profile (Bier et al., 2016; Bottari et al., 2009); and

- The Perceive, Recall, Plan, and Perform System of Task Analysis (Aubin et al., 2009; Nott & Chapparo, 2012).

Many additional measures discussed in later chapters of this text have been refined and validated for different populations.

As in other clinical situations where professional roles are blurred, the distinct professional lens and emphasis differentiate the contribution of occupational therapists from that of other disciplines (AOTA, 2019). Clinical neuropsychologists typically attempt to isolate specific cognitive deficits, understand specific neuropsychological mechanisms of multitasking and strategy-application disorders, or link performance with brain structures (Lezak et al., 2012). For example, Burgess and colleagues (2006; Marcotte et al., 2010) have used their work with the MET to go from "function to construct"—that is, seeking to backtrack from functional performance to the neurological mechanisms involved in task performance (Burgess et al., 2006).

Occupational therapists, conversely, use performance-based tests to determine how real-world performance breaks down and use more observable global processes (e.g., planning, initiation, organizing, sequencing) to find avenues to support functional performance. This distinct focus on real-world performance is central to the construct of functional cognition as developed by occupational therapists.

Characteristics of Performance-Based Tests of Functional Cognition

Performance-based measures of functional cognition are intended to capture aspects of cognitive ability that support performance of both simple and complex everyday activities. These standardized measures are essentially ***top-down measures:*** They allow for the direct observation of the individual's ability to perform tasks and to infer specific performance abilities. They may also be related to specific cognitive abilities (Al-Heizen et al., 2018; Baum & Katz, 2010; Douglas et al., 2007; Gillen, 2009). Occupation is the mediator of the assessments, which are presented in the form of activities with varying levels of complexity.

The assessment task is usually structured so that global cognitive processes (e.g., initiating, planning, multitasking) and strategy use can be evaluated. The latter may relate to either discrete cognitive steps, such as using mnemonics to improve memory components, or to global performance, which may include compensatory techniques. There is often a focus on novel problem-solving ability, and, in general, there may be more than 1 route to satisfactory performance. Functional–cognitive assessments have a greater emphasis on cognitive rather than physical skills, and they require the integration of multiple sources of information, the sequencing of multiple actions, or both, for goal completion (Giles et al., 2017).

Functional–cognitive abilities are influenced by habits and routines (e.g., self-organizational routines) that individuals develop through experience. The degree of familiarity with or novelty of the tasks or elements can differ among assessments. In many instances, the specific task used is likely to be novel, but some aspect of the activity may be familiar. Attempts to account for familiarity must be included in test interpretation, and some tests require the participant to rate their familiarity with the particular task or the testing environment.

For example, individuals taking the MET may be asked to rate their familiarity with the specific testing environment (e.g., hospital, shopping area). When being administered the ACLS, test takers are asked whether they have performed similar tasks before. Some people are familiar with sewing, but few have performed leather lacing or the specific complex stitch that is part of the test. Many participants taking the EFPT (Baum et al., 2008) have cooked pasta before, but none likely have done so using the particular equipment and instructions that are provided for the test.

In all cases, practitioners must consider previous experience when interpreting test results, because it may be related to level of independence (Morrison et al., 2013). Prior experience with an activity or with a location where testing takes place may support better test performance, suggesting greater competency than is actually present. Sometimes test takers must inhibit *prepotent* (i.e., overlearned, familiar, or frequent) response tendencies to perform the task adequately (Reason, 1990). In such scenarios, familiarity may be a disadvantage. For these reasons, the occupational profile is a central component of functional–cognitive assessment; it is necessary to select appropriate measures and to adequately interpret performance (see Chapter 5, "Occupational Profile").

Metacognition, or a person's self-awareness and regulation of their cognitive competencies, is also regarded as an important factor in mediating occupational performance. Individuals' own awareness of their competencies (or lack thereof), as derived from prior experience, has been termed ***intellectual self-awareness*** (Toglia, 2018b; Toglia & Kirk, 2000). This is a general awareness that exists and relates to overall functioning and is seen as contributing to individuals' strategy use. The ability to accurately assess the demands of an assessment task and to anticipate, monitor, and regulate ongoing task performance has been termed ***online self-awareness*** (Toglia, 2018b; Toglia & Kirk, 2000). Many performance-based tests of functional cognition map both intellectual self-awareness and online self-awareness of performance errors.

Occupational therapy practitioners can assess intellectual and online self-awareness by asking test takers to rate the degree of perceived difficulty, either before or after performing the assessment task. When test takers perceive the task as easily within their competency, they may be less likely to use strategies. Some functional cognition measures include a score for strategy use, and others have an after-test interview in which strategy use is explored but not scored.

Complexity is an element that is central to functional cognition measures, whether they are screening tools or in-depth assessments. Complex tasks are those that require integration of multiple sources of information or the completion of multiple action steps that are unfamiliar and necessitate problem solving. Practitioners can vary a measure's complexity by manipulating several parameters of the assessment itself or the conditions under which it is administered. These parameters may include

- The task and the number and sequencing of subtasks;

- Interactions between the test taker and test administrator, including instructions and rules;

- The test stimuli; and

- The testing environment.

The degree of variation in these parameters may be influenced by the purpose and context of the test, the clinical setting, and the population for whom the measure is intended. Increased complexity in an assessment affects the information-processing demands of the task, or the **cognitive load.** The complexity and cognitive load of the task together have an impact on the individual's ability to use strategies effectively (Toglia, 2018a): If the load is too high, then strategy use may be impaired.

Comparing different performance-based tests highlights various ways that practitioners manage complexity and cognitive load, by adjusting test instructions, task sequencing, and structure. To increase test complexity, practitioners can manipulate the type and amount of information that is provided initially and that the test taker has to retain "online" in working memory, alongside the amount of concurrently competing information (i.e., multitasking). For example, the PASS Medication Management Task instructions are presented serially, and the task therefore has less cognitive load (or complexity) than either the Weekly Calendar Planning Activity (WCPA; Toglia, 2015) or the MET (Chisholm et al., 2014).

In both the WCPA and the MET, all task requirements are presented at the beginning, and the test taker has to independently organize the overlapping and, in some cases, competing task demands (Morrison et al., 2013; Toglia, 2015). This has the effect of requiring more self-organization from the test taker. For example, adequate performance on the WCPA requires test takers to enter the "fixed" appointment first, but they must recognize and adopt this strategy without any guidance from the test instructions.

Further along this "structure" continuum, some performance-based tests are designed to reduce the type of inherent structure that is present in most tabletop tests. As a result, these less structured tests may achieve superior assessment of real-world functioning (Chaytor et al., 2006). Such minimally structured performance-based tests, which require test takers to create or impose their own organization, include the IADL Profile (Bottari et al., 2009, 2010) and the MET (Morrison et al., 2013; Shallice & Burgess, 1991). Evidence indicates that greater strategy use has been associated with superior task performance in several populations (Bottari, Wai Shun, et al., 2014; Tomaszewski Farias et al., 2018).

Practitioners can also increase the cognitive load by manipulating the rules of the assessment to constrain task performance and make it more challenging. These rules may be

familiar, naturally occurring, implicit conditions that arise within the test activities and therefore do not require inhibition of customary behaviors. However, some assessments add explicit rules that do require such inhibition (e.g., not talking to the test administrator), and others add unfamiliar rules that require inhibition and further complicate task performance (e.g., the MET rule for purchasing multiple items but not entering the same store twice; Morrison et al., 2013; Shallice & Burgess, 1991). Adequate performance in this example requires test takers to constrain actions and incorporate multiple rules, which they must consciously attend to as they perform the test activities, thereby increasing cognitive load.

Another factor that can influence the complexity of tasks in performance-based testing is the degree to which test administrators interact with test takers. When tasks are presented serially, there may be significant interaction with the test administrator, but some of the most complex assessments restrict communication with the test administrator, and there may even be a specific instruction not to speak to the administrator (e.g., WCPA, MET). Should this rule be broken, scoring penalties may be applied in a graded manner. Test administrators may also attempt to have test takers violate the prohibition against speaking to them—for example, by asking test takers questions. The intent of this strategy is to evaluate the extent to which test takers exercise inhibitory control by not answering (e.g., WCPA).

The materials used in assessments may also increase or decrease test complexity. Some assessments allow test takers to use their own familiar, everyday equipment and include potentially familiar and relevant activities (e.g., the AMPS). Although the majority use standardized items contained in a test battery or kit, some tests have a combination of both approaches (e.g., the PASS Medication Management Task has a home or clinic version using either test takers' own medications or clinic-based, simulated medications).

Familiarity with specific test items or appliances may impede or facilitate performance, as implicit knowledge structures (based on similarity with overlearned patterns and the frequency of performance) interact with the environment. For example, a cooking task with unfamiliar utensils, locations, and appliances may impose more cognitive load for someone with poorer functional cognition than the same cooking task in their own kitchen with familiar items and technology. This lack of familiarity may significantly disrupt task performance (Toglia, 2018a).

Assessments of functional cognition vary in how much they use the environmental context to increase cognitive load. Ensuring a stable testing environment is 1 way to limit load. For example, in some tests, test takers remain in a seated position, similar to traditional neuropsychological, tabletop testing, which is traditionally done at a bedside or in a quiet office space. This approach reduces the demands on cognitive-processing ability.

Other measures require some movement in a defined or limited space, such as a room—a kitchen is used commonly (e.g., PASS Cooking Task, EFPT Cooking Task). Other assessments may take place in a broader setting, such as a hospital lobby or a local shopping center, so that test takers have to move around in a (known or unknown) environment and interact with others, such as retail employees (e.g., purchasing items for the MET, going to the grocery store in the IADL Profile). In these cases, the potentially unpredictable social element is part of the test, and it may draw on some very general adaptive processes (Reason, 1990). This ability to manage novel and unpredictable situations is required for community independence (Toglia, 2018a).

Timed performance is a variable common to most neuropsychological assessments, but many performance-based tests of functional cognition do not penalize test takers for slow performance. In this case, the goal of an evaluation is generally to assess safety and independence rather than speed of processing per se. The time taken for individuals to perform the tasks may be recorded and may be included in a calculation of performance efficiency—but this may be seen as secondary, not the primary indicator of performance competency. (*Performance efficiency* considers the number of activities performed correctly in relation to time to test completion—e.g., locations visited in the MET–Revised—and allows for an integration of 2 factors that may indicate adequate or superior performance; Toglia, 2015.)

However, some functional–cognitive assessments record time, and these may have particular relevance to certain diagnostic groups. For example, studies show that individuals with mild neurocognitive disorders have impaired speed of performance (Tuokko et al., 2005; Wadley et al., 2008). In this context, specifying error types in performance, including taking excessive time, has been suggested as enabling therapists to "identify more specific areas of functional decline" (Belchior, Holmes, et al., 2015, p. 7).

A final element that is common to many performance-based tests of functional cognition is an evaluation of performance skills. The dynamic nature of performance-based tests often necessitates that test takers make regular adjustments to both motor and cognitive processes simultaneously to optimize performance. Cognitive habits and routines, such as an individual's approach to organization, also form part of the evaluation of performance skills. For example, an individual might have developed the lifelong habit of checking their work before completion.

In terms of quantifying ability, there are 2 distinct approaches used in performance-based tests of functional cognition, which can be classified as either categorical or dimensional (Streiner et al., 2015). The *categorical approach* involves a straightforward count of the number of correct responses, with parameters described for adequate performance. The attribute is categorized as either present or absent (i.e., the response was correct or incorrect).

The *dimensional approach* provides different information and has origins in the educational and developmental psychology theories of Lev Vygotsky, a Soviet psychologist in the first decades of the 1900s (Holm & Rogers, 2008; Vygotsky, 2000). The dimensional approach requires test administrators to be interactive during test administration. That is, test administrators use a *dynamic–interactive assessment* approach, noting the points of performance breakdown and providing the test takers with standardized cues to allow for successful task completion. When performing a dynamic–interactive assessment, occupational therapists establish the client's current level of performance without assistance, then provide necessary assistance in a hierarchical manner to improve task performance, thus determining the conditions and type of assistance that facilitate optimal performance in the context of existing cognitive impairment (Chisholm et al., 2014; Holm & Rogers, 2008).

This dimensional approach provides more information about the extent of impairment and the amount of support necessary to enable adequate performance (Chisholm et al., 2014; Holm & Rogers, 2008). It reflects the view that functional performance capacity is on a continuum, but the approach requires greater skill from test administrators (e.g., see Chapter 7 for the cueing hierarchy used systematically in the EFPT). In addition, scoring systems are usually more complex than assessments that use a categorical approach to testing.

Some assessments take this dynamic assessment approach (Toglia, 2018a) a step further and build in a cumulative assessment of individuals' ability to use feedback effectively. For example, the PASS Medication Management Task has test takers distribute pills from a pill box into an organizer twice. Test administrators can observe any change in performance on the 2nd pill distribution after any cueing that was required on the first distribution.

Toglia (2015) used a different method in the WCPA. The assessment is presented in standard form. Then a post-assessment interview is used as an opportunity for guided discovery (to probe strategy use and self-awareness) and to explore different strategies that test takers might use to complete the test requirements. The practitioner can then administer an alternative form of the test to examine any change in task performance as a result of the prior experience and guided discovery. Morrison et al. (2013) noted how the process of guided discovery through open-ended questions about task performance on the MET can inform post-assessment treatment. Repeat assessment on an alternative form can evaluate the integration of adaptive strategy use (Toglia, 2018a).

Performance-based measures of functional cognition can be used either for screening or for in-depth assessment (see Chapter 6, "Baseline Cognitive Screening Tools"). A performance-based screening tool is intended to indicate whether a particular individual is at high risk for deficits in functional cognition that are significant enough to impair occupational performance (Sedgwick, 2014). This may guide the selection of a specific measure, depending on the target population and the purpose of the evaluation (see Chapter 5, "Occupational Profile"), which is then reflected in the degree of complexity of the test or the evaluation approach overall.

Work by Hartman-Maeir, Katz, and Baum (2009) has helped provide a practical and synthesized approach to assessment of individuals with cognitive impairment. The Cognitive–Functional Evaluation (Bar-Haim Erez & Katz, 2018; Hartman-Maeir, Katz, & Baum, 2009; see Chapter 4, "The Cognitive–Functional Evaluation Framework") provides a framework for occupational therapists to combine different assessment processes to gain a comprehensive picture of individuals' functional–cognitive performance in everyday life.

Many performance-based measures have a particular theoretical conceptualization of occupational performance, and results of assessments are thus interpreted within this framework, which then guides intervention. For example, the Cognitive Performance Test (Burns, 2018; see Chapter 14) provides theoretical information about cognitive decline in the context of occupational performance, and a specific hierarchy of ability is used to interpret test results.

Interventions for functional cognition depend primarily on activity demands and the life context of the individuals being assessed, and the need for support is also influenced by individuals' level of self-awareness and potential for learning and change. Support may also be provided by others in the client's world (e.g., care partners for the person living with dementia modify the environment and ensure that tasks are set up); intervention is not always directed at the client with impaired functional cognition (Jensen & Padilla, 2017).

Common Observations of Performance During Functional–Cognitive Evaluation

Functional cognition is an attribute all individuals possess. Like the range of abilities observed for other skills and attributes, there is a continuum of functional cognition. Some individuals, depending on diagnosis and developmental processes, have limited ability to manage deviations from routine behaviors and to manage change. Others may seem to have strong self-awareness; good self-organizational and adaptive abilities; and the ability to successfully manage novel task demands, even those with a high cognitive load. The following discussion highlights some of the behaviors individuals may demonstrate during an evaluation of functional cognition.

Performance-based tests of functional cognition evaluate goal-directed behavior. At the most fundamental level, these assessments describe a goal state and ask test takers to perform certain actions to achieve it. This requires the ability to understand either a concrete or an abstract representation of the stated outcome or goal. Cognitive processes needed to achieve the goal may range from abstract conceptualizations to development of a series of straightforward actions.

The occupational therapist, or test administrator, observes whether test takers seem to understand the scope of task requirements, including the goal. They may evaluate whether the test taker develops and follows a plan and whether the plan was adequate. They may also look for "derailments"

where overlearned behaviors may override other intended actions. Additonally, if test takers make performance errors, the administrator evaluates their ability to notice these errors and to respond to cueing to correct their performance.

During testing, individuals with impaired functional cognition may demonstrate the following characteristics:

- *Fail to comprehend the goal.* The test taker may be unable to grasp the desired goal state and therefore may fail to understand the process of working toward the outcome. These individuals are not able to demonstrate goal-directed behavior and tend to be action focused rather than activity focused.

- *Fail to plan.* The test taker may impulsively engage in the behavioral components of the task prematurely without developing a plan. They may fail to listen to or follow instructions and so may never grasp key task parameters related to the outcome.

- *Oversimplify the task.* Test takers may simplify, miss, or omit key components of the task and fail to respond adequately. They again may seem to ignore parameters that are necessary for adequate task performance.

- *Fail to recognize errors or to monitor for errors.* Test takers may proceed with the task without checking whether actions comply with the desired outcome. That is, they may engage in behaviors that are incompatible with the goal state or deviate from a plan that they made but consider their performance complete without noticing errors or correcting them.

- *Recognize errors, but not self-correct.* Test takers may also "refuse" to correct errors when cued (often because they lack the capacity to correct them). They may still resist changing responses even when given direct assistance on how to do so.

- *Plan adequately but have poor execution and become derailed, often by preestablished behavior patterns.* Test takers may lose track of key steps in the task, missing necessary information or steps in the task, or may jump from 1 step to another in a haphazard or unpredictable order, which indicates inability to retain the goal state.

- *Reject the complexity of the task.* Test takers may seem overwhelmed by task demands. Responses may include a rapid or haphazard approach, with no or little attention paid to outcome or accuracy of performance (which is a form of task rejection based on being overwhelmed by perceived load).

Sometimes correct performance requires the use of novel stimuli or information. Some individuals are unable to generate suitable responses or to override previous learning or embedded routines to adapt to the new situation. In addition, some individuals may insert their own material into the testing environment (e.g., test takers enter their own routine appointments into the calendar in the WCPA or insist during the ACLS that the complex single cordovan stitch is a blanket stitch and proceed to produce the latter). Such individuals may be reliant on overlearned skills and habits to participate in everyday activities. Their behavior is procedurally based, demonstrating an inability to adapt to changes encountered in novel environments and situations.

Behaviors associated with good performance on assessment are generally related to metacognition, adequate plan development, and the consistent use of strategies that refine understanding and implementation of the actions required to obtain the specified goal state (Toglia, 2018b). When individuals perform well, test administrators may observe them to

- Ask clarifying questions,

- Take time to plan before initiating a response,

- Check and recheck instructions, and

- Compare intermediate states with task requirements frequently during task performance.

Despite impaired ability to adapt to novel task demands and circumstances, individuals with impaired functional cognition are still able to participate in everyday activities to a greater or lesser extent—people still "do things" and may manage to cope despite highly inefficient performance. Some people may not see a problem with their limitations, and, in fact, very mild impairments may be considered normative function for some of the population. Depending on individuals' life roles and expectations, some impairments may not be seen as barriers to community living by either the individuals or their family. The degree of functional cognition required by an individual depends greatly on their life roles. Therefore, it is crucial that occupational therapists consider the context and purpose of the functional–cognitive evaluation: The assessments they select should vary accordingly.

For example, it would be inappropriate to use the MET with someone who is moving into a supervised living setting—it has too high a floor to provide the clinical information that is required. The assessment should relate to the relevant occupational performance. In this example, that may include whether the individual can prepare their own food or needs help managing their medications. The functional cognition required to perform these skills may be more appropriately evaluated by a measure such as the PASS or the EFPT.

The Future of Functional Cognition

Functional cognition is a construct that has come of age, and a confluence of factors both within and outside occupational therapy support the profession's distinct approach to strengthening the occupational performance of individuals with impaired functional cognition. Internationally, government agencies are increasingly implementing consumer-directed care, and understanding functional cognition will help justify remuneration packages designed to support these individuals.

Changes in health care reimbursement practices will likely continue to move in the direction of supporting quality outcomes for individuals and move away from models that are based on procedures conducted by practitioners.

Research has demonstrated that occupational therapists using a functional–cognitive approach have been successful in improving quality outcomes for individuals. For example, Gitlin and her colleagues (2010, 2018) have worked with older adults living with dementia in the community and their care partners, incorporating a specific functional–cognitive approach to enhance activity engagement and improve care partners' well-being. Participants showed a reduction in the occurrence of behaviors known to precipitate nursing home placement and better ADL and IADL performance, and care partners demonstrated improved well-being. A recent report in the United States suggests that occupational therapy is the only health care discipline for which increasing expenditure reduces hospital readmissions (Rogers et al., 2017).

Also in the United States, in response to the Improving Medicare Post-Acute Care Transformation Act of 2014 (IMPACT Act; Pub. L. 113–185), the Centers for Medicare and Medicaid Services (CMS) are examining alternative data-collection processes. AOTA has been working with CMS to develop tools to identify people with less severe impairment who are at risk for hospital recidivism. The goal of this work is to allow occupational therapists to provide services to these individuals (Giles et al., 2017; see Chapter 3, "Principles of Functional–Cognitive Assessment").

AOTA has designated functional cognition as a research priority since 2015 (AOTA, 2017), and the Accreditation Council for Occupational Therapy Education (2012, 2018) in the United States has added functional cognition to the educational standards, so that occupational therapy training programs will need to include functional cognition in their curricula. National and international meetings of occupational therapists increasingly include presentations about functional cognition, and a recent survey of occupational therapy practitioners suggests that measures of functional cognition are finding their way into therapists' assessment practices (J. Furniss, personal communication, August 13, 2018).

Conclusion

Functional cognition represents a synthesis of ideas that have deep historical roots in the professional practice of occupational therapy. Many of the principles and practices described in this text are shared with other disciplines, but their combination represents a distinct occupational therapy approach to assessment and intervention. Assessment is performed through an examination of how individuals approach functional tasks, and intervention addresses ADL and IADL performance directly, to provide the supports that the individual needs.

Central to functional cognition is the recognition that occupational performance deficits need to be addressed directly, not indirectly through attempts to rehabilitate cognition as if cognitive processes were akin to a mental muscle. Despite apparent changes on brain scans and laboratory-based measures showing improvements after interventions that address cognition directly, evidence that these approaches translate to improved occupational performance is slight (AOTA, 2019; Bahar-Fuchs et al., 2013; Toglia, 2018b). Interventions that teach strategies, train skills, or improve occupational performance through changing the environment are receiving increased attention across professional disciplines (AOTA, 2019; Padilla, 2011).

Finally, using a functional–cognitive approach mitigates against devaluing individuals with cognitive limitations. It allows for the provision of cognitive support in ways that parallel the support provided to those managing physical challenges, by identifying specific strategies and environmental supports that enable occupational performance: It helps therapists better understand how to provide "universal cognitive access" for all. A functional–cognitive approach makes sense for everyone involved.

References

Accreditation Council for Occupational Therapy Education. (2012). 2011 Accreditation Council for Occupational Therapy Education (ACOTE®) standards. *American Journal of Occupational Therapy, 66*(6, Suppl.), S6–S74. https://doi.org/10.5014/ajot.2012.66S6

Accreditation Council for Occupational Therapy Education. (2018). 2018 Accreditation Council for Occupational Therapy Education (ACOTE®) standards and interpretative guide (effective July 31, 2020). American *Journal of Occupational Therapy, 72*(Suppl.2), 7212410005. https://doi.org/10.5014/ajot.2018.72S217

Alderman, N., Burgess, P. W., Knight, C., & Henman, C. (2003). Ecological validity of a simplified version of the Multiple Errands Shopping Test. *Journal of the International Neuropsychological Society, 9*, 31–44. https://doi.org/10.1017/S1355617703910046

Al-Heizen, M. O., Giles, G. M., Wolf, T. J., & Edwards, D. F. (2018). The construct validity of a new screening measure of functional cognitive ability: The Menu Task. *Neuropsychological Rehabilitation*, e-published ahead of print. https://doi.org/10.1080/09602011. 2018.1531767

Allen, C. K. (1982). Independence through activity: The practice of occupational therapy (psychiatry). *American Journal of Occupational Therapy, 36*, 731–739. https://doi.org/10.5014/ajot.36.11.731

Allen, C. K. (1985). *Occupational therapy for psychiatric diseases: Measurement and management of cognitive disabilities*. Boston: Little, Brown.

Allen, C. K., & Allen, R. E. (1987). Cognitive disabilities: Measuring the social consequences of mental disorders. *Journal of Clinical Psychiatry, 48*, 185–190.

Allen, C. K., Austin, S. L., David, S. K., Earhart, C. A., McCraith, D. B., & Riska-Williams, L. (2007). *Manual for the Allen Cognitive Level Screen–5 (ACLS–5) and Large Allen Cognitive Level Screen–5 (LACLS–5)*. Camarillo, CA: ACLS & LACLS Committee.

Allen, C. K., Earhart, C. A., & Blue, T. (1992). *Occupational therapy treatment goals for the physically and cognitively disabled*. Rockville, MD: AOTA Press.

American Occupational Therapy Association. (2014). Occupational therapy practice framework: Domain and process (3rd ed.). *American Journal of Occupational Therapy, 68*(Suppl. 1), S1–S48. https://doi.org/10.5014/ajot.2014.682006

American Occupational Therapy Association. (2017). *Role of occupational therapy in assessing functional cognition*. Retrieved from https://www.aota.org/Advocacy-Policy/Federal-Reg-Affairs/Medicare/Guidance/role-OT-assessing-functional-cognition.aspx

American Occupational Therapy Association. (2019). Cognition, cognitive rehabilitation, and occupational performance. *American Journal of Occupational Therapy*.

Arnadottir, G. (1990). *Brain and behavior: Assessing cortical dysfunction through activities of daily living (ADL)*. St. Louis: Mosby.

Arnadottir, G. (2011). Impact of neurobehavioral deficits on activities of daily living. In G. Gillen (Ed.), *Stroke rehabilitation: A function-based approach* (3rd ed., pp. 456–500). St. Louis: Elsevier/Mosby.

Aubin, G., Chapparo, C., Gélinas, I., Stip, E., & Rainville, C. (2009). Use of the Perceive, Recall, Plan and Perform System of Task Analysis for persons with schizophrenia: A preliminary study. *Australian Occupational Therapy Journal, 56*, 189–199. https://doi.org/10.1111/j.1440-1630.2007.00725.x

Bahar-Fuchs, A., Clare, L., & Woods, B. (2013). Cognitive training and cognitive rehabilitation for mild to moderate Alzheimer's disease and vascular dementia. *Cochrane Database of Systematic Reviews, 6*, CD003260. https://doi.org/10.1002/14651858.CD003260.pub2

Bar-Haim Erez, A., & Katz, N. (2018). Cognitive Functional Evaluation. In N. Katz & J. Toglia (Eds.), *Cognition, occupation, and participation across the lifespan: Neuroscience, neurorehabilitation, and models of intervention in occupational therapy* (4th ed., pp. 69–85). Bethesda, MD: AOTA Press.

Baum, C. M., Connor, L. T., Morrison, T., Hahn, M., Dromerick, A. W., & Edwards, D. F. (2008). Reliability, validity, and clinical utility of the Executive Function Performance Test: A measure of executive function in a sample of people with stroke. *American Journal of Occupational Therapy, 62*, 446–455. https://doi.org/10.5014/ajot.62.4.446

Baum, C., & Edwards, D. F. (1993). Cognitive performance in senile dementia of the Alzheimer's type: The Kitchen Task Assessment. *American Journal of Occupational Therapy, 47*, 431–436. https://doi.org/10.5014/ajot.47.5.431

Baum, C. M., & Katz, N. (2010). Occupational therapy approach to assessing the relationship between cognition and function. In T. D. Marcotte & I. Grant (Eds.), *Neuropsychology of everyday functioning* (pp. 63–90). New York: Guilford.

Baum, C. M., Morrison, T., Hahn, M., & Edwards, D. F. (2003). *Executive Function Performance Test: Test protocol booklet*. St Louis: Washington University School of Medicine.

Belchior, P., Holmes, M., Bier, N., Bottari, C., Mazer, B., Robert, A., & Kaur, N. (2015). Performance-based tools for assessing functional performance in individuals with mild cognitive impairment. *Open Journal of Occupational Therapy, 3*(3). https://doi.org/10.15453/2168-6408.1173

Belchior, P., Korner-Bitensky, N., Holmes, M., & Robert, A. (2015). Identification and assessment of functional performance in mild cognitive impairment: A survey of occupational therapy practices. *Australian Occupational Therapy Journal, 62*, 187–196. https://doi.org/10.1111/1440-1630.12201

Bier, N., Belchior, P. C., Paquette, G., Beauchemin, É., Lacasse-Champagne, A., Messier, C., . . . Bottari, C. (2016). The Instrumental Activity of Daily Living Profile in aging: A feasibility study. *Journal of Alzheimer's Disease, 52*, 1361–1371. https://doi.org/10.3233/JAD-150957

Bottari, C., Dassa, C., Rainville, C., & Dutil, E. (2009). The factorial validity and internal consistency of the Instrumental Activities of Daily Living Profile in individuals with a traumatic brain injury. *Neuropsychological Rehabilitation, 19*, 177–207. https://doi.org/10.1080/09602010802188435

Bottari, C., Dassa, C., Rainville, C., & Dutil, E. (2010). A generalizability study of the Instrumental Activities of Daily Living Profile. *Archives of Physical Medicine and Rehabilitation, 91*, 734–742. https://doi.org/10.1016/j.apmr.2009.12.023

Bottari, C., & Dawson, D. R. (2011). Executive functions and real-world performance: How good are we at distinguishing people with acquired brain injury from healthy controls? *OTJR: Occupation,*

Participation and Health, 31(Suppl.), S61–S68. https://doi.org/10.3928/15394492-20101108-10

Bottari, C., Iliopoulos, G., Wai Shun, P. L., & Dawson, D. R. (2014). The clinical reasoning that guides therapists in interpreting errors in real-world performance. *Journal of Head Trauma Rehabilitation, 29,* E18–E30. https://doi.org/10.1097/HTR.0000000000000029

Bottari, C., Wai Shun, P. L., Dorze, G. L., Gosselin, N., & Dawson, D. (2014). Self-generated strategic behavior in an ecological shopping task. *American Journal of Occupational Therapy, 68,* 67–76. https://doi.org/10.5014/ajot.2014.008987

Brown, C. L., & Finlayson, M. L. (2013). Performance measures rather than self-report measures of functional status predict home care use in community-dwelling older adults. *Canadian Journal of Occupational Therapy, 80,* 284–294. https://doi.org/10.1177/0008417413501467

Burgess, P. W., Alderman, N., Forbes, C., Costello, A., Coates, L. M., Dawson, D. R., . . . Channon, S. (2006). The case for the development and use of "ecologically valid" measures of executive function in experimental and clinical neuropsychology. *Journal of the International Neuropsychological Society, 12,* 194–209. https://doi.org/10.1017/S1355617706060310

Burns, T. (2018). *Cognitive Performance Test (revised manual).* Pequannock, NJ: Maddak.

Burns, T., McCarten, J. R., Adler, G., Bauer, M., & Kuskowski, M. A. (2004). Effects of repetitive work on maintaining function in Alzheimer's disease patients. *American Journal of Alzheimer's Disease and Other Dementias, 19,* 39–44. https://doi.org/10.1177/153331750401900109

Burton, C. L., Strauss, E., Bunce, D., Hunter, M. A., & Hultsch, D. F. (2009). Functional abilities in older adults with mild cognitive impairment. *Gerontology, 55,* 570–581. https://doi.org/10.1159/000228918

Chaytor, N., & Schmitter-Edgecombe, M. (2003). The ecological validity of neuropsychological tests: A review of the literature on everyday cognitive skills. *Neuropsychology Review, 13,* 181–197. https://doi.org/10.1023/B:NERV.0000009483.91468.fb

Chaytor, N., Schmitter-Edgecombe, M., & Burr, R. (2006). Improving the ecological validity of executive functioning assessment. *Archives of Clinical Neuropsychology, 21,* 217–227. https://doi.org/10.1016/j.acn.2005.12.002

Chisholm, D., Toto, P., Raina, K., Holm, M., & Rogers, J. (2014). Evaluating capacity to live independently and safely in the community: Performance Assessment of Self-Care Skills. *British Journal of Occupational Therapy, 77,* 59–63. https://doi.org/10.4276/030802214X13916969447038

Clark, A. J., Anderson, N. D., Nalder, E., Arshad, S., & Dawson, D. R. (2017). Reliability and construct validity of a revised Baycrest Multiple Errands Test. *Neuropsychological Rehabilitation, 27,* 667–684. https://doi.org/10.1080/09602011.2015.1117981

Coster, W. J., Haley, S. M., Ludlow, L. H., Andres, P. L., & Ni, P. S. (2004). Development of an applied cognition scale to measure rehabilitation outcomes. *Archives of Physical Medicine and Rehabilitation, 85,* 2030–2035. https://doi.org/10.1016/j.apmr.2004.05.002

Dawson, D. R., Anderson, N. D., Burgess, P., Cooper, E., Krpan, K. M., & Stuss, D. T. (2009). Further development of the Multiple Errands Test: Standardized scoring, reliability, and ecological validity for the Baycrest version. *Archives of Physical Medicine and Rehabilitation, 90*(Suppl.), S41–S51. https://doi.org/10.1016/j.apmr.2009.07.012

Desai, A. K., Grossberg, G. T., & Sheth, D. N. (2004). Activities of daily living in patients with dementia: Clinical relevance, methods of assessment and effects of treatment. *CNS Drugs, 18,* 853–875. https://doi.org/10.2165/00023210-200418130-00003

Doble, S. E., Fisk, J. D., & Rockwood, K. (1999). Assessing the ADL functioning of persons with Alzheimer's disease: Comparison of family informants' ratings and performance-based assessment findings. *International Psychogeriatrics, 11,* 399–409. https://doi.org/10.1017/S1041610299006018

Donovan, N. J., Kendall, D. L., Heaton, S. C., Kwon, S., Velozo, C. A., & Duncan, P. W. (2008). Conceptualizing functional cognition in stroke. *Neurorehabilitation and Neural Repair, 22,* 122–135. https://doi.org/10.1177/1545968307306239

Douglas, A. M., Letts, L. J., Richardson, J. A., & Eva, K. W. (2013). Validity of predischarge measures for predicting time to harm in older adults. *Canadian Journal of Occupational Therapy, 80,* 19–27. https://doi.org/10.1177/0008417412473577

Douglas, A., Liu, L., Warren, S., & Hopper, T. (2007). Cognitive assessments for older adults: Which ones are used by Canadian therapists and why. *Canadian Journal of Occupational Therapy, 74,* 370–381. https://doi.org/10.2182/cjot.07.010

Earhart, C. A. (2006). *Allen Diagnostic Module: Manual* (2nd ed.). Colchester, CT: S&S Worldwide.

Farias, S. T., Mungas, D., & Jagust, W. (2005). Degree of discrepancy between self and other-reported everyday functioning by cognitive status: Dementia, mild cognitive impairment, and healthy elders. *International Journal of Geriatric Psychiatry, 20,* 827–834. https://doi.org/10.1002/gps.1367

Fisher, A. G., & Jones, K. B. (2010a). *Assessment of Motor and Process Skills: Vol. 1: Development, standardization, and administration manual* (7th ed.). Ft. Collins, CO: Three Star Press.

Fisher, A. G., & Jones, K. B. (2010b). *Assessment of Motor and Process Skills: Vol. 2: User manual* (7th ed.). Ft. Collins, CO: Three Star Press.

Giles, G. M., Edwards, D. F., Morrison, M. T., Baum, C., & Wolf, T. J. (2017). Screening for functional cognition in postacute care and the Improving Medicare Post-Acute Care Transformation (IMPACT) Act of 2014. *American Journal of Occupational Therapy, 71,* 7105090010. https://doi.org/10.5014/ajot.2017.715001

Gillen, G. (2009). *Cognitive and perceptual rehabilitation: Optimizing function.* St. Louis: Elsevier/Mosby.

Gillen, G. (2013). A fork in the road: An occupational hazard? *American Journal of Occupational Therapy, 67,* 641–652. https://doi.org/10.5014/ajot.2013.676002

Giovannetti, T., Bettcher, B. M., Brennan, L., Libon, D. J., Burke, M., Duey, K., . . . Wambach, D. (2008). Characterization of everyday functioning in mild cognitive impairment: A direct assessment approach. *Dementia and Geriatric Cognitive Disorders, 25,* 359–365. https://doi.org/10.1159/000121005

Gitlin, L. N., Arthur, P., Piersol, C., Hessels, V., Wu, S. S., Dai, Y., & Mann, W. C. (2018). Targeting behavioral symptoms and functional decline in dementia: A randomized clinical trial. *Journal of the American Geriatrics Society, 66,* 339–345. https://doi.org/10.1111/jgs.15194

Gitlin, L. N., Winter, L., Burke, J., Chernett, N., Dennis, M. P., & Hauck, W. W. (2008). Tailored activities to manage neuropsychiatric behaviors in persons with dementia and reduce caregiver burden: A randomized pilot study. *American Journal of Geriatric Psychiatry, 16,* 229–239. https://doi.org/10.1097/01.JGP.0000300629.35408.94

Gitlin, L. N., Winter, L., Dennis, M. P., Hodgson, N., & Hauck, W. W. (2010). Targeting and managing behavioral symptoms in individuals with dementia: A randomized trial of a nonpharmacological intervention. *Journal of the American Geriatrics Society, 58,* 1465–1474. https://doi.org/10.1111/j.1532-5415.2010.02971.x

Gold, D. A. (2012). An examination of instrumental activities of daily living assessment in older adults and mild cognitive impairment. *Journal of Clinical and Experimental Neuropsychology, 34,* 11–34. https://doi.org/10.1080/13803395.2011.614598

Hartman-Maeir, A., Harel, H., & Katz, N. (2009). Kettle Test—A brief measure of cognitive functional performance: Reliability and validity in stroke rehabilitation. *American Journal of Occupational Therapy, 63,* 592–599. https://doi.org/10.5014/ajot.63.5.592

Hartman-Maeir, A., Katz, N., & Baum, C. M. (2009). Cognitive Functional Evaluation (CFE) process for individuals with suspected cognitive disabilities. *Occupational Therapy in Health Care, 23,* 1–23. https://doi.org/10.1080/07380570802455516

Holm, M. B., & Rogers, J. C. (2008). The Performance Assessment of Self-Care Skills (PASS). In B. Hemphill-Pearson (Ed.), *Assessments in occupational therapy mental health* (2nd ed., pp. 101–110). Thorofare, NJ: Slack.

Improving Medicare Post-Acute Care Transformation Act of 2014, Pub. L. 113–185, 42 U.S.C. § 1305 et seq.

Jekel, K., Damian, M., Wattmo, C., Hausner, L., Bullock, R., Connelly, P. J., . . . Frölich, L. (2015). Mild cognitive impairment and deficits in instrumental activities of daily living: A systematic review. *Alzheimer's Research and Therapy, 7,* 17. https://doi.org/10.1186/s13195-015-0099-0

Jensen, L., & Padilla, R. (2017). Effectiveness of environment-based interventions that address behavior, perception, and falls in people with Alzheimer's disease and related major neurocognitive disorders: A systematic review. *American Journal of Occupational Therapy, 71,* 7105180030. https://doi.org/10.5014/ajot.2017.027409

Jonas, C., Schiffczyk, C., Lahmeyer, C., Mueller, F., & Riepe, M. W. (2011). Staging dementia using proxy-reported activities of daily living. *Dementia and Geriatric Cognitive Disorders, 32,* 111–117. https://doi.org/10.1159/000331420

Katz, N. (2006). *Routine Task Inventory–Expanded (RTI–E) manual.* Retrieved from http://www.allen-cognitive-network.org/images/stories/pdf_files/rtimanual2006.pdf

Labi, M. L. C., Brentjens, M., Shaffer, K., Weiss, C., & Zielezny, M. A. (1998). Functional Cognition Index©: A new instrument to assess cognitive disability after traumatic brain injury. *Journal of Neurologic Rehabilitation, 12,* 45–51. https://doi.org/10.1177/154596839801200201

Lezak, M. D., Howieson, D. B., Bigler, E. D., & Tranel, D. (2012). *Neuropsychological assessment* (5th ed.). New York: Oxford University Press.

Loewenstein, D., & Acevedo, A. (2010). The relationship between instrumental activities of daily living and neuropsychological performance. In T. D. Marcotte & I. Grant (Eds.), *Neuropsychology of everyday functioning* (pp. 93–112). New York: Guilford.

Marcotte, T. D., Scott, J. C., Kamat, R., & Heaton, R. K. (2010). Neuropsychology and the prediction of everyday functioning. In T. D. Marcotte & I. Grant (Eds.), *Neuropsychology of everyday functioning* (pp. 5–38). New York: Guilford.

Martyr, A., & Clare, L. (2018). Awareness of functional ability in people with early-stage dementia. *International Journal of Geriatric Psychiatry, 33,* 31–38. https://doi.org/10.1002/gps.4664

Mayer, M. A. (1988). Analysis of information processing and cognitive disability theory. *American Journal of Occupational Therapy, 42,* 176–183. https://doi.org/10.5014/ajot.42.3.176

McAlister, C., Schmitter-Edgecombe, M., & Lamb, R. (2016). Examination of variables that may affect the relationship between cognition and functional status in individuals with mild cognitive impairment: A meta-analysis. *Archives of Clinical Neuropsychology, 31,* 123–147. https://doi.org/10.1093/arclin/acv089

McCraith, D., Austin, S., & Earhart, C. (2011). The cognitive disabilities model in 2011. In N. Katz (Ed.), *Cognition, occupation, and participation across the lifespan: Neuroscience, neurorehabilitation, and models of intervention in occupational therapy* (3rd ed., pp. 383–406). Bethesda, MD: AOTA Press.

Morrison, M. T., Edwards, D. F., & Giles, G. M. (2015). Performance-based testing in mild stroke: Identification of unmet opportunity for occupational therapy. *American Journal of Occupational Therapy, 69,* 6901360010. https://doi.org/10.5014/ajot.2015.011528

Morrison, M. T., Giles, G. M., Ryan, J. D., Baum, C. M., Dromerick, A. W., Polatajko, H. J., & Edwards, D. F. (2013). Multiple Errands Test–Revised (MET–R): A performance-based measure of executive function in people with mild cerebrovascular accident. *American Journal of Occupational Therapy, 67,* 460–468. https://doi.org/10.5014/ajot.2013.007880

Nott, M. T., & Chapparo, C. (2012). Exploring the validity of the Perceive, Recall, Plan and Perform System of Task Analysis: Cognitive strategy use in adults with brain injury. *British Journal of Occupational Therapy, 75,* 256–263. https://doi.org/10.4276/030802212X13383757345067

Padilla, R. (2011). Effectiveness of interventions designed to modify the activity demands of the occupations of self-care and leisure for people with Alzheimer's disease and related dementias. *American Journal of Occupational Therapy, 65,* 523–531. https://doi.org/10.5014/ajot.2011.002618

Penny, N. H., Mueser, K. T., & North, C. T. (1995). The Allen Cognitive Level Test and social competence in adult psychiatric patients. *American Journal of Occupational Therapy, 49,* 420–427. https://doi.org/10.5014/ajot.49.5.420

Pollard, D., & Olin, D. W. (2005). *Allen's cognitive levels: Meeting the challenges of client focused services: A guide for health care professionals working in acute care, skilled nursing facilities and home care settings* (2nd ed.). Monona, WI: SelectOne Rehab.

Puente, A. N., Terry, D. P., Faraco, C. C., Brown, C. L., & Miller, L. S. (2014). Functional impairment in mild cognitive impairment evidenced using performance-based measurement. *Journal of Geriatric Psychiatry and Neurology, 27,* 253–258. https://doi.org/10.1177/0891988714532016

Rabin, L. A., Burton, L. A., & Barr, W. B. (2007). Utilization rates of ecologically oriented instruments among clinical neuropsychologists. *Clinical Neuropsychologist, 21,* 727–743. https://doi.org/10.1080/13854040600888776

Reason, J. T. (1990). *Human error.* Cambridge, England: Cambridge University Press. https://doi.org/10.1017/CBO9781139062367

Robertson, I. H., Ward, T., Ridgeway, V., & Nimmo-Smith, I. (1994). *The Test of Everyday Attention.* Bury St. Edmunds, England: Thames Valley Test Company.

Rodakowski, J., Skidmore, E. R., Reynolds, C. F., III, Dew, M. A., Butters, M. A., Holm, M. B., . . . Rogers, J. C. (2014). Can performance on daily activities discriminate between older adults with normal cognitive function and those with mild cognitive impairment? *Journal of the American Geriatrics Society, 62,* 1347–1352. https://doi.org/10.1111/jgs.12878

Rogers, A. T., Bai, G., Lavin, R. A., & Anderson, G. F. (2017). Higher hospital spending on occupational therapy is associated with lower readmission rates. *Medical Care Research and Review, 74,* 668–686. https://doi.org/10.1177/1077558716666981

Rogers, J. C., & Holm, M. B. (1989). *Performance Assessment of Self-Care Skills.* Pittsburgh: University of Pittsburgh.

Rogers, J. C., Holm, M. B., & Chisholm, D. (2016). *Performance Assessment of Self-Care Skills (PASS–Clinic; Version 4.1).* Pittsburgh: University of Pittsburgh.

Rojo-Mota, G., Pedrero-Pérez, E. J., Huertas-Hoyas, E., Merritt, B., & MacKenzie, D. (2017). Allen Cognitive Level Screen for the classification of subjects treated for addiction. *Scandinavian Journal of Occupational Therapy, 24,* 290–298. https://doi.org/10.3109/11038128.2016.1161071

Royall, D. R., Lauterbach, E. C., Kaufer, D., Malloy, P., Coburn, K. L., & Black, K. J. (2007). The cognitive correlates of functional status: A review from the Committee on Research of the American Neuropsychiatric Association. *Journal of Neuropsychiatry and Clinical Neurosciences, 19,* 249–265. https://doi.org/10.1176/jnp.2007.19.3.249

Scanlan, J. N., & Still, M. (2013). Functional profile of mental health consumers assessed by occupational therapists: Level of independence and associations with functional cognition. *Psychiatry Research, 208,* 29–32. https://doi.org/10.1016/j.psychres.2013.02.032

Schmitter-Edgecombe, M., McAlister, C., & Weakley, A. (2012). Naturalistic assessment of everyday functioning in individuals with mild cognitive impairment: The Day-Out Task. *Neuropsychology, 26,* 631–641. https://doi.org/10.1037/a0029352

Schmitter-Edgecombe, M., & Parsey, C. M. (2014). Cognitive correlates of functional abilities in individuals with mild cognitive impairment: Comparison of questionnaire, direct observation, and performance-based measures. *Clinical Neuropsychologist, 28,* 726–746. https://doi.org/10.1080/13854046.2014.911964

Schutz, L. E., & Wanlass, R. L. (2009). Interdisciplinary assessment strategies for capturing the elusive executive. *American Journal of Physical Medicine and Rehabilitation, 88,* 419–422. https://doi.org/10.1097/PHM.0b013e3181a0e2d3

Schwartz, M. F., Buxbaum, L. J., Ferraro, M., Veramonti, T., & Segal, M. (2003). *The Naturalistic Action Test.* Bury St. Edmunds, England: Thames Valley Test Company.

Secrest, L., Wood, A. E., & Tapp, A. (2000). A comparison of the Allen Cognitive Level Test and the Wisconsin Card Sorting Test in adults with schizophrenia. *American Journal of Occupational Therapy, 54*, 129–133. https://doi.org/10.5014/ajot.54.2.129

Sedgwick, P. (2014). Measuring the perfomance of screening tests. *BMJ, 348*, g4438. https://doi.org/10.1136/bmj.g4438

Seidel, G. A., Giovannetti, T., Price, C. C., Tanner, J., Mitchell, S., Eppig, J., & Libon, D. J. (2013). Neuroimaging correlates of everyday action in dementia. *Journal of Clinical and Experimental Neuropsychology, 35*, 993–1005. https://doi.org/10.1080/13803395.2013.844773

Shallice, T., & Burgess, P. W. (1991). Deficits in strategy application following frontal lobe damage in man. *Brain, 114*, 727–741. https://doi.org/10.1093/brain/114.2.727

Sikkes, S. A., De Lange-de Klerk, E. S., Pijnenburg, Y. A., Scheltens, P., & Uitdehaag, B. M. (2009). A systematic review of instrumental activities of daily living scales in dementia: Room for improvement. *Journal of Neurology, Neurosurgery, and Psychiatry, 80*, 7–12. https://doi.org/10.1136/jnnp.2008.155838

Streiner, D. L., Norman, G. R., & Cairney, J. (2015). *Health measurement scales: A practical guide to their development and use* (5th ed.). Oxford, England: Oxford University Press. https://doi.org/10.1093/med/9780199685219.001.0001

Toglia, J. P. (1998). A dynamic interactional model to cognitive rehabilitation. In N. Katz (Ed.), *Cognition and occupation in rehabilitation: Cognitive models for intervention in occupational therapy* (pp. 5–50). Bethesda, MD: American Occupational Therapy Association.

Toglia, J. (2015). *Weekly Calendar Planning Activity (WCPA): A performance test of executive function.* Bethesda, MD: AOTA Press.

Toglia, J. (2018a). The Dynamic Interactional Model and the Multicontext Approach. In N. Katz & J. Toglia (Eds.), *Cognition, occupation, and participation across the lifespan: Neuroscience, neurorehabilitation, and models of intervention in occupational therapy* (4th ed., pp. 355–385). Bethesda, MD: AOTA Press.

Toglia, J. (2018b). Self-awareness and metacognition: Effect on occupational performance and outcome across the lifespan. In N. Katz & J. Toglia (Eds.), *Cognition, occupation, and participation across the lifespan: Neuroscience, neurorehabilitation, and models of intervention in occupational therapy* (4th ed., pp. 143–163). Bethesda, MD: AOTA Press.

Toglia, J., & Kirk, U. (2000). Understanding awareness deficits following brain injury. *NeuroRehabilitation, 15*, 57–70.

Tomaszewski Farias, S., Schmitter-Edgecombe, M., Weakley, A., Harvey, D., Denny, K. G., Barba, C., . . . Willis, S. (2018). Compensation strategies in older adults: Association with cognition and everyday function. *American Journal of Alzheimer's Disease and Other Dementias, 33*, 184–191. https://doi.org/10.1177/1533317517753361

Tuokko, H., Morris, C., & Ebert, P. (2005). Mild cognitive impairment and everyday functioning in older adults. *Neurocase, 11*, 40–47. https://doi.org/10.1080/13554790490896802

Turnure, J. E. (1985). Communication and cues in the functional cognition of the mentally retarded. *International Review of Research in Mental Retardation, 13*, 43–77. https://doi.org/10.1016/S0074-7750(08)60232-3

Vygotsky, L. S. (2000). *Thought and language.* Cambridge, MA: MIT Press.

Wadley, V. G., Okonkwo, O., Crowe, M., & Ross-Meadows, L. A. (2008). Mild cognitive impairment and everyday function: Evidence of reduced speed in performing instrumental activities of daily living. *American Journal of Geriatric Psychiatry, 16*, 416–424. https://doi.org/10.1097/01.JGP.0000310780.04465.13

Wesson, J., Clemson, L., Brodaty, H., & Reppermund, S. (2016). Estimating functional cognition in older adults using observational assessments of task performance in complex everyday activities: A systematic review and evaluation of measurement properties. *Neuroscience and Biobehavioral Reviews, 68*, 335–360. https://doi.org/10.1016/j.neubiorev.2016.05.024

Willis, S. L. (1996). Everyday cognitive competence in elderly persons: Conceptual issues and empirical findings. *Gerontologist, 36*, 595–601. https://doi.org/10.1093/geront/36.5.595

Wilson, B. A., Alderman, N., Burgess, A. W., Emslie, H., & Evans, J. J. (1996). *Behavioural Assessment of the Dysexecutive Syndrome.* Bury St. Edmunds, England: Thames Valley Test Company.

Wilson, B. A., Cockburn, J., & Baddeley, A. (1991). *The Rivermead Behavioural Memory Test.* Bury St. Edmunds, England: Thames Valley Test Company.

Wilson, B. A., Cockburn, J., & Baddeley, A. D. (2003). *The Rivermead Behavioural Memory Test* (2nd ed.). London: Pearson Assessment.

Wilson, B. A., Cockburn, J., & Halligan, P. W. (1987). *Behavioural Inattention Test: Manual.* London: Thames Valley Test Company.

2

Functional Cognition in the Health Care System

SHARMILA SANDHU, JD,
AND JEREMY FURNISS, OTD, MS, OTR/L, BCG

LEARNING OBJECTIVES

After completing this chapter, readers should be able to

- Describe the relationship of the Patient Protection and Affordable Care Act of 2010 and the Triple Aim to current Medicare reimbursement,
- Discuss how functional cognition can affect the quality of occupational therapy evaluation and intervention, and
- Identify Medicare standardized data elements that are related to cognition.

KEY TERMS AND CONCEPTS

- Bundled payment • Improving Medicare Post-Acute Care Transformation Act of 2014 • Medicare Access and CHIP Reauthorization Act of 2015 • National Quality Strategy • Patient-driven groupings model • Patient-driven payment model • Patient Protection and Affordable Care Act of 2010 • Prospective payment systems • Quadruple Aim • Triple Aim

Overview

The U.S. health care system is experimenting with a reimbursement shift from rewarding the volume of services provided to rewarding the value of services provided. Beginning almost 2 decades ago, 2 major Institute of Medicine reports (IOM, 2000, 2002) highlighted the need to focus on the quality of care and value of services rather than the quantity. In these reports, the IOM called for a redesign of the U.S. health care system and fundamental changes to improve the quality of care provided. These documents also outlined overarching principles and specific strategies that could be used to accomplish these goals.

Although value-based payment is a relatively simple concept—reimburse providers for high-value care—implementing a value-based health care reimbursement system across the highly fragmented U.S. health care system is a monumental challenge. Providers, purchasers, and health plans are all experimenting with ways to increase the value of services—to pay more for better health care and to pay less (or nothing) for worse health care (Conrad et al., 2014).

Medicare, Medicaid, and insurers have reconfigured payments to providers to incentivize value in 2 ways:

1. Reimbursing a bundled payment or flat fee on the basis of client characteristics

2. Reimbursing a differential payment on the basis of the reporting of quality measures at either the individual practitioner or the institutional level.

A *bundled payment* is when an organization receives a single payment for all services provided (Finkelstein et al., 2018). Both strategies are intended to enhance the quality of care and to deincentivize the overutilization of health care services.

These shifts in reimbursement policies provide new opportunities for occupational therapy practitioners. By assessing and addressing impairments in functional cognition, practitioners can demonstrate added value to patient outcomes by helping clients achieve improved functional independence. In addition, occupational therapists can demonstrate the value of their professional services to the health system as a whole by

* Providing more cost-efficient care,

* Reducing caregiver burden, and

* Decreasing overall resource utilization.

This chapter reviews functional cognition in the context of Medicare reimbursement policy.

Essential Considerations

In an effort to drive quality improvement and increase the value of health care services to Medicare beneficiaries, Congress recently passed 3 major pieces of legislation. These bills have created significant changes in Medicare policies and clinical processes. The **Patient Protection and Affordable Care Act of 2010** (ACA; Pub. L. 111–148) restructured the way health care coverage is administered, offered, and accepted. It emphasized a systematic approach to focusing on the value of health care services.

The **Improving Medicare Post-Acute Care Transformation Act of 2014** (IMPACT Act; Pub. L. 113–185) changed the way Medicare Part A services are provided in postacute care (PAC) settings, including skilled nursing facilities, home health agencies, inpatient rehabilitation facilities, and long-term care hospitals. The act fueled changes in Medicare Part A PAC services. In addition to implementing the changes required by the IMPACT Act, the Centers for Medicare and Medicaid Services (CMS) are also making significant changes to the **prospective payment systems,** which determine reimbursement for services in PAC settings before the service is furnished to a client, on the basis of a specific set of assessment characteristics.

Furthermore, the **Medicare Access and CHIP [Children's Health Insurance Program] Reauthorization Act of 2015** (MACRA; Pub. L. 114–10), which was intended to further the effects of an earlier Medicare program called the *Physician Quality Reporting System* (PQRS), reshaped the way that Medicare Part B outpatient services are reimbursed (Leland et al., 2015). Each of these acts and the resulting regulations created opportunity for occupational therapy practitioners to engage and demonstrate value in the area of functional cognition.

ACA: Setting the Stage for Value

In 2010, enactment of the ACA demonstrated the U.S. government's strong commitment to quality health care by requiring that the secretary of the U.S. Department of Health and Human Services (HHS) establish the **National Quality Strategy** (NQS; Agency for Healthcare Research and Quality [AHRQ], 2016), an approach to unite stakeholders from the public and private sectors to make higher quality health care available to all Americans. The NQS pursues 3 broad aims, referred to as the **Triple Aim:**

1. *Better care:* Make health care more patient centered, reliable, accessible, and safe.

2. *Healthy people and healthy communities:* Improve the health of the U.S. population by supporting proven interventions to address behavioral, social, and environmental determinants of health, in addition to delivering higher quality care.

3. *Affordable care:* Reduce the cost of quality health care for individuals, families, employers, and the government.

Many organizations acknowledge that focusing on these areas will also have an impact on providers and have now adopted the **Quadruple Aim,** which adds a 4th goal to the Triple Aim: improving the provider experience (Sikka et al., 2015).

The NQS created a framework that guided the development of the IMPACT Act, MACRA, and many other reimbursement and provider changes. In particular, the NQS identified key points of control "levers" that can be used to advance the Triple Aim. Among others, these levers include

* Measurement,

* Public reporting, and

* Payment (AHRQ, 2016).

Each of these levers is put into practice through the enactment of the legislation and regulations discussed below.

The ACA also established accountable care organizations (ACOs) to incentivize physicians and other providers to work together to provide more coordinated care to their patients. ACOs agree

* To take responsibility for the cost and quality of their patients' care,

* To improve care coordination and safety, and

* To promote appropriate use of preventive health services, with any subsequent financial savings being shared with the ACO.

Recently, a report from CMS (2016) found mixed results with the Pioneer ACO models. Other alternative health care payment models that potentially affect occupational therapists include

* Episode-based and bundled payments,

* Shared savings programs,

* Pay for performance,

* Medical homes, and

* Comprehensive primary care initiatives (Miller, 2018).

These models have potential for occupational therapy, especially as they continue to develop. See Box 2.1 for definitions of each of these models.

IMPACT Act: Emphasizing Client Characteristics

On September 18, 2014, Congress passed the IMPACT Act, which focuses on the measurement lever identified in the NQS. In an effort to standardize a series of measures, including

BOX 2.1. Alternative Payment Models for Health Care

- *Bundled payments:* A single payment for all services provided related to a specific condition (Finkelstein et al., 2018). Bundled payments are a type of episode-based payment and include a "group of services that tend to belong together clinically, potentially making care redesign for bundles easier for health systems to implement" (Navathe et al., 2017, p. 2371).
- *Comprehensive primary care initiatives:* Originally 1 of the largest public–private alternative payment models tested. CMS partnered with private payers to provide care management fees to primary care organizations and to share savings between payers and providers (Anglin et al., 2017).
- *Episode-based payments:* A fixed payment for all services over a period of time (e.g., 90 days, 120 days; Navathe et al., 2017).
- *Medical homes:* A patient-centered medical home is a concept of health care delivery that emphasizes "patients' ongoing relationship with a personal physician; team approaches to care; a whole-person orientation; mechanisms to support care integration, quality, safety and access; and payment for added value" (Crabtree et al., 2010, p. S80).
- *Pay for performance:* A program whereby a payer provides additional payment to organizations that meet or exceed benchmarks in quality improvement. The program may also apply penalties to organizations that do not meet benchmarks in quality improvement (Ryan et al., 2014).
- *Shared savings programs:* A program that includes an agreement between a provider and a payer. The provider agrees to monitor quality of care and reduce costs for the payer. If successful, the provider receives a portion of the savings as an additional payment (McWilliams et al., 2018).

functional cognition, across PAC offerings, the act requires the submission of standardized data by

- Long-term care hospitals (LTCHs),
- Skilled nursing facilities (SNFs),
- Home health agencies, and
- Inpatient rehabilitation facilities (IRFs).

The IMPACT Act requires, among other significant activities, the reporting of standardized patient-assessment data with regard to quality measures, resource use, and other measures.

In addition to "function, cognitive function, and changes in function and cognitive function" (Section 2[c][1][a]), the IMPACT Act identifies 7 other domains to be standardized by CMS:

1. Skin integrity and changes in skin integrity
2. Medication reconciliation
3. Incidence of major falls
4. Transfer of health information and care preferences when an individual transitions from 1 facility to another facility or to the community
5. Resource-use measures, including total estimated Medicare spending per beneficiary

6. Discharge to the community
7. All-condition risk-adjusted potentially preventable hospital readmissions rates.

Each PAC provider must report standardized patient-assessment data to CMS at admission and discharge. In addition to defining the 7 newly standardized domains, the IMPACT Act also

- Requires PAC providers to report common and consistent data with existing and new assessment tools. These data are necessary for reporting patient assessment, quality comparisons, resource-use measurement, and payment reform.
- Protects the patient's choice and access to care while encouraging use of quality data in discharge planning. This approach allows for comparable data across PAC settings to inform future PAC payment reforms.
- Provides Congress with detailed information about new payment models to consider for future PAC payment reforms, including a site-neutral unified payment model.

To date, CMS has made significant progress in measuring function and changes in function that are sensitive to the practice of occupational therapy. The organization has introduced standardized data elements in Section GG of each PAC assessment instrument based on items from the Continuity Assessment

Record and Evaluation (CARE) tool (Gage et al., 2012). These instruments include

- The Inpatient Rehabilitation Facility Patient Assessment Instrument,

- The Minimum Data Set (CMS, 2018b) in SNFs,

- The Outcome and Assessment Information Set (OASIS; CMS, 2018a) for home health agencies, and

- The Long-Term Care Hospital Continuity Assessment Record and Evaluation (Sandhu et al., 2018).

Read more about these self-care and mobility items and American Occupational Therapy Association (AOTA) engagement at www.aota.org/care.

CMS focused on the use of a particular set of assessment items, or data elements, originally developed as part of the Post-Acute Care Payment Reform Demonstration Project, called the CARE Item Set (CMS, n.d.). However, AOTA argued in a series of meetings with CMS and CMS's contractor, RAND Corporation, that there are considerable limitations in the proposed CARE Item Set. Without augmentation, the item set would provide only limited data on individuals with mild but functionally significant cognitive and IADL impairment.

AOTA, along with a work group of member experts, met with CMS and RAND officials beginning in May 2015. The association has been actively involved in discussions, including through appointments to 7 critical CMS technical expert panel meetings, to provide expertise and feedback regarding the profession's clinical and administrative implementation concerns.

The Medicare assessments currently include the Confusion Assessment Method (CAM) for delirium (Wei et al., 2008) and the Brief Interview for Mental Status (BIMS) for moderate to severe problems with memory and orientation (Saliba et al., 2012). The CAM is Item C1310 in the Minimum Data Set for SNFs and Item C1610 in the Long-Term Care Hospital Continuity Assessment Record and Evaluation. The CAM and the BIMS both do a nice job of meeting these goals.

The BIMS and CAM data elements are not sufficient to understand whether a person is able to use cognitive capacities to complete tasks needed to live independently, such as IADLs (Giles et al., 2017). AOTA and member experts are participating in an ongoing dialogue with CMS regarding these policy issues (Giles et al., 2017).

CMS has also established common data elements for cognition. The language of the IMPACT Act states that cognition is specifically referenced in relation to the required collection of standardized patient-assessment data in several key domains. In Section 2(b)[B](ii), cognitive function is described as the "ability to express ideas and to understand." The same paragraph describes mental status using the examples of "dementia and depression."

It is important for occupational therapy practitioners to understand what data are collected by CMS on cognition and to contribute when possible. In Section GG, as of the date of publication of this chapter, the assessments require documentation of prior functioning for functional cognition. Although this may be an easy element for occupational therapy practitioners to overlook, it is critical because it is used to risk-adjust reimbursement and quality measures.

CMS uses a relatively limited definition of *functional cognition*: the person's "need for assistance with planning regular tasks, such as shopping or remembering to take medication" (ID No. GG0100D; CMS, 2018b, p. 17). The item is to be scored on the basis of the person's ability "prior to the current illness, exacerbation, or injury" (CMS, 2018b, p. 17). The item can be coded as "independent," "needed some help," "dependent," "unknown," or "not applicable."

Note that the exact terminology used by CMS may change from year to year. In this chapter, when we refer to the terminology used in the CMS assessments, we also provide the item number. Readers can find the current terminology used by visiting the CMS Data Element Library (https://del.cms.gov) and searching by ID. In this example, the ID used to look up the data element is GG0100D.

Each PAC assessment instrument also includes unique variables to assess cognitive function. These important data elements are discussed below. Functional cognition is a critical element that is not fully captured by the CMS instruments. Occupational therapy practitioners should be familiar with the data elements for cognition but also should have an in-depth understanding of how functional cognition affects a person's ability to participate in meaningful activities. Being able to provide the right interventions at the right time to the right people in the area of functional cognition provides distinct value.

Prospective Payment Systems: New Reimbursement Models in PAC

Another lever identified by the NQS is payment. Medicare, 1 of the nation's largest payers for health care, is making significant changes to the way that Part A inpatient services are reimbursed. The data elements that capture information about the client's cognition play an increasingly important role in determining payment rates. Perhaps the best examples of these changes are the recent overhauls CMS has made to the prospective payment systems that pay for SNFs and home health agencies.

SNFs

SNFs have most recently been reimbursed on the basis of resource utilization groups, which are calculated on the basis of the resources used to care for the beneficiaries during the Part A SNF stay. The more rehabilitation minutes, including occupational therapy, a person received while in the SNF, the higher the reimbursement.

In 2019, SNFs will transition to the new *patient-driven payment model,* which only uses the patient's characteristics to determine payment (Acumen, 2018). In this new model, the SNF will no longer be reimbursed at a higher rate on the basis of the volume of therapy, including occupational therapy, that each client receives. This transition was driven by several factors, not the least of which was reports of SNF fraud and abuse.

SNF billing practices in the highest reimbursement category indicated that patients might have received therapy services that were not medically necessary. SNFs also might have billed Medicare for therapy services that were never actually provided to clients so that the highest possible reimbursement level could be obtained. Several HHS Office of Inspector General investigations were launched, resulting in a number of lawsuits and settlements with SNFs.

Under the patient-driven payment model, reimbursement is determined by a number of factors, including

- The beneficiary's condition that caused the original acute care admission,

- Cognitive status, and

- Functional ability.

The shift to paying for the Medicare Part A SNF benefit on the basis of patients' clinical characteristics rather than services means that providers, including occupational therapy practitioners, must be able to demonstrate value to the clients. They can do this by demonstrating improved quality measure scores (e.g., self-care, mobility) and by demonstrating that the services are benefitting the clients on the basis of their goals.

Home Health Agencies
To qualify for the Medicare Part A home health benefit, the patient must

- Be homebound;

- Be under the care of a physician; and

- Need skilled nursing or therapy services, which must be certified by a physician.

The prospective payment system for home health uses the OASIS to gather quality information and to calculate payment rates. The OASIS gathers data on the patient's

- Discharge needs,

- ADLs,

- Living arrangements,

- Support systems,

- Equipment management,

- Medications,

- Diagnosed conditions,

- Psychosocial status, and

- Physical status.

On the basis of the data submitted from the OASIS, software made available to providers by CMS calculates the appropriate home health resource group for payment. The resource group is partially determined by the number of therapy visits provided to the beneficiary.

In 2019, it is expected that home health will move away from payment that is partially defined by the services provided and toward payment that is defined by characteristics of the beneficiary with the ***patient-driven groupings model*** (PDGM). The PDGM determines reimbursement entirely on the basis of the patient characteristics, similar to the new SNF payment model, and is no longer tied in any meaningful way to the Medicare beneficiary's need for therapy services, including occupational therapy.

Before the implementation of PDGM, reimbursement was partially determined by the number of therapy visits a beneficiary received: If a client received visits over a certain threshold, reimbursement increased. Under PDGM, the number of therapy visits has no impact on reimbursement. The agency receives the same payment no matter how many occupational therapy visits are provided.

IRFs
The prospective payment system for IRFs uses a standard base rate that is adjusted by various factors. This system uses medical diagnoses to establish the reimbursement rate on the basis of a case mix group. Adjustments to the payment rate are made on the basis of age and comorbidities, in addition to the diagnosed psychiatric condition. Payments also are adjusted on the basis of length of stay. Beneficiaries who are admitted to an IRF are required to receive at least 3 hours of therapy 5 days a week. The reimbursement level does not change on the basis of the amount of therapy provided.

LTCHs
LTCHs treat patients who are clinically very complex and need 25 or more days of skilled service. These patients have very acute or chronic conditions that require extended services, including rehabilitation, respiratory therapy, pain management, treatment of traumatic brain injury (TBI), and close medical management. Payment is based on a Medicare Severity Diagnosis Related Group system on a per-discharge basis. The LTCH prospective payment system also considers

- Patient demographics,

- Discharge status,

- Principal diagnosis, and

- Additional diagnoses and medical procedures

to determine the reimbursement rate. Occupational therapy must be available in an LTCH, but, unlike in IRFs, there is no requirement that a beneficiary receive therapy.

MACRA: The Quality Payment Program and Community-Based Practice
CMS's implementation of MACRA has significant implications for outpatient occupational therapy payment. MACRA laid out the new Medicare Part B Quality Payment Program (QPP).

Although occupational therapy practitioners were not originally eligible for QPP payment in the first year of the program (i.e., 2017), occupational and physical therapy professionals are required to report as of January 1, 2019. On the basis of reporting performance in the program in 2019, occupational therapists can receive upward or downward payment adjustments in Payment Year 2021. QPP includes 2 pathways to Part B reimbursement:

1. Using the Merit-Based Incentive Payment System (MIPS), or

2. Participating in an advanced alternative payment model (APM).

MIPS

MIPS replaced PQRS. PQRS required Medicare Part B providers to report quality measures to CMS to avoid decreased reimbursement. QPP combines PQRS and other physician-focused quality programs into 4 new categories that carry a weighted score to result in a 100% total composite score:

1. Quality

2. Advancement of care information

3. Clinical practice improvement activities

4. Resource use measures.

APMs and Advanced APMs

An APM is a payment approach that gives added incentive payments to provide high-quality and cost-efficient care. APMs can apply to a specific clinical condition, a care episode, or a population. Examples of APMs are the Medicare Shared Savings Program ACO (Track 1) or the Comprehensive Care for Joint Replacement Model.

An advanced APM is a subset of an APM that allows practices to earn more for taking on some risk related to their patients' outcomes (Halpern et al., 2017). Clinicians may earn an incentive payment by increasing the share of financial risk related to improving patient care through an advanced APM. The advanced APM alternative represents different quality and eligibility criteria because of the heightened financial risk that the advanced APM entity must assume.

To qualify, the entity must

- Use certified electronic health record technology,

- Develop a quality measures reporting component using measures comparable to those required under MIPS, and

- Either bear financial risk for monetary losses that are in excess of a nominal amount or be designated a Medical Home Model under a specific Social Security Act definition.

Qualifying as an advanced APM entity exempts clinicians from MIPS. Clinicians and groups that participate in APMs and advanced APMs have the opportunity to rewrite reimbursement rules.

Practical Applications in Occupational Therapy

New payment models create challenges and opportunities for occupational therapy practitioners. Occupational therapy can take this opportunity to demonstrate high value to the health system, payers, and clients by understanding and advocating for the role of the profession in the changing health care system. Practitioners must be able to identify the right people who will benefit from services and the right services to provide. Understanding how to screen and assess functional cognition and how this critical factor affects participation is a key step in this process.

Why Must Occupational Therapy Address Cognition?

According to AOTA's (2019) statement on cognition, cognitive rehabilitation, and occupational performance, the assessment of cognition should be in context and should examine the ability of an individual to function, not just recall or perform a single cognitive task. Thus, after the passage of the IMPACT Act, AOTA recommended that CMS consider broadening the assessment of cognition in PAC settings. The assessment of cognition and functional status, as described in the IMPACT Act, does not meet the objectives intended by the law.

AOTA worked closely with subject matter experts to propose that new measures of functional cognition be included in the CMS IMPACT Act Data Element Library and used in PAC settings. This perspective sets the stage for reinforcement of occupational therapy's contribution to PAC outcomes.

Functional cognition is "how an individual uses and integrates thinking and processing skills to accomplish everyday activities in clinical and community living environments" (Giles et al., 2017, p. 2). Giles and colleagues explained that occupational therapy practitioners assess and treat cognition in performance and context, which is a different approach than isolating individual, specific cognitive constructs. Occupational therapists assess functional cognition in context to ascertain the ability of someone to live independently by using performance-based tests (Moore et al., 2007; Poulin et al., 2013; Wesson et al., 2016).

Opportunities for Occupational Therapy in PAC Settings

Occupational therapy practitioners can demonstrate distinct value by addressing functional cognition in the context of performance. Practitioners should know what data elements related to function and functional cognition are collected by CMS and how these data elements relate to occupational therapy. When possible, practitioners can contribute to the collection of these data elements and should highlight when the practice of occupational therapy is related to the quality measures being captured by CMS.

Occupational therapy practitioners should also understand where the data elements and measures fall short. The data elements used to capture cognition at this time are not sufficient to identify challenges or changes in functional cognition. This is especially true for people who have a milder but functionally significant form of cognitive impairment. Practitioners should use the strategies identified in this book to clearly articulate to administration and management the importance of functional cognition for a person's ability to maintain independence in the community.

It is important that occupational therapy practitioners provide the right care at the right time to the right people. Identifying impairments in occupational performance and client factors is a critical first step to identifying the right people and providing the right services. Understanding clients' cognition may help prevent a range of adverse events, including falls and hospital readmission (Leland et al., 2012; Roberts & Robinson, 2014).

When possible, practitioners should use the CMS data elements described in this chapter, in addition to more sensitive and comprehensive assessments, to demonstrate clients' needs and progress toward meaningful goals. It is more important than ever to fully document the skill, reason, and impact of occupational therapy intervention to demonstrate the impact of services.

The new payment models are just beginning to take shape. Current 3rd-party payer coverage policies are frequently inconsistent in regard to coverage for occupational therapy services related to key cognitive conditions, such as TBI, stroke, Alzheimer's disease, and other related dementias.

AOTA staff and member experts have spent significant time and resources advocating against problematic Medicare administrative contractor local coverage determinations (i.e., coverage policies that may differ from region to region across the country), including advocating for the role of occupational therapy in Medicare maintenance therapy programs. AOTA continues to advocate for more advanced and meaningful data elements and measures for functional cognition. Using the strategies in this book to evaluate, treat, and document functional cognition in the context of functional performance will support the efforts to establish data elements and measures that more accurately describe a person's cognition as it relates to occupational performance.

Opportunities for Community-Based Practice and Outpatient Therapy

The QPP provides new opportunities for occupational therapy practitioners in outpatient and community-based practice. Although the QPP still allows for traditional fee-for-service occupational therapy, there is an increased focus on quality. Practitioners who bill Medicare Part B fee for service will also have to submit quality measures and improvement activities to show that they are diligently working to provide better, more efficient care through MIPS.

The American Academy of Neurology and PCPI have developed quality measures specific to cognition. Occupational therapists were part of the quality measure development. Although the measures are specific to persons with major neurocognitive disorders and dementia, therapists can use a registry to report the following quality measures related to cognition:

- MIPS 281 Dementia: Cognitive Assessment
- MIPS 282 Dementia: Functional Status Assessment
- MIPS 283 Dementia: Associated Behavioral and Psychiatric Symptoms Screening and Management
- MIPS 286 Dementia: Safety Concerns Screening and Mitigation Recommendations or Referral for Patients With Dementia.

More details about these measures can be found online at https://qpp.cms.gov.

APMs are aimed at providing the most effective care at lower cost and with demonstrable data-driven outcomes. The advanced APMs provide another pathway for participation in QPP. Occupational therapy practitioners must be able to clearly identify and demonstrate value to be significant participants in an APM (Halle et al., 2018; Miller, 2018).

Summary

The health care system is shifting from paying for the volume of services to purchasing high-value health care. This presents new opportunities for occupational therapy practitioners who are able to clearly identify their value by providing the right services to the right people at the right time. Assessing and addressing functional cognition and the impact on occupational performance can be an important part of this process.

Occupational therapy practitioners should identify when functional cognition is impairing occupational performance. Assessing functional cognition can identify the right persons for occupational therapy intervention. This is especially true for those with mild but functionally significant cognitive impairment, who may not be identified by mechanisms used by CMS.

Identifying when functional cognition is impaired drives the choices of the right interventions. The plan of care and intervention strategies is different for those with impaired functional cognition than for those without. The strategies in this book can add another tool in the occupational therapy toolkit to articulate the distinct value.

References

Acumen. (2018). *Skilled nursing facilities patient-driven payment model technical report.* Baltimore: Centers for Medicare & Medicaid Services.

Agency for Healthcare Research and Quality. (2016). *The National Quality Strategy: Fact sheet.* Rockville, MD: Author.

American Occupational Therapy Association. (2019). Cognition, cognitive rehabilitation, and occupational performance. *American Journal of Occupational Therapy.*

Anglin, G., Tu, H., Liao, K., Sessums, L., & Taylor, E. F. (2017). Strengthening multipayer collaboration: Lessons from the Comprehensive Primary Care Initiative. *Milbank Quarterly, 95,* 602–633. https://doi.org/10.1111/1468-0009.12280

Centers for Medicare & Medicaid Services. (2016). *Pioneer ACO final report.* Baltimore: Author.

Centers for Medicare & Medicaid Services. (2018a). *Home Health Agency Outcome and Assessment Information Set Version D (OASIS–D).* Retrieved from https://www.cms.gov/Medicare/Quality-Initiatives-Patient-Assessment-Instruments/HomeHealthQualityInits/OASIS-Data-Sets.html

Centers for Medicare & Medicaid Services. (2018b). *Minimum Data Set (MDS) Version 3.0: Resident Assessment and Care Screening Nursing Home Comprehensive (NC) Item Set.* Retrieved from https://www.cms.gov/Medicare/Quality-Initiatives-Patient-Assessment-Instruments/NursingHomeQualityInits/MDS30RAIManual.html

Centers for Medicare & Medicaid Services. (n.d.). *Continuity Assessment Record and Evaluation (CARE) Item Set* (developed as part of the Medicare Post-Acute Care Payment Reform Demonstration (PAC–PRD). Retrieved from https://www.cms.gov/Medicare/Quality-Initiatives-Patient-Assessment-Instruments/Post-Acute-Care-Quality-Initiatives/CARE-Item-Set-and-B-CARE.html

Conrad, D. A., Grembowski, D., Hernandez, S. E., Lau, D., & Marcus-Smith, M. (2014). Emerging lessons from regional and state innovation in value-based payment reform: Balancing collaboration and disruptive innovation. *Milbank Quarterly, 92,* 568–623. https://doi.org/10.1111/1468-0009.12078

Crabtree, B. F., Nutting, P. A., Miller, W. L., Stange, K. C., Stewart, E. E., & Jaén, C. J. (2010). Summary of the National Demonstration Project and recommendations for the patient-centered medical home. *Annals of Family Medicine, 8*(Suppl. 1), S80–S90. https://doi.org/10.1370/afm.1107

Finkelstein, A., Ji, Y., Mahoney, N., & Skinner, J. (2018). Mandatory Medicare bundled payment program for lower extremity joint replacement and discharge to institutional postacute care: Interim analysis of the first year of a 5-year randomized trial. *JAMA, 320,* 892–900. https://doi.org/10.1001/jama.2018.12346

Gage, B., Deutsch, A., Smith, L., Schwartz, C., Ross, J., Coots, L., . . . Mallinson, T. (2012). *The development and testing of the Continuity Assessment Record and Evaluation (CARE) Item Set: Final report on CARE Item Set and current assessment comparisons* (Vol. 3). Washington, DC: George Washington University.

Giles, G. M., Edwards, D. F., Morrison, M. T., Baum, C., & Wolf, T. J. (2017). Screening for functional cognition in postacute care and the Improving Medicare Post-Acute Care Transformation (IMPACT) Act of 2014. *American Journal of Occupational Therapy, 71,* 7105090010. https://doi.org/10.5014/ajot.2017.715001

Halle, A. D., Mroz, T. M., Fogelberg, D. J., & Leland, N. E. (2018). Occupational therapy and primary care: Updates and trends. *American Journal of Occupational Therapy, 72,* 7203090010. https://doi.org/10.5014/ajot.2018.723001

Halpern, V. J., Shireman, P. K., Woo, K., Rathbun, J., & Johnson, B. (2017). What is an advanced alternative payment model? *Journal of Vascular Surgery, 66,* 1299. https://doi.org/10.1016/j.jvs.2017.07.099

Improving Medicare Post-Acute Care Transformation Act of 2014, Pub. L. 113–185, 42 U.S.C. §§ 1305 et seq.

Institute of Medicine. (2000). *To err is human: Building a safer health system.* Washington, DC: National Academies Press.

Institute of Medicine. (2001). *Crossing the quality chasm: A new health system for the 21st century.* Washington, DC: National Academies Press.

Leland, N. E., Crum, K., Phipps, S., Roberts, P., & Gage, B. (2015). Advancing the value and quality of occupational therapy in health service delivery. *American Journal of Occupational Therapy, 69,* 6901090010. https://doi.org/10.5014/ajot.2015.691001

Leland, N. E., Elliott, S. J., O'Malley, L., & Murphy, S. L. (2012). Occupational therapy in fall prevention: Current evidence and future directions. *American Journal of Occupational Therapy, 66,* 149–160. https://doi.org/10.5014/ajot.2012.002733

McWilliams, J. M., Hatfield, L. A., Landon, B. E., Hamed, P., & Chernew, M. E. (2018). Medicare spending after 3 years of the Medicare Shared Savings Program. *New England Journal of Medicine, 379,* 1139–1149. https://doi.org/10.1056/NEJMsa1803388

Medicare Access and CHIP Reauthorization Act of 2015, Pub. L. 114–10, 42 U.S.C. § 1305 et seq.

Miller, C. (2018). Accountable care organizations and occupational therapy. *American Journal of Occupational Therapy, 72,* 7205090010. https://doi.org/10.5014/ajot.2018.725003.

Moore, D. J., Palmer, B. W., Patterson, T. L., & Jeste, D. V. (2007). A review of performance-based measures of functional living skills. *Journal of Psychiatric Research, 42,* 97–118. https://doi.org/10.1016/j.jpsychires.2005.10.008

Navathe, A. S., Song, Z., & Emanuel, E. J. (2017). The next generation of episode-based payments. *JAMA, 317,* 2371–2372. https://doi.org/10.1001/jama.2017.5902

Patient Protection and Affordable Care Act, Pub. L. 111–148, 42 U.S.C. §§ 18001–18121 (2010).

Poulin, V., Korner-Bitensky, N., & Dawson, D. R. (2013). Stroke-Specific Executive Function Assessment: A literature review of performance-based tools. *Australian Occupational Therapy Journal, 60,* 3–19. https://doi.org/10.1111/1440-1630.12024

Roberts, P. S., & Robinson, M. R. (2014). Occupational therapy's role in preventing acute readmissions. *American Journal of Occupational Therapy, 68,* 254–259. https://doi.org/10.5014/ajot.2014.683001

Ryan, A., Sutton, M., & Doran, T. (2014). Does winning a pay-for-performance bonus improve subsequent quality performance? Evidence from the Hospital Quality Incentive Demonstration. *Health Services Research, 49,* 568–587. https://doi.org/10.1111/1475-6773.12097

Saliba, D., Buchanan, J., Edelen, M. O., Streim, J., Ouslander, J., Berlowitz, D., & Chodosh, J. (2012). MDS 3.0: Brief Interview for Mental Status. *Journal of Post-Acute and Long-Term Care Medicine, 13,* 611–617. https://doi.org/10.1016/j.jamda.2012.06.004

Sandhu, S., Furniss, J., & Metzler, C. (2018). Using the new postacute care quality measures to demonstrate the value of occupational therapy. *American Journal of Occupational Therapy, 72,* 7202090010. https://doi.org/10.5014/ajot.2018.722002

Sikka, R., Morath, J. M., & Leape, L. (2015). The Quadruple Aim: Care, health, cost and meaning in work. *BMJ Quality and Safety, 24,* 608–610. http://doi.org/10.1136/bmjqs-2015-004160

Wei, L. A., Fearing, M. A., Sternberg, E. J., & Inouye, S. K. (2008). The Confusion Assessment Method: A systematic review of current usage. *Journal of the American Geriatrics Society, 56,* 823–830. https://doi.org/10.1111/j.1532-5415.2008.01674.x

Wesson, J., Clemson, L., Brodaty, H., & Reppermund, S. (2016). Estimating functional cognition in older adults using observational assessments of task performance in complex everyday activities: A systematic review and evaluation of measurement properties. *Neuroscience and Biobehavioral Reviews, 68,* 335–360. https://doi.org/10.1016/j.neubiorev.2016.05.024

Assessment

Introduction to Principles of Assessment

Occupational therapy practitioners work in many contexts in which it is not possible to achieve extensive naturalistic observation of the full range of functional performance necessary for independent community functioning. Similarly, they often have limited time to administer assessments. For these reasons, practitioners may develop an occupational profile and, whenever possible, use information from the profile and from brief screening measures to establish where the focus should be in the assessment process.

Section II begins with an overview of the principles of assessment as they apply to functional cognition (Chapter 3). Many of these principles apply to all forms of occupational therapy assessment; however, the particular focus of this section is performance-based assessment, which is the primary way that functional cognition is assessed. The next chapter (Chapter 4) reviews Cognitive–Functional Evaluation (C–FE), which is a framework for the assessment of functional cognition. The C–FE provides a typology for the most frequently used types of cognitive assessment and for how these different forms of assessment fit together to provide the occupational therapist with the information necessary to develop a treatment plan that addresses functional cognition.

The remaining chapters in Section II (Chapters 5–16) follow the stages of the C–FE and provide examples of assessments that can be used at each stage of the C–FE process. The majority of the chapters (Chapters 7–15) describe specific performance-based assessments. Each chapter follows a similar format, the primary focus of which is the pragmatic application of each of the assessments in practice. For each assessment, an introduction discusses how and why the assessment was developed, with the majority of the chapter focused on clients for whom the assessment is appropriate, how it is administered, information related to training on the assessment (if necessary), how to obtain the assessment, how to score the assessment, and finally, how to document results of the assessment. These chapters have associated video content to demonstrate administration of at least portions of the assessments to supplement information provided in the text.

Principles of Functional–Cognitive Assessment

3

GORDON MUIR GILES, PhD, OTR/L, FAOTA; TIMOTHY J. WOLF, OTD, PhD, OTR/L, FAOTA; AND DOROTHY FARRAR EDWARDS, PhD

LEARNING OBJECTIVES

After completing this chapter, readers should be able to

- Describe the purpose of performance-based testing of functional cognition,
- Explain why assessment through observation alone is insufficient, and
- Describe the important parameters for evaluating the psychometric characteristics of performance-based testing of functional cognition.

KEY TERMS AND CONCEPTS

- Alternate form reliability • Ceiling effects • Clinical utility • Concurrent validity • Construct validity
- Content validity • Convergent validity • Criterion validity • Divergent validity • Face validity • Floor effects
- Internal consistency • Interrater reliability • Intrarater reliability • Performance-based tests • Predictive validity
- Rasch analysis • Reliability • Sensitivity • Specificity • Test–retest reliability • Validity

Introduction

Cognition is a complex construct that overlaps the scope of practice of several professions. Each discipline has a particular focus and, as a result, has a distinct contribution to the assessment of cognitive function. Occupational therapy's distinct contribution is the use of performance-based testing to explain functional cognition.

Performance-based tests of functional cognition examine the *how* of performance but, unlike neuropsychological tests, are not intended to identify brain dysfunction (either the consequences of brain damage in general or specific neuropsychological functions that may be impaired). Performance-based testing of functional cognition examines the behavior produced by the test taker, not the hypothesized brain functions or the client's diagnoses seen as causing the behavior (Fava et al., 2012; Feinstein, 1983).

The emphasis of functional cognition as a measure of ADL and IADL competency is on occupational performance because many routes can lead to adequate performance, and many different abilities may contribute to adequate execution of functional activities. The goal of performance-based testing is the assessment and characterization of functional cognition and occupational performance, not identification of disease.

Occupational therapists approach the assessment process very differently from professionals in some other disciplines. Testing has a different place in the profession of occupational therapy than it has in psychology or neuropsychology. Before neuroimaging largely supplanted all other approaches in identification of the presence or the localization of brain damage, these were major roles ascribed to clinical neuropsychological testing (Lezak et al., 2012). The time allocated to testing was often extensive, and the generation of a test report delineating strengths and weaknesses of different cognitive functions was often the primary reason the client was seen (Lezak et al., 2012). The neuropsychologist's report often concludes with a summary of impairments and perhaps treatment recommendations to be carried out by other disciplines.

However, neither the presence of brain damage nor the specification of areas of strength and weakness in cognitive functioning necessarily predicts the ADL or IADL capacity of the individual client. Cognition and function are best considered as interrelated but separate constructs, with neither being wholly derivable from the other (Giles, 2010). Rather than trying to isolate specific cognitive functions (e.g., attention, memory), occupational therapists assess the individual's ability to apply the totality of his or her metacognitive (i.e., self-awareness of cognitive ability), cognitive, and performance-based capacities or skills to achieve occupational performance goals (Giles et al., 2017).

Paradoxically, although neuropsychological measures attempt to isolate specific cognitive deficits, when predicting real-world performance, combined measures (i.e., a global composite index of impairment, based on summed scores of test sections or items that assess multiple cognitive domains) typically show the greatest relationship to performance. This suggests that global measures may be the most predictive of functional cognition and IADL competency (Chelune & Moehle, 1986; Heaton & Pendleton, 1981).

The assessment of functional cognition does not obviate the need for neuropsychology assessment to identify the specific cognitive processes that are impaired, knowledge of which can inform therapeutic interventions. Many factors may contribute to a person's functional–cognitive ability, and many performance-based tests of functional cognition allow the deconstruction of performance to identify the types of performance-based errors that test takers make. The identification of such errors, in addition to the understanding based on neuropsychological testing, can provide insight into how performance might be rehabilitated or supported.

There are many ways to assess ADL and IADL competency, including self- and proxy report and inferring competency from neuropsychological testing. However, performance-based testing of IADL skills is emerging as the method that is possibly most predictive of community functioning. Performance-based testing of functional cognition relies on the notion that a sample of performance of a novel, complex psychomotor task indicates the test taker's ability to perform other novel psychomotor tasks (i.e., it will allow inferences to be made regarding occupational performance more generally).

Assessment of functional cognition is intended to capture information about the test taker's common responses to the cognitive demands of everyday situations. The performance-based testing of functional cognition may also reveal the way individuals attempt the task. When performance is impaired, such testing may suggest avenues to shore up performance.

The test results are interpreted in the context of other sources of information from the occupational profile:

- The nature of the errors

- The test taker's awareness of errors and their reaction to them

- The impact of errors on daily life functions and social relationships.

Additionally, when appropriate, the results obtained by the occupational therapist should be integrated with those obtained by other professional disciplines so that occupational therapy maintains its discipline-specific role and enriches the interdisciplinary understanding of the client and his or her needs.

Need for a Framework

Testing in occupational therapy practice occurs in the context of a strong preference for client-centered goal setting (American Occupational Therapy Association, 2014) and typically occurs within the context of the development of an occupational profile. The Cognitive–Functional Evaluation (C–FE) framework (see Chapter 4) provides a systematic process for assessment in occupational therapy. This framework was used to structure the content for the remaining chapters of this text related to assessment. The C–FE framework provides a context for how cognitive assessment information from multiple sources (e.g., screening, performance-based testing, neuropsychological testing) can be incorporated into an occupational therapy treatment plan.

Importance of Performance-Based Testing: Why Observation Is Not Enough

Occupational therapists recognize that spending a sustained period of time observing a client perform daily activities can reveal a great deal about his or her occupational performance ability. However, there are many circumstances in which the extensive naturalistic observation of basic ADLs and IADLs is not possible because of time constraints or because the environment (e.g., the acute hospital) constrains the activities that can be observed (Morrison et al., 2015). Similarly, the accuracy of a hospitalized patient's self-report is limited by the patient's own lack of experience with their new self after illness or injury or by lack of awareness of deficit (Morrison et al., 2015). In these circumstances, qualitative observation of ADLs (usually available in a hospital environment) is insufficient to identify milder forms of functional–cognitive impairment or to judge the severity of IADL impairments when present.

Although many occupational therapists may assume that they know cognitive deficits when they see them, evidence suggests that this is not always the case (Bottari & Dawson, 2011; Edwards et al., 2006). As a result, therapists may fail to identify individuals with cognitive impairments who could be assisted by occupational therapy interventions. There are also advantages to the use of standardized measures that are not present with naturalistic observation or with other forms of testing (Giles et al., 2017). As a result, there are strong theoretical and practical reasons why therapists should adopt standardized measures, the results of which can be used to infer the likely presence of occupational performance deficits.

Assessment Considerations

There are now a range of measures of functional cognition, and the occupational therapist can select a measure according to the specific purpose of the testing and the needs of the test taker. Screening measures are used if there is a question regarding the appropriateness of more comprehensive assessment; they are intended to be rapid and applied to a population. The selection of measures for comprehensive testing is influenced by

- The occupational profile,
- The expected face validity of the test to the test taker, and
- The specific goals of testing.

Performance-based tests vary in their novelty and degree of cognitive load, and they particularly differ in the demands placed on the test taker's executive functions (EFs; Toglia, 2015, 2018). In a study of individuals with self-reported difficulties in community functioning after stroke, Morrison et al. (2013) found that the FIM® (Hamilton et al., 1987) was the least sensitive measure in detecting participants who self-identified as having difficulty after stroke. The Executive Function Performance Test (EFPT; Baum et al., 2008) was more sensitive to self-identified impairment than the FIM, and the Multiple Errands Test–Revised (MET–R) was found to be the most sensitive to self-reported deficits after mild stroke (Morrison et al., 2013).

Occupational therapists are called on to answer a range of questions regarding functional independence in ADLs, IADLs, and work environments. The heterogeneity of client characteristics—with differing interests, goals, and questions—means that a variety of measures with different formats and levels of complexity are required to meet the needs of testing. If, for example, the test taker will be returning to a high-pressure occupation in which they are required to handle a high degree of novel information in a social context, then the practitioner might select a performance-based test that contains these elements (e.g., the MET). In contrast, if the test taker needs to be able to manage safely in a familiar environment, the practitioner might select a measure that focuses on safety awareness, such as the EFPT or the Performance Assessment of Self-Care Skills (PASS; Rogers et al., 2016).

The following are common uses of performance-based tests of functional cognition:

- Identification of the presence of impaired functional cognition (both screening and more comprehensive assessment)
- Questions about placement, often relating to safety and the degree of support the individual will need to maintain a specific living situation (including prediction of specific long-term care needs)
- Legal or compensation claims used in costs prediction for ongoing support

- Assessment of self-awareness during task performance
- Identification of how the test taker attempts to address task demands, with implications for intervention
- Evaluation of response to intervention
- Evaluation of the use of strategies
- Specific questions about how functional cognition supports or fails to support specific IADL functions
- Specific questions about how functional cognition supports or fails to support specific questions about return to work.

Psychometric Characteristics of Performance-Based Testing

Individuals taking performance-based tests of functional cognition must be able to sustain arousal to participate in the testing (i.e., they have to register sensory information necessary for the test). They have to engage in the activity. For the individual to participate in testing of functional cognition, they have to understand that they are being posed a problem and that the end state that is to be accomplished is different from the current state.

Many impaired individuals lose the "set" and fail to maintain the recognition that they are taking a test; continuous awareness of participating in a test is not a prerequisite for testing. For most performance-based testing of functional cognition, the individual has to be able to understand language. Most, but not all, tests involve reading and writing. For many very cognitively impaired individuals, performance-based testing of functional cognition may be unnecessary, because the severity of their deficits is readily apparent with other, simpler forms of testing.

Elsewhere we have proposed a stepwise procedure for the assessment of cognitive functions in acute and postacute care settings (Giles et al., 2017; Morrison et al., 2015). The Confusion Assessment Method scale is used to identify individuals in delirium (Inouye et al., 1990; Wei et al., 2008). For those not in delirium, the Brief Interview for Mental Status (Saliba et al., 2012), the Mini-Cog (Borson et al., 2000), or other cognitive screening measures are used to identify individuals with severe cognitive impairment.

In contrast, we propose to further use a performance-based measure of functional cognition that is more sensitive to milder deficits for individuals who do not show deficits on the measures of more significant cognitive impairment. We note, however, that even individuals who score as unimpaired on standard cognitive screening measures (e.g., ≥26 on the Montreal Cognitive Assessment; Nasreddine et al., 2005) may nonetheless evidence impaired functional performance (Toglia et al., 2017). Therefore, individuals who do not seem to have impaired cognition should, at minimum, be screened for deficits in functional cognition before discharge.

Estimations of the effects of impaired functional cognition are based on the probability that an event with a negative outcome may occur. Specific dangerous or adverse events are not predictable, but the testing may answer questions about whether the test taker can adjust behavior to the prevailing circumstances to avoid reasonably predictable negative outcomes. What these negative outcomes will be depends on

- The person's specific characteristics,
- The task demands they are likely to encounter, and
- The environment that they need to manage.

The interpretation of a test's results depends on the level of difficulty posed by the test and what is being assessed.

Although it is relatively new, standardized performance-based testing of functional cognition has benefited from the advances in test development made over the last 100 years in education and in clinical psychology (Anastasi & Urbina, 1997). All the measures described in this text have standardized methods of administration. However, many of the measures lack extensive normative data (normative data may be absent, limited in number of participants, or limited in terms of the diagnostic groups included). Test developers have frequently opted to make the measures free or very low cost. As a result, the large-scale testing programs required for the development of extensive normative data cannot be funded by test publishers, as has been the case with the tests produced by other disciplines.

When deciding on a test for a particular client or group of clients, the therapist should examine the psychometric characteristics of the measure. Data relevant to test selection that are reported for the majority of the performance-based measures of functional cognition in Chapters 6–16 of this text include

- Forms of reliability and validity,
- Internal consistency,
- Ceiling and floor effects,
- Sensitivity and specificity, and
- Data related to the use of the test with specific populations.

Reliability

The *reliability* of a measure is the consistency of test takers' scores obtained under similar testing conditions. Measures are said to be reliable if the obtained test scores are accurate, reproducible, and consistent from 1 testing occasion to another (i.e., if the testing process were repeated with the same group of test takers, similar results would be obtained). Because no measurement process is perfect, all forms of measurement include random error.

Various forms of reliability relate to the changes in testing conditions and the degree to which the measures are affected by random error. Random error results from a variety of factors, including

- Random variations in the state of the test taker (e.g., fatigue, discomfort, distraction),
- The ambiguity of items in the test itself,
- The strictness of the test administrator in test rule interpretation (Anastasi & Urbina, 1997), and
- Variation in the testing environment.

Reliability in its various forms indicates the degree to which differences of scores on a test can be interpreted as representing the true differences (i.e., not random error) within or between test takers or between test takers and expected scores on a test. If a measure is not reliable, different scores may result from errors related to testing, not from true differences within or between test takers or over time in the same test.

A measure of the degree to which error may contribute to differences in scores on a measure is the standard error of measurement (SEM; Anastasi & Urbina, 1997). The SEM can be computed when the standard deviation and the reliability of the test are known. On the basis of the parameters of the normal distribution, it is then possible to estimate the chances that the test taker's true score is within a certain range of their obtained score.

Rater Reliability

Intrarater reliability is the observed agreement between the ratings of the same rater using the same measure with the same group of test takers (i.e., it is a rating of whether the same rater using the same measure on the same individual obtains the same results). **Interrater reliability** is the observed agreement between different raters using the same measure with the same group of test takers (i.e., it is an indication of whether findings are consistent on the measure when used by different raters).

Both intrarater and interrater reliability can be assessed statistically in a variety of ways, but interrater reliability is most frequently reported as the correlation coefficient of 2 sets of raters. When using Pearson product–moment correlations for parametric data and Spearman rank order correlations for nonparametric data, researchers consider coefficients in the .80s and .90s to be desirable (Anastasi & Urbina, 1997). The kappa statistic can be used to assess the reliability of scales that have a small number of response options, because it controls for chance agreement (Cohen, 1988).

Test–Retest Reliability

Test–retest reliability is the degree of agreement between the results of successive applications of a measure with the same test takers. The measurements are typically taken twice, with an intervening period of defined duration (usually a relatively short period to limit maturation effects), and show the extent to which scores can be generalized across administrations. The test–retest reliability is usually reported as the correlation coefficient for the 2 administrations of the test.

Test–retest reliability (like any repeat administration of a test) is potentially affected by practice. In some instances, what is being tested changes on repeat administration. This is likely to be a particular problem with tests that examine novel problem solving, as is the case with many tests of functional cognition. The test taker may carry over to subsequent testing information or strategies developed during the first test session. Therefore, test–retest reliability may be low or may not be reported by test developers who see reporting it as misleading.

Alternate Form Reliability

Alternate form reliability is 1 method used to avoid the problems of reduced novelty or of practice effects with repeat administration of the same test (Anastasi & Urbina, 1997). With alternate forms of the same test, the same test taker can be tested without practice or novelty effects obscuring any change in competency.

However, although parallel forms of tests of vocabulary or word-list learning are relatively straightforward to construct, parallel forms of measures of functional cognition that involve IADLs are far more problematic. Tests such as the EFPT or PASS, for which the intercorrelations among subtests are known, may be used as alternate forms. Nonetheless, in some circumstances repeat administration of performance-based tests of functional cognition may be used to assess intervention effectiveness (e.g., changes in strategy use can be assessed with repeat administration of the Weekly Calendar Planning Activity; Toglia, 2015).

Internal Consistency

Researchers can examine **internal consistency** by assessing a measure's interitem correlations (or the interitem correlation of items on the same subscale of a multiscale test). Internal consistency is intended to evaluate the degree of homogeneity of the various items in a measure and the degree to which the various items relate to the latent variable or construct that the test is purporting to measure. For example, if a test taker scored as independent on multiple items relating to distributing medications in a mediset, but failed items relating to counting the number of pills that were being distributed, this might indicate that different constructs were being measured. A test intended to assess different constructs would be expected to have low internal consistency—a finding that would not necessarily indicate error variance.

Cronbach's alpha is the statistical procedure used most often to measure internal consistency. Cronbach's alpha is higher for tests measuring narrow constructs and lower when more general constructs are measured. Very high internal consistency may indicate that the items are measuring exactly the same construct. This suggests that items can be eliminated and the test shortened without loss of test integrity. The number of items in a test also strongly influences its internal consistency, so shorter tests often have lower Cronbach's alpha yet still are preferable in some circumstances because of their lower test taker and test administrator burden.

Validity

Validity is the extent to which a test measures what it is intended to measure and relates to what can be inferred from the test taker's performance on the test with respect to the construct being measured or assessed. Practitioners should exercise caution in accepting either the test name or the activity that is used in the test as an indication of what can be inferred from the test. A clock drawing test may provide a lot more information than whether an individual can draw a clock.

Tests of functional cognition are intended to assess the processes that test takers use to achieve the goal state required by the test and relate to more than the test taker's competency in the activity that is used as the medium of the test. Validity concerns the relationship between test takers' performance on a test and their other performance characteristics, and these are often only marginally related to the surface characteristics of the test. This is the principal advantage of the use of validated tests: The relationship of performance on the test to other aspects of individuals' performance in their daily lives (i.e., IADL competency) has been empirically established for a particular population.

Construct Validity

Construct validity relates to the degree to which a test operationalizes a theoretical construct or trait (e.g., the degree to which a particular test that is purported to measure functional cognition actually measures the construct functional cognition).

Convergent and Divergent Validity

Convergent and divergent validity are related constructs. **Convergent validity** is the degree to which the outcome of the testing is related to other tests to which it should be related theoretically (e.g., a measure of functional cognition should be related to IADL competency). **Divergent validity** is the extent to which theoretically unrelated constructs should have limited correlations with the measure of interest.

Content Validity

Content validity relates to whether the content of the test is representative of the domain of interest. Content validity evidence involves the degree to which the content of the test matches a content domain associated with the construct. Given the limited time allotted for testing in occupational therapy, performance-based tests of functional cognition usually include 1 or a limited number of functional tasks and do not have the content validity that could be achieved by an ADL or IADL self-report measure. Self-report ADL and IADL measures may be far more comprehensive in their coverage of the domain of interest (Gold, 2012) yet less accurate in their ability to predict functional competence in context.

Performance-based tests of functional cognition are likely to be approached in different ways by different test takers, who may use different skills and strategies in responding to the same test. Thus, an identical test may draw on very different skills and strategies for different test takers. It therefore is not possible to determine the skills a test taker used in performing the test by looking simply at the particular set of tasks that the person has to perform to pass the test (Anastasi & Urbina, 1997).

Face Validity

To maximize rapport, buy-in, and appropriate effort from the test taker, the surface characteristics of the test should be such that test takers can recognize the test's relevance to the problems they are facing. *Face validity* is an estimate of whether a test seems to measure a certain criterion, not whether the test actually measures phenomena in that domain. A measure may have high predictive validity, but when the test content does not seem to be measuring material relevant to the test taker or is perceived as demeaning in some way, it has low face validity.

As a practical matter, face validity is closely related to content validity. For example, Chapter 6, "Baseline Cognitive Screening Tools," describes functional–cognitive screening measures involving medication management tasks. These tasks have high content validity and face validity for the assessment of the ability to manage medications. However, there is no necessary relationship between content and face validity, on the one hand, and the actual medication management ability, on the other hand. It is, for example, quite possible that an appointment scheduling or money management task might be more predictive of the test taker's ability to manage complex medication schedules than a simple medication management task. Face validity also affects the currency of a measure outside of the profession, such as in judicial or legislative arenas (Anastasi & Urbina, 1997).

Criterion Validity

Criterion validity indicates the effectiveness of a test in establishing a test taker's competency in other specified activities. The performance of the test is established against a criterion variable, usually another measure of known validity or an outcome variable.

Concurrent and Predictive Validity

Concurrent validity is when the new test data and the criterion variable or measure data are collected at the same time. *Predictive validity* is when data on the test are collected at Time 1 and the data on the criterion variable or measure are collected at Time 2. The finding that individuals with more-severe impairment on the PASS require more home care services in the 30 months following hospital discharge than those with less-severe impairment is an example of predictive validity (Brown & Finlayson, 2013).

Clinical Utility

Although clinical utility is not a psychometric property of a test, it is an important factor to consider when selecting a measure (Hand et al., 2018). *Clinical utility* is the clinical effectiveness of a measure, as reflected in the value provided and the ease with which it can be incorporated into everyday practice (Smart, 2006). Considerations include

- The amount of training needed;
- Administration time;
- Clear, concise, and thorough manuals; and
- Simple scoring and interpretation.

Ceiling and Floor Effects

Ceiling effects relate to a test's ability to indicate changes in the test taker's ability above a certain level of functioning. For example, an individual recovering from a traumatic brain injury who is independent in ADLs may show no improvement on the FIM (Uniform Data System for Medical Rehabilitation, 1997) or the Barthel Index (Mahoney & Barthel, 1965) despite continued improvement, because neither scale assesses IADLs. The measures are insensitive to the true capacity of the test taker above the "ceiling" of ADL independence. A *floor effect* is a similar insensitivity, but at the other end of the test's range, where the measure becomes insensitive below a certain obtained value and fails to differentiate levels of capacity below the "floor" of the scale (Portney & Watkins, 2009).

Sensitivity and Specificity

Sensitivity and specificity are statistical measures of the ability of a test to classify a condition or state as present or absent. *Sensitivity* is the degree to which a test identifies the true positive rate and the proportion of actual positives that are correctly identified (e.g., the percentage of individuals with impaired functional cognition who are correctly identified). *Specificity* is the degree to which a test identifies the true negative rate (e.g., the proportion of individuals without impaired functional cognition who are correctly identified).

The sensitivity of a test is often inversely related to its specificity (i.e., as sensitivity goes up, specificity goes down). The relative importance of sensitivity or specificity depends on the purpose of the test. Screening tests are likely to emphasize sensitivity over specificity, because it is important when screening not to fail to identify individuals with the condition, and a test that emphasizes sensitivity can be followed up with measures of greater specificity.

Sensitivity and specificity are also related to base rates. When a condition occurs frequently in a population (e.g., in 50% of a population), a reasonably sensitive measure will yield a relatively low proportion of individuals scoring as having the condition who actually do not have it. However, when the frequency of the occurrence of the condition in the population is low, a test that has even high specificity will yield a high number of false positives.

Rasch Analysis

Rasch analysis is a statistical approach to test development that addresses the assumption that each test item is of equal difficulty. This assumption allows test developers to sum item scores to create a total test score. If the assumption of equal difficulty is inaccurate and some scale items are, on average, more challenging than other test items, the summed score will not accurately reflect the test taker's true performance on the test.

Rasch analysis is a special case of item-response analysis that places each item on a continuum of difficulty in relation to the underlying latent construct that the test is assumed to be measuring. As a result, it allows the test to be calibrated for item difficulty, test taker ability, and test administrator strictness. The Assessment of Motor and Process Skills (Fisher & Jones, 2010) is the only functional cognition measure that has been subjected to Rasch analysis.

Sample Populations

When one considers the applicability of a test result to an actual client or population, it is important to remember that a test's measurement properties (reliability and validity) relate specifically to the measure's performance in the sample population that has been tested. This is why when a test administrator is reading reports on research studies, it is important to evaluate whether the sample population studied is similar in important characteristics to the population to which the test administrator is considering applying the test. Additionally, the reliability of a test depends on the heterogeneity of the sample population. If, for example, a specific measure was standardized on a more heterogeneous sample than the target sample, the test's reliability is likely to be lower in the target sample than in the population used to assess reliability (Anastasi & Urbina, 1997).

Conclusion

Assessment is an essential element of the occupational therapy process. This chapter addresses the challenge of determining a test's ability to denote an individual's capacity to safely and effectively manage complex life tasks (i.e., IADLs). Many assessment methods currently are directed at achieving this goal, including

- Self-report,

- Unstructured observations,

- Neuropsychological testing,

- Proxy or informant reports, and

- Performance-based assessment.

Occupational therapy's distinct contribution is related to the use of performance-based testing. The emergence of performance-based testing and the availability of reliable and valid performance measures have informed occupational therapy's understanding of the contribution of functional cognition to independence in IADLs and engagement in complex occupations. The superiority of performance-based testing for identification of impaired functional cognition is also reflected in the ability to match intervention strategies to the problems

identified through observation of performance of real-world tasks in dynamic settings.

Performance-based tests are designed to enhance ecological validity and thus the assessment's applicability to the test taker's real-world abilities. The information provided by performance-based assessments complements the information obtained from other forms of testing (e.g., neuropsychological testing). When used together, they can help guide more effective treatment and discharge planning, including more directed caregiver and family education; environmental modification; and ongoing, supportive community-based services.

References

American Occupational Therapy Association. (2014). Occupational therapy practice framework: Domain and process (3rd ed.). *American Journal of Occupational Therapy, 68*(Suppl. 1), S1–S48. https://doi.org/10.5014/ajot.2014.682006

Anastasi, A., & Urbina, S. (1997). *Psychological testing* (7th ed.). Upper Saddle River, NJ: Prentice Hall.

Baum, C. M., Connor, L. T., Morrison, T., Hahn, M., Dromerick, A. W., & Edwards, D. F. (2008). Reliability, validity, and clinical utility of the Executive Function Performance Test: A measure of executive function in a sample of people with stroke. *American Journal of Occupational Therapy, 62,* 446–455. https://doi.org/10.5014/ajot.62.4.446

Borson, S., Scanlan, J., Brush, M., Vitaliano, P., & Dokmak, A. (2000). The Mini-Cog: A cognitive "vital signs" measure for dementia screening in multi-lingual elderly. *International Journal of Geriatric Psychiatry, 15,* 1021–1027.

Bottari, C., & Dawson, D. R. (2011). Executive functions and real-world performance: How good are we at distinguishing people with acquired brain injury from healthy controls? *OTJR: Occupation, Participation and Health, 31*(Suppl.), S61–S68. https://doi.org/10.3928/15394492-20101108-10

Brown, C. L., & Finlayson, M. L. (2013). Performance measures rather than self-report measures of functional status predict home care use in community-dwelling older adults. *Canadian Journal of Occupational Therapy, 80,* 284–294. https://doi.org/10.1177/0008417413501467

Chelune, G. J., & Moehle, K. A. (1986). Neuropsychological assessment and everyday function. In D. Wedding, A. M. Horton, & J. Webster (Eds.), *The neuropsychology handbook* (pp. 489–525). New York: Springer.

Cohen, J. (1988). *Statistical power analysis for the behavioral sciences.* Hillside, NJ: Erlbaum.

Edwards, D. F., Hahn, M. G., Baum, C. M., Perlmutter, M. S., Sheedy, C., & Dromerick, A. W. (2006). Screening patients with stroke for rehabilitation needs: Validation of the Post-Stroke Rehabilitation Guidelines. *Neurorehabilitation and Neural Repair, 20,* 42–48. https://doi.org/10.1177/1545968305283038

Fava, G. A., Tomba, E., & Sonino, N. (2012). Clinimetrics: The science of clinical measurements. *International Journal of Clinical Practice, 66*(1), 11–15. https://doi.org/10.1111/j.1742-1241.2011.02825.x

Feinstein, A. R. (1983). An additional basic science for clinical medicine: IV. The development of clinimetrics. *Annals of Internal Medicine, 99,* 843–848. https://doi.org/10.7326/0003-4819-99-6-843

Fisher, A. G., & Jones, K. B. (2010). *Assessment of Motor and Process Skills: Vol. 2: User manual* (7th ed.). Ft. Collins, CO: Three Star Press.

Giles, G. M. (2010). Cognitive versus functional approaches to rehabilitation after traumatic brain injury: Commentary on a randomized controlled trial. *American Journal of Occupational Therapy, 64,* 182–185. https://doi.org/10.5014/ajot.64.1.182.

Giles, G. M., Edwards, D. F., Morrison, M. T., Baum, C., & Wolf, T. J. (2017). Screening for functional cognition in postacute care and the Improving Medicare Post-Acute Care Transformation (IMPACT)

Act of 2014. *American Journal of Occupational Therapy, 71,* 7105090010. https://doi.org/10.5014/ajot.2017.715001

Gold, D. A. (2012). An examination of instrumental activities of daily living assessment in older adults and mild cognitive impairment. *Journal of Clinical and Experimental Neuropsychology, 34,* 11–34. https://doi.org/10.1080/13803395.2011.614598

Hamilton, B. B., Granger, C. V., Sherwin, F. S., Zielezny, M., & Tashman, J. S. (1987). A uniform national data system for medical rehabilitation. In M. J. Fuhrer (Ed.), *Rehabilitation outcomes: Analysis and measurement* (pp. 137–147). Baltimore: Brookes.

Hand, B. N., Darragh, A. R., & Persch, A. C. (2018). Thoroughness and psychometrics of fidelity measures in occupational and physical therapy: A systematic review. *American Journal of Occupational Therapy, 72,* 7205205050. https://doi.org/10.5014/ajot.2018.025510

Heaton, R. K., & Pendleton, M. G. (1981). Use of neuropsychological tests to predict adult patients' everyday functioning. *Journal of Consulting and Clinical Psychology, 49,* 807–821. https://doi.org/10.1037/0022-006X.49.6.807

Inouye, S. K., Van Dyck, C. H., Alessi, C. A., Balkin, S., Siegal, A. P., & Horwitz, R. I. (1990). Clarifying confusion: The Confusion Assessment Method. A new method for detection of delirium. *Annals of Internal Medicine, 113,* 941–948. https://doi.org/10.7326/0003-4819-113-12-941

Lezak, M. D., Howieson, D. B., Bigler, E. D., & Tranel, D. (2012). *Neuropsychological assessment* (5th ed.). New York: Oxford University Press.

Mahoney, F. I., & Barthel, D. W. (1965). Functional evaluation: The Barthel Index. *Maryland State Medical Journal, 14,* 61–65.

Morrison, M. T., Edwards, D. F., & Giles, G. M. (2015). Performance-based testing in mild stroke: Identification of unmet opportunity for occupational therapy. *American Journal of Occupational Therapy, 69*(1), 6901360010. https://doi.org/10.5014/ajot.2015.011528

Morrison, M. T., Giles, G. M., Ryan, J. D., Baum, C. M., Dromerick, A. W., Polatajko, H. J., & Edwards, D. F. (2013). Multiple Errands Test–Revised (MET–R): A performance-based measure of executive function in people with mild cerebrovascular accident. *American Journal of Occupational Therapy, 67,* 460–468. https://doi.org/10.5014/ajot.2013.007880

Nasreddine, Z. S., Phillips, N. A., Bédirian, V., Charbonneau, S., Whitehead, V., Collin, I., . . . Chertkow, H. (2005). The Montreal Cognitive Assessment, MoCA: A brief screening tool for mild cognitive impairment. *Journal of the American Geriatrics Society, 53,* 695–699. https://doi.org/10.1111/j.1532-5415.2005.53221.x

Portney, L. G., & Watkins, M. P. (2009). *Foundations of clinical research: Applications to practice.* Upper Saddle River, NJ: Pearson/Prentice Hall.

Rogers, J. C., Holm, M. B., & Chisholm, D. (2016). *Performance Assessment of Self-Care Skills—Version 4.1.* Pittsburgh: University of Pittsburgh.

Saliba, D., Buchanan, J., Edelen, M. O., Streim, J., Ouslander, J., Berlowitz, D., & Chodosh, J. (2012). MDS 3.0: Brief Interview for Mental Status. *Journal of Post-Acute and Long-Term Care Medicine, 13,* 611–617. https://doi.org/10.1016/j.jamda.2012.06.004

Smart, A. (2006). A multi-dimensional model of clinical utility. *International Journal for Quality in Health Care, 18,* 377–382. https://doi.org/10.1093/intqhc/mzl034

Toglia, J. (2015). *Weekly Calendar Planning Activity (WCPA): A performance test of executive function.* Bethesda, MD: AOTA Press.

Toglia, J. (2018). The Dynamic Interactional Model and the Multicontext Approach. In N. Katz & J. Toglia (Eds.), *Cognition, occupation, and participation across the lifespan: Neuroscience, neurorehabilitation, and models of intervention in occupational therapy* (4th ed., pp. 355–385). Bethesda, MD: AOTA Press.

Toglia, J., Askin, G., Gerber, L. M., Taub, M. C., Mastrogiovanni, A. R., & O'Dell, M. W. (2017). Association between 2 measures of cognitive instrumental activities of daily living and their relation to the Montreal Cognitive Assessment in persons with stroke. *Archives of Physical Medicine and Rehabilitation, 98,* 2280–2287. https://doi.org/10.1016/j.apmr.2017.04.007

Uniform Data System for Medical Rehabilitation. (1997). *Guide for the Uniform Data Set for Medical Rehabilitation (including the FIM® instrument),* version 5.1. Buffalo, NY: Author.

Wei, L. A., Fearing, M. A., Sternberg, E. J., & Inouye, S. K. (2008). The Confusion Assessment Method: A systematic review of current usage. *Journal of the American Geriatrics Society, 56,* 823–830. https://doi.org/10.1111/j.1532-5415.2008.01674.x

4

The Cognitive–Functional Evaluation Framework

SHLOMIT ROTENBERG, PhD, OT,
AND ADINA MAEIR, PhD, OT

LEARNING OBJECTIVES

After completing this chapter, readers should be able to

- Understand the distinct occupational therapy perspective on cognition evaluation,
- Describe the 5 domains of the Cognitive–Functional Evaluation (C–FE),
- Describe the methods of evaluation and their application to the C–FE domains, and
- Understand the clinical implications of the C–FE for the treatment process.

KEY TERMS AND CONCEPTS

- Cognition • Cognitive–Functional Evaluation • Ecological validity • Functional cognition

Distinct Occupational Therapy Perspective on Cognitive Evaluation

The distinct role of occupational therapists in the assessment of clients with suspected deficits in functional cognition is to understand the clients' cognitive profile in relation to occupation. *Functional cognition* is how an individual uses and integrates their thinking and processing skills to accomplish everyday activities in clinical and community living settings. Functional cognition can also be termed *cognition in everyday life,* which reflects the interactions among cognition, contextual variables, and occupations.

Deficits in functional cognition are a consequence of many health conditions and present significant barriers to participation. Therefore, deficits in functional cognition are relevant in all occupational therapy practice areas. Occupational therapists assess the impact of cognitive factors on everyday functioning.

Functional outcomes of cognitive deficits depend only in part on the nature and severity of the cognitive impairment. The distinct occupational therapy perspective maintains that occupational performance cannot be explained by cognitive factors

in isolation. Instead, the key is how they interact with the whole person in their lived environment. Therefore, contextual factors of the person (e.g., self-awareness, beliefs) and their environment (e.g., demands, supports) play an important role and affect how cognition interplays with functioning.

The purpose of a cognitive–functional assessment is

- To determine the implications of cognitive deficits on everyday life for people with suspected cognitive disabilities;

- To determine clients' capacity to live in their home, work, or do any daily task that is important and meaningful for them in a safe and efficient manner; and

- To guide the clinical reasoning process for interventions that enable participation in meaningful occupations.

The *Cognitive–Functional Evaluation* (C–FE) framework was introduced by Hartman-Maeir, Katz, and Baum (2009) to provide a systematic approach to evaluating the implications of cognitive deficits in everyday life. The C–FE's original stages included interview and background information, cognitive screening and baseline status tests, general measures of cognition and executive functions (EFs) in occupation, cognitive tests for specific domains, measures of specific cognitive domains in occupations, and environmental assessment.

This model was recently updated and expanded by Bar-Haim Erez and Katz (2018). The extended C–FE includes measures of quality of life and well-being as the ultimate outcomes in occupational therapy interventions. The current C–FE framework, presented in this chapter, further conceptualizes the C–FE and differentiates the domains from the methods of the evaluation. The domains denote the content, or the "what," of the evaluation, with each domain contributing a distinctive facet to understanding the client's cognitive profile and its impact on everyday life.

The methods refer to the "how" of the evaluation process, explicating the procedures and the means that may be used to obtain the information. The overall C–FE represents an integrative approach to obtaining a comprehensive understanding of functional cognition. In this chapter, the term **cognition** is used to describe cognitive abilities (e.g., attention, memory, EF) or process skills that support or fail to support occupational performance. The term *functional cognition* is used to describe the broader concept of cognition as it interacts with personal and environmental factors to affect everyday functioning.

C–FE: Domains and Methods

The C–FE comprises 5 domains that reflect the occupational therapist's understanding of factors involved in the interaction between cognition and everyday functioning and that provide a comprehensive account of cognition in context. The 5 domains are

1. The client's cognitive occupational narrative,

2. Cognitive factors,

3. Functional cognition observed during occupational performance,

4. Self-awareness and beliefs regarding cognitive deficits and functional cognition, and

5. Evaluation of environmental factors.

The 3 methods of assessment are

1. Interviews,

2. Self-reports and informant reports regarding everyday functioning, and

3. Performance-based assessments.

Figure 4.1 illustrates the C–FE domains and methods. The assessment process typically starts with an interview regarding the client's occupational narrative, followed by brief screening of cognitive factors. The administration order of the other domains is more flexible and is decided on the basis of situational clinical reasoning. Because of the complexity of functional cognition and interactions among domains, some domains

FIGURE 4.1. The Cognitive–Functional Evaluation Framework.

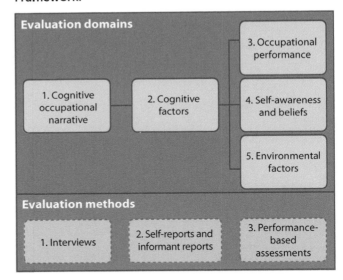

might be evaluated simultaneously or might be embedded in other domains. For example, occupational therapy practitioners may infer awareness and beliefs from observing clients' behaviors during any stage of the evaluation.

The following sections of this chapter provide a comprehensive description of the 5 C–FE domains. The possible applications of the 3 assessment methods are presented in each domain to illustrate their contribution to the evaluation process. The methods of assessment are not linked with 1 specific domain and therefore are described in more than 1 domain in the following sections.

Cognitive Occupational Narrative

Individuals construct their narratives through an ongoing process of reflecting on and interpreting life experiences over time. The *cognitive occupational narrative* represents the way clients understand their cognitive profile and the way they interpret its impact on their occupational experiences. The narrative captures the individual's experience as it is shaped by subjective personal factors, values, priorities, and choices. The evaluation of the narrative is a dynamic process that addresses how the client perceives the effects of cognitive factors in various occupations and contexts.

The ways cognitive deficits are represented in clients' narratives depend not only on self-awareness but also on the nature of their occupational demands and on personal and environmental factors. For example, the effect of executive deficits may be experienced differently by a person employed in a supervisory position than by a person whose work requires routine, habitual tasks. A person's values and self-efficacy may influence the way they interpret performance difficulties, ranging from extreme distress to empowered motivation. These interpretations may be reflected in diverse narrative statements, such as, "Forgetting people's names is unacceptable and means I am worthless," or, "I forget people's names, but I focus on important aspects of our relationship and explain my difficulties to them, so my forgetfulness doesn't get in the way of our relationship."

Furthermore, the narrative is affected by social–environmental factors, such as attitudes, stigma, and degree of support. For example, a work environment that embraces human diversity and allows for variations in performance styles will most likely result in better work performance for a person with cognitive deficits.

Understanding the client's subjective perception of their functional cognition is an essential component of the client-centered approach in occupational therapy. Therefore, in parallel with the American Occupational Therapy Association's *Occupational Therapy Practice Framework: Domain and Process* (3rd ed.; AOTA, 2014) occupational profile, the narrative is typically the first stage of the C–FE. In addition, initiating the evaluation process with the client's narrative has an added value for establishing rapport with the client. This is especially helpful before the occupational therapy practitioner administers potentially challenging and often frustrating screening and performance tests.

The methods for evaluating the client's narrative include semistructured interviews as well as standardized questionnaires targeting the implications of cognition on everyday life. It is important to provide the client with an opportunity to express not only their problems and concerns but also their strengths and resources related to functional cognition. This may be achieved through nonstandardized interviews as well as generic occupational performance measures, such as the Occupational Questionnaire (Smith et al., 1986), the Canadian Occupational Performance Measure (Law et al., 2005), and the Occupational Performance History Interview (Kielhofner et al., 1989).

In addition, occupational therapy practitioners may use standardized self-report questionnaires targeting a specific area of cognitive functioning to further probe the client's difficulties related to functional cognition. Examples are the Cognitive Failures Questionnaire (Broadbent et al., 1982), the Everyday Memory Questionnaire (Sunderland et al., 1983), the Behavior Rating Inventory of Executive Function (BRIEF; Roth et al., 2005), and the Multifactorial Memory Questionnaire (Troyer & Rich, 2002).

Measures of health-related quality of life specific to health conditions involving neurocognitive factors (e.g., stroke, traumatic brain injury [TBI], attention deficit hyperactivity disorder [ADHD], major neurocognitive disorder [dementia]) are also conceptualized as part of the occupational narrative. To this end, practitioners may use measures such as the Stroke Impact Scale (Duncan et al., 1999), the Adult ADHD Quality of Life Scale (Brod et al., 2005), and the Dementia Quality of Life Instrument (Brod et al., 1999).

The addition of health-related quality of life is in line with the recent recommendations of the extended C–FE (Bar-Haim Erez & Katz, 2018). The application of an interview or self-report questionnaires may sometimes be compromised by severe language or other cognitive impairments. When a person cannot adequately express their narrative, the practitioner gathers this information, as best as possible, from informants who know the client well.

Cognitive Factors

Occupational therapists use cognitive tests to screen for cognitive deficits. These tests address multiple cognitive factors, such as perception, attention, orientation, memory, language, praxis, and EFs. The scores are norm referenced and are indicative of the presence or absence of cognitive deficits.

The use of these tests is not unique to occupational therapy; they have been universally adopted by health professionals caring for individuals with suspected cognitive disabilities (e.g., physicians, psychologists, speech–language pathologists). The assessment method is based on the performance of a decontextualized task, typically involving relatively short pen-and-paper tests. These include tests, such as the Mini-Mental State Examination (Folstein et al., 1975) or the Montreal Cognitive Assessment (Nasreddine et al., 2005), or computerized cognitive batteries, such as the Cambridge Neuropsychological Test Automated Battery (Fray & Robbins, 1996).

In the C–FE process, cognitive tests provide a baseline cognitive profile indicating areas of cognitive deficits and strengths. However, it has been suggested that laboratory- and clinic-based tests may lack *ecological validity,* defined as the extent to which an assessment produces data representing an individual's interactions with their surroundings in authentic contexts (Robertson et al., 2017; Wallisch et al., 2018). Therefore, these tests cannot provide a comprehensive account of the implications of cognition for everyday life.

Occupational Performance

This domain of the C–FE relates to the evaluation of functional cognition during the performance of a task, activity, or occupation. As opposed to evaluating cognitive factors in isolation (as presented in the previous section), this domain focuses on the client's observable behaviors during their performance of activities. The purpose of assessing occupational performance in the C–FE is to understand how the interactions of cognitive factors with occupational and contextual factors affect performance. To this end, occupational therapists use their expertise in activity analyses to design standardized, ecologically valid assessments that target general or specific cognitive abilities.

Several aspects of the observable behaviors attributed to cognitive factors can be analyzed and scored. These aspects include process skills, errors and clients' responses to errors, strategic behaviors, and the level of assistance required.

Process skills are observable actions related to cognitive abilities that people use to manage and modify their actions during the performance of daily occupations (Fisher & Keilhofner, 1995). The evaluation of process skills is based on the observation of clients as they select, interact with, and use tools and materials; carry out individual actions and steps; and modify their performance when they encounter problems (Boyt Schell et al., 2014).

Occupational task performance can also be analyzed on the basis of the types of errors clients make while performing tasks. Doig et al. (2017) defined 4 types of error categories:

1. Errors of omission are made when actions necessary to complete the task are not performed or are incompletely performed.

2. Errors of addition are actions that are not necessary to complete the defined task.

3. Errors of repetition are unnecessary repetitions of an action or sequence of actions required to complete the task.

4. Errors of accuracy are made when actions are performed incorrectly, out of sequence, too slowly, or too quickly.

These errors can lead to both difficulties in task completion and poor performance outcomes. The client's verbal and behavioral responses, such as comments, gestures, or actions, can inform the understanding of their online awareness, as explained in the next section, "Self-Awareness and Beliefs."

Strategic behaviors are defined as mental plans of action that allow a person to approach a new task or problem systematically. They support performance in terms of efficiency, speed, accuracy, and consistency (Toglia et al., 2012). People use strategic behaviors to prepare for anticipated difficulties during performance or as a response to performance errors. The occupational therapist observes the frequency and types of strategies used, the flexibility of use, and, most important, the strategies' effectiveness in supporting performance.

Finally, the level of assistance required is derived from the interaction between the task demands and client's cognitive abilities and resources. Hierarchical cueing systems embedded in performance tests (e.g., indirect verbal guidance, direct verbal guidance, gestural guidance, physical assistance, performance of the task step for the client) allow the examiner to evaluate the minimal level of assistance the client requires to enable performance. This aspect of the evaluation is especially important for understanding the client's ability to function independently in daily life.

The methods for evaluating cognition in performance of a task, activity, or occupation vary in the degree to which the tasks and the settings they use reflect performance in real life. Performance-based assessment methods range from observations of occupational performance in naturalistic settings to standardized, in-lab tasks that share some attributes with real-world occupations. Tools such as the Model of Human Occupation Screening Tool (Parkinson et al., 2006) and Routine Task Inventory (Allen et al., 1989) allow clinicians to assess cognition in occupational functioning in a standardized yet flexible manner that can be applied to a variety of occupations performed in naturalistic settings. However, real-life observations are not always feasible because of limited resources in the clinical settings, which may restrict access to various occupational contexts.

An alternative approach is to assess occupational performance through standardized, simulated real-life tasks. Assessments such as the Multiple Errands Test (MET; Shallice & Burgess, 1991), the Kettle Test (Hartman-Maeir, Harel, & Katz 2009), and the Executive Function Performance Test (EFPT; Baum et al., 2007) assess functional cognition during the performance of predefined tasks that are designed to simulate everyday life tasks, including shopping, cooking, and taking medication. These types of assessments can be carried out in a real-world environment (e.g., MET), in a more controlled clinical setting (e.g., EFPT, Kettle Test), or in a virtual environment (e.g., virtual MET; Rand et al., 2009).

Virtual reality provides a highly standardized yet ecologically valid environment, which is useful for the assessment of functional cognition in tasks that entail potential risk when performed in natural environments (e.g., crossing the street; see Kim et al., 2010). Recently, Goverover and Deluca (2018) introduced the Actual Reality, a performance-based approach that uses real-world tasks, such as using the Internet to order airline tickets, cookies, and pizza. This approach allows the therapist to examine functional cognition with an up-to-date performance method, and it offers a real-world context in the clinical setting.

Performance-based assessments that use simulated real-life tasks have the potential to achieve a high level of ecological validity (Wallisch et al., 2018). For example, the MET had good to strong correlations with everyday functioning among people with acquired brain injury (Dawson et al., 2009). In another study, it predicted participation in everyday life activities 3 months after discharge from a neurorehabilitation facility (Maeir et al., 2011).

Subjective reports of functional cognition that use self-report or informant-report standardized questionnaires (e.g., Everyday Memory Questionnaire, BRIEF) provide an additional method to assess the impact of specific cognitive abilities in everyday functioning. Although observations provide an objective account of the client's ability to perform a task, they are limited to a specific time and place and may not account for the inherent variations that occur in cognitive performance.

Personal factors, such as emotional status and motivational resources, may influence performance. The heightened emotional demands associated with cognitive functioning in the real world can create a discrepancy whereby a person may report difficulties in everyday life that are not observed in simulated task performance (Carrigan et al., 2017). Furthermore, these questionnaires provide an opportunity to assess self-initiated performance, which is often masked in structured observations, because the instructions and presence of the therapist may preclude the assessment of self-initiated performance. Therefore, self-reports and informant reports add a unique perspective that is necessary to gain a representative portrayal of functional cognition.

Self-Awareness and Beliefs

The client's awareness of their cognitive profile and its impact on occupational performance is central to the clinical reasoning process guiding the choice of treatment approach (Toglia & Maeir, 2018). Cognitive problems are often elusive and difficult for the client to grasp, because of neurogenic and psychogenic mechanisms (Toglia & Maeir, 2018). An additional metacognitive factor that is related to awareness concerns beliefs about cognitive abilities and their implications for everyday life (Toglia & Kirk, 2000). Because cognition is typically highly valued by individuals as an expression of their self-worth, negative beliefs may trigger severe occupational withdrawal. Conversely, positive beliefs and social support may enable constructive coping and limit the negative impact on occupational performance. Therefore, the assessment of awareness and beliefs regarding cognition is an essential part of the C–FE.

According to the Dynamic Comprehensive Model of Awareness (Toglia & Kirk, 2000), which guides neurorehabilitation practice, there are 2 major components of awareness. The first is *metacognitive knowledge*, or intellectual awareness that exists before a task or situation. The 2nd, *online awareness*, refers to self-monitoring and evaluation of performance in the context of an activity.

In the C–FE process, it is necessary to evaluate both components of awareness that mediate the impact of cognitive deficits on occupational performance. Both awareness components affect the degree of the client's safety and engagement in the therapeutic process, as well as the implementation of strategies to improve occupational performance.

Intellectual awareness typically is evaluated in a semistructured interview and through comparison of self-reports with reports by an informant on cognitive–functional questionnaires. The Self-Awareness of Deficits Interview (Fleming et al., 1996) and the Awareness Questionnaire (Sherer et al., 1998) are examples of measures used to evaluate intellectual awareness. Questionnaires such as the BRIEF and the Dysexecutive Questionnaire (Wilson et al., 1996) have 2 versions for self-report and informant report, and comparing any discrepancy between the 2 provides information about intellectual awareness.

Online awareness is evaluated within the performance of a specific task. Practitioners conduct these evaluations throughout the C–FE process by observing the client's responses to errors. Doig et al. (2017) differentiated between responses that indicate the client identified an error (verbal or nonverbal) and actual attempts to correct errors in performance.

In addition, practitioners can assess online awareness by asking clients to predict their performance before the task or evaluate their performance afterward. The client can be asked questions about aspects related to task demands, quantitative attributes of performance (e.g., time, accuracy), or qualitative aspects (e.g., difficulty, strategy use, satisfaction, safety). The Weekly Calendar Planning Activity (Toglia, 2015) is an example of a measure that incorporates a standardized assessment of online awareness in a functional test of EFs.

In addition to intellectual and online awareness, it is important to evaluate the client's beliefs about their cognitive profile and its impact on functioning. This personal contextual factor may vary among clients with a wide range of beliefs, from acceptance, hope, and self efficacy (e.g., "There is something I can do about this") to self-criticism, blame, pessimism, and helplessness. Practitioners may elicit clients' beliefs about their functional cognition through standard questionnaires, such as the Contentment scale of the Multifactorial Memory Questionnaire, as well as through open-ended questions at different stages of the C–FE.

Environmental Factors

Occupational performance occurs in a person's everyday life environment, including the physical setting, social network, and cultural context. Environmental factors significantly mediate the impact of cognitive deficits in everyday life. A supportive physical and social environment can optimize functioning for individuals with cognitive impairments. Therefore, it is critical to evaluate the environment in which the client functions.

Evaluation of the physical environment is focused on the extent to which the home or community environments support safe and satisfying occupational performance. Occupational therapy practitioners conduct this aspect of the evaluation by observing the impact of environmental factors on the client's performance of everyday occupations in their natural environment (e.g., home).

When evaluating the environment, it is important to assess the client's ability to use environmental supports rather than merely assessing their presence in the home. For example, a calendar may be present at home as a cognitive support for daily planning of tasks, but it will not be beneficial to the client if they do not actually use it. In some cases, training to use existing environmental supports is the key to their impact on everyday functioning. The In-Home Occupational Performance Evaluation (Stark et al., 2010) is an example of a standardized measure that provides an assessment of environmental barriers to occupational performance in the home.

In addition to the physical environment, the evaluation of environmental factors addresses the impact of the social environment on occupational performance. The occupational therapist should explore not only the availability of social support but also the client's view on the adequacy of support for their needs. For example, some clients may view tangible assistance from people close to them as enabling and supportive, whereas others may describe the same assistance as threatening their independence and autonomy (Rotenberg-Shpigelman, 2017). The therapist is obligated to report cases of client neglect or abuse.

In addition, the occupational therapist should use clinical judgment to determine whether social involvement is preventing the client from engaging in occupations according to their abilities and desires. The therapist evaluates aspects of tangible and emotional social support using open-ended questions and standardized questionnaires, such as the Medical Outcomes Study Social Support Survey (Sherbourne & Stewart, 1991).

Clinical Implications for Intervention

The product of the evaluation is a cognitive–functional profile that provides a description of the client's cognitive strengths and weaknesses and their implications for occupational performance. This includes recommendations concerning the type and amount of assistance currently required for safe and meaningful occupational performance, and it affords the basis for clinical reasoning in selecting the treatment approach.

Occupational therapy intervention typically draws on change mechanisms in the person or the environment. Practitioners can enable occupation by modifying person factors (e.g., knowledge, belief, abilities, skills, strategies) and environmental factors (e.g., removing social and physical barriers, designing optimal supports for performance). The choice of intervention approach is guided by the person's ability to learn and adapt (determined to a large extent by the severity of cognitive deficit), awareness and beliefs, and environmental resources, as well as the demands of their occupations and life roles.

The following 3 case examples demonstrate the complex interactions among the C–FE domains that are unique to each client. **Alex** and **Bob** (both age 50) were referred to occupational therapy after a mild head injury. When cognitive factors were assessed, both clients demonstrated similar mild cognitive deficits in attention, memory, and EFs.

However, the implications of the cognitive deficits on their real-world occupational functioning and narrative differ significantly. Alex's cognitive occupational narrative reveals a profound impact of his cognitive deficits on all his life roles. He lives alone, shares custody of his 2 young children (ages 3 and 5 years) with his ex-wife, and is the owner and manager of a small business. Since his injury, he describes a breakdown in his ability to meet his occupational demands. Alex reported these difficulties in standardized ecological questionnaires that capture occupational performance.

Alex feels he can no longer manage his household tasks or keep track of his business budget. He sadly talks about the loss of joyful engagement with his children, which has been replaced by feeling overwhelmed and resentful of their needs. Alex is aware of his cognitive difficulties and expresses the belief that his occupational identity as an able, independent individual has been compromised.

In relation to environmental factors, Alex reports having minimal social support, mainly from 1 long-distance friend. In summary, Alex demonstrates good self-awareness with only mild cognitive deficits, but he has limited social support and high cognitive demands in his occupations. Therefore, Alex is at risk for occupational malfunction, withdrawal, and disability. He requires an integrative approach that uses environmental adaptations and support to promote occupational functioning in the short term, as well as a declarative metacognitive learning approach to foster acquisition and transfer of strategies that will support independent future performance.

Bob's cognitive occupational narrative reveals a notably lower impact of his cognitive deficits on his current occupational functioning. Bob's major productive role is as a homemaker. He is experiencing some difficulties managing IADLs, but he has discovered some strategies, such as "1 at a time," that he finds useful.

In addition, Bob has begun to use more public transportation after experiencing difficulties and stress while driving. He describes the feeling of relief in using public transportation and the opportunity it provides him to meet other people. Bob describes being content with his occupational performance. The assessment of environmental factors reveals that Bob lives with a supportive partner and has ongoing positive interactions with friends and family.

During the assessment of occupational performance, Bob became more aware of his impairments, and he expressed surprise as to how difficult some of the occupational performance tests were for him. He requested assistance in learning more about his cognitive profile and in discovering additional strategies to cope with more-challenging tasks. Given Bob's emerging awareness and learning ability, he is also a good candidate for a metacognitive approach to promote awareness and strategy use that will enable engagement in complex tasks. However, given his current occupational performance and satisfaction, he does not require environmental adaptations or supports.

Carol, age 45, was referred to occupational therapy after a severe TBI resulting from a car accident. Before the accident, Carol was a music teacher. She was in charge of household management and was enthusiastic about entertaining and going out with friends. Her cognitive occupational narrative reveals great frustration with her doctors, who do not permit her to return to work, and with her husband for taking over some of her household responsibilities, such as financial management.

During the assessment of cognitive factors, Carol demonstrates severe impairments in multiple cognitive areas, including attention, memory, and EFs. She also demonstrates severe difficulties in occupational performance, both in everyday tasks and in standardized simulated tasks, but is unaware of her cognitive deficits and performance difficulties. Her husband describes significant changes in her functioning, including difficulties in cooking and using simple electrical appliances, such as the washing machine. However, Carol attributes these occupational difficulties to fatigue, further demonstrating deficits in awareness.

Because of her severe impairments and lack of awareness, Carol is likely to benefit from a treatment approach that combines a neurofunctional model (Giles, 2018) based on procedural learning; environmental adaptations, including modifications of the physical environment; and significant, ongoing social support.

Summary

Occupational performance cannot be explained by cognitive factors in isolation but rather as they interact with the whole person in their lived environment. The purpose of a C–FE is to determine the implication of cognitive deficits on everyday life among people with suspected cognitive disabilities, to determine the client's capacity to live in their home. Therefore, the C–FE is designed to be an ecologically valid, multidomain process that represents the complexity of functional cognition. The domains of the C–FE, including narrative, cognitive factors, occupational performance, self-awareness, and environmental factors, represent the unique occupational therapy perspective, integrating cognition into daily life.

References

Allen, C., Heimann, N., & Yerxa, E. (1989). The Routine Task Inventory: A tool for describing the functional behavior of the cognitively disabled. *OT Practice, 1,* 67–74.

American Occupational Therapy Association. (2014). Occupational therapy practice framework: Domain and process (3rd ed.). *American Journal of Occupational Therapy, 68*(Suppl. 1), S1–S48. https://doi.org/10.5014/ajot.2014.682006

Bar-Haim Erez, A., & Katz, N. (2018). Cognitive Functional Evaluation. In N. Katz & J. Toglia (Eds.), *Cognition, occupation, and participation across the lifespan: Neuroscience, neurorehabilitation, and models of intervention in occupational therapy* (4th ed., pp. 69–86). Bethesda, MD: AOTA Press.

Baum, C., Morrison, T., Hahn, M., & Edwards, D. (2007). *Executive Function Performance Test: Test protocol booklet.* St. Louis: Program in Occupational Therapy, Washington University School of Medicine.

Boyt Schell, B. A., Gillen, G., & Scaffa, M. (2014). Glossary. In B. A. Boyt Schell, G. Gillen, & M. Scaffa (Eds.), *Willard and Spackman's occupational therapy* (12th ed., pp. 1229–1243). Philadelphia: Lippincott Williams & Wilkins.

Broadbent, D. E., Cooper, P. F., FitzGerald, P., & Parkes, K. R. (1982). The Cognitive Failures Questionnaire (CFQ) and its correlates. *British Journal of Clinical Psychology, 21,* 1–16. https://doi.org/10.1111/j.2044-8260.1982.tb01421.x

Brod, M., Perwien, A., Adler, L., & Spencer, T. (2005). Conceptualization and assessment of quality of life for adults with attention deficit disorder. *Primary Psychiatry, 12,* 58–64.

Brod, M., Stewart, A. L., Sands, L., & Walton, P. (1999). Conceptualization and measurement of quality of life in dementia: The Dementia Quality of Life Instrument (DQoL). *Gerontologist, 39,* 25–36. https://doi.org/10.1093/geront/39.1.25

Carrigan, N., Barkus, E., Ong, A., & Wei, M. (2017). Do complaints of everyday cognitive failures in high schizotypy relate to emotional working memory deficits in the lab? *Comprehensive Psychiatry, 78,* 115–129. https://doi.org/10.1016/j.comppsych.2017.06.016

Dawson, D. R., Anderson, N. D., Burgess, P., Cooper, E., Krpan, K. M., & Stuss, D. T. (2009). Further development of the Multiple Errands Test: Standardized scoring, reliability, and ecological validity for the Baycrest version. *Archives of Physical Medicine and Rehabilitation, 90*(Suppl.), S41–S51. https://doi.org/10.1016/j.apmr.2009.07.012

Doig, E., Fleming, J., Ownsworth, T., & Fletcher, S. (2017). An occupation-based, metacognitive approach to assessing error performance and online awareness. *Australian Occupational Therapy Journal, 64,* 137–148. https://doi.org/10.1111/1440-1630.12322

Duncan, P. W., Lai, S. M., Wallace, D., Embretson, S., Johnson, D., & Studenski, S. (1999). *Stroke Impact Scale* (Version 3.0). Kansas City: University of Kansas Medical Center.

Fisher, A., & Keilhofner, G. (1995). Skill in occupational performance. In G. Keilhofner (Ed.), *A model of human occupation theory and application* (pp. 113–137). Baltimore: Williams & Wilkins.

Fleming, J. M., Strong, J., & Ashton, R. (1996). Self-awareness of deficits in adults with traumatic brain injury: How best to measure? *Brain Injury, 10,* 1–16. https://doi.org/10.1080/026990596124674

Folstein, M. F., Folstein, S. E., & McHugh, P. R. (1975). "Mini-Mental State": A practical method for grading the cognitive state of patients for the clinician. *Journal of Psychiatric Research, 12*(3), 189–198. https://doi.org/10.1016/0022-3956(75)90026-6

Fray, P. J., & Robbins, T. W. (1996). CANTAB Battery: Proposed utility in neurotoxicology. *Neurotoxicology and Teratology, 18,* 499–504. https://doi.org/10.1016/0892-0362(96)00027-X

Giles, G. M. (2018). Neurofunctional Approach to rehabilitation after brain injury. In N. Katz & J. Toglia (Eds.), *Cognition, occupation, and participation across the lifespan: Neuroscience, neurorehabilitation, and models of intervention in occupational therapy* (4th ed., pp. 419–442). Bethesda, MD: AOTA Press.

Goverover, Y., & Deluca, J. (2018). Assessing everyday life functional activity using Actual Reality in persons with MS. *Rehabilitation Psychology, 63,* 276–285. https://doi.org/10.1037/rep0000212

Hartman-Maeir, A., Harel, H., & Katz, N. (2009). Kettle Test—A brief measure of cognitive functional performance: Reliability and validity in stroke rehabilitation. *American Journal of Occupational Therapy, 63,* 592–599. https://doi.org/10.5014/ajot.63.5.592

Hartman-Maeir, A., Katz, N., & Baum, C. M. (2009). Cognitive Functional Evaluation (CFE) process for individuals with suspected cognitive disabilities. *Occupational Therapy in Health Care, 23,* 1–23. https://doi.org/10.1080/07380570802455516

Kielhofner, G., Henry, A., & Walens, D. (1989). *A user's guide to the Occupational Performance History Interview.* Rockville, MD: American Occupational Therapy Association.

Kim, D. Y., Ku, J., Chang, W. H., Park, T. H., Lim, J. Y., Han, K., . . . Kim, S. I. (2010). Assessment of post-stroke extrapersonal neglect using a three-dimensional immersive virtual street crossing program. *Acta Neurologica Scandinavica, 121,* 171–177. https://doi.org/10.1111/j.1600-0404.2009.01194.x

Law, M., Baptiste, S., Carswell, A., McColl, M. A., Polatajko, H., & Pollock, N. (2005). *The Canadian Occupational Performance Measure manual* (4th ed.). Ottawa: CAOT Publications.

Maeir, A., Krauss, S., & Katz, N. (2011). Ecological validity of the Multiple Errands Test (MET) on discharge from neurorehabilitation hospital. *OTJR: Occupation, Participation and Health, 31*(Suppl. 1), S38–S46. https://doi.org/10.3928/15394492-20101108-07

Nasreddine, Z. S., Phillips, N. A., Bédirian, V., Charbonneau, S., Whitehead, V., Collin, I., . . . Chertkow, H. (2005). The Montreal Cognitive Assessment, MoCA: A brief screening tool for mild cognitive impairment. *Journal of the American Geriatrics Society, 53,* 695–699. https://doi.org/10.1111/j.1532-5415.2005.53221.x

Parkinson, S., Forsyth, K., & Kielhofner, G. (2006). *User's manual for the Model of Human Occupation Screening Tool (MOHOST)* (Version 2.0). Chicago: Model of Human Occupation Clearinghouse, Department of Occupational Therapy, College of Applied Health Sciences, University of Illinois at Chicago.

Rand, D., Basha-Abu Rukan, S., Weiss, P. L., & Katz, N. (2009). Validation of the Virtual MET as an assessment tool for executive functions. *Neuropsychological Rehabilitation, 19,* 583–602. https://doi.org/10.1080/09602010802469074

Robertson, K., Schmitter-Edgecombe, M., Weeks, D., & Pimentel, J. (2017). Naturalistic assessment using a simulated environment: Cognitive correlates and relationship to functional status in individuals with neurologic conditions. *Archives of Clinical Neuropsychology, 33,* 1024–1039. https://doi.org/10.1093/arclin/acx136

Rotenberg-Shpigelman, S. (2017). *Older adults seeking help for subjective memory complaints: Psycho-social characteristics and implications on participation and quality-of-life informed the development of an occupation-based meta-cognitive group intervention.* Jerusalem: Hebrew University of Jerusalem.

Roth, R., Isquith, P., & Gioia, G. (2005). *Behavior Rating Inventory of Executive Function—Adult version.* Lutz, FL: Psychological Assessment Resources.

Shallice, T., & Burgess, P. W. (1991). Deficits in strategy application following frontal lobe damage in man. *Brain, 114,* 727–741. https://doi.org/10.1093/brain/114.2.727

Sherbourne, C. D., & Stewart, A. L. (1991). The MOS Social Support Survey. *Social Science and Medicine, 32,* 705–714. https://doi.org/10.1016/0277-9536(91)90150-B

Sherer, M., Bergloff, P., Boake, C., High, W., Jr., & Levin, E. (1998). The Awareness Questionnaire: Factor structure and internal consistency. *Brain Injury, 12,* 63–68. https://doi.org/10.1080/026990598122863

Smith, N. R., Kielhofner, G., & Watts, J. H. (1986). The relationships between volition, activity pattern, and life satisfaction in the elderly. *American Journal of Occupational Therapy, 40,* 278–283. https://doi.org/10.5014/ajot.40.4.278

Stark, S. L., Somerville, E. K., & Morris, J. C. (2010). In-Home Occupational Performance Evaluation (I-HOPE). *American Journal of Occupational Therapy, 64,* 580–589. https://doi.org/10.5014/ajot.2010.08065

Sunderland, A., Harris, J. E., & Baddeley, A. D. (1983). Do laboratory tests predict everyday memory? A neuropsychological study. *Journal of Verbal Learning and Verbal Behavior, 22,* 341–357. https://doi.org/10.1016/S0022-5371(83)90229-3

Toglia, J. (2015). *Weekly Calendar Planning Activity (WCPA): A performance test of executive function.* Bethesda, MD: AOTA Press.

Toglia, J., & Kirk, U. (2000). Understanding awareness deficits following brain injury. *NeuroRehabilitation, 15,* 57–70.

Toglia, J., & Maeir, A. (2018). Self-awareness and metacognition: Effect on occupational performance and outcome across the lifespan. In N. Katz & J. Toglia (Eds.), *Cognition, occupation, and participation across the lifespan: Neuroscience, neurorehabilitation, and models of intervention in occupational therapy* (4th ed., pp. 143–164). Bethesda, MD: AOTA Press.

Toglia, J. P., Rodger, S. A., & Polatajko, H. J. (2012). Anatomy of cognitive strategies: A therapist's primer for enabling occupational performance. *Canadian Journal of Occupational Therapy, 79,* 225–236. https://doi.org/10.2182/cjot.2012.79.4.4

Troyer, A. K., & Rich, J. B. (2002). Psychometric properties of a new metamemory questionnaire for older adults. *Journals of Gerontology, Series B: Psychological Sciences, 57,* 19–27. https://doi.org/10.1093/geronb/57.1.P19

Wallisch, A., Little, L. M., Dean, E., & Dunn, W. (2018). Executive function measures for children: A scoping review of ecological validity. *OTJR: Occupation, Participation and Health, 38,* 6–14. https://doi.org/10.1177/1539449217727118

Wilson, B., Alderman, N., Burgess, P., Emslie, H., & Evans, J. (1996). *Behavioural Assessment of the Dysexecutive Syndrome.* Bury St. Edmunds, England: Thames Valley Test Company.

Occupational Profile: The Anchor of Functional–Cognitive Assessment

TIMOTHY J. WOLF, OTD, PhD, OTR/L, FAOTA,
AND CAROLYN M. BAUM, PhD, OTR/L, FAOTA

LEARNING OBJECTIVES

After completing this chapter, readers should be able to

- Understand the importance of the occupational profile in functional–cognitive evaluation,
- Describe the key elements obtained from an occupational profile that are necessary to understand and interpret occupational performance changes,
- Understand how a care support partner may help with developing an occupational profile, and
- Describe how to use the results from the occupational profile to help establish treatment goals and select performance-based assessments.

KEY TERMS AND CONCEPTS

- Habitual tasks • Motivation • Novel tasks • Occupational profile • Saliency

Introduction

When one explores functional–cognitive evaluation, it should not come as a surprise that the foundation for the evaluation is the occupational profile. This is highlighted not only in the description of the Cognitive–Functional Evaluation (C–FE) that is used as the framework in this text (see Chapter 4) but also in the *Occupational Therapy Practice Framework: Domain and Process* (3rd ed., *OTPF–3*; American Occupational Therapy Association [AOTA], 2014). According to the *OTPF–3*, the ***occupational profile*** is "a summary of a client's occupational history and experiences, patterns of daily living, interests, values, and needs. Developing the occupational profile provides the occupational therapy practitioner with an understanding of a client's perspective and background" (AOTA, 2014, p. S13).

Additionally, the occupational profile helps the occupational therapist understand

- How the client's level of engagement in specific occupations might have changed over time,

- What is important to the client (i.e., saliency),
- The client's level of familiarity with occupations (habitual vs. novel tasks), and
- What motivates the client.

In general, this information is essential for client-centered care, which focuses on the specific needs, wants, and goals of the client. This chapter reviews specific methods to obtain an occupational profile and then further discusses the key concepts (i.e., saliency, habitual vs. novel tasks, motivation) as they relate to informing the assessment, setting goals, and guiding the treatment process when the focus is functional cognition.

Methods and Tools to Obtain an Occupational Profile

As with all other forms of assessment, there are 2 primary methods to obtain an occupational profile: informal interview and formal assessment. Some of the formal assessments use interview methodology with the client, the care partner, or both. The sections that follow describe some of the methods and tools practitioners use to obtain an occupational profile. These are provided for illustrative purposes and are not intended to be an exhaustive list.

Informal Interview

Often, occupational therapists conduct an informal interview with the client, care partner, or both to obtain an occupational history to build the occupational profile. This is most often the case in very time-restricted health care settings (e.g., acute care). Efficiency is the primary justification for this approach. The disadvantage is that it is possible and somewhat likely that elements of the occupational history will be missed.

Formal Measures

AOTA Occupational Profile Template

AOTA (2017) developed the *AOTA Occupational Profile Template* as a semistructured interview to establish a client's occupational profile. Based on the *OTPF–3,* the template provides page numbers that link each construct to the practice framework. Questions are posed in the template related to the client's

- Perceptions of why they need occupational therapy services,

- Occupational performance strengths and weaknesses,

- Values and beliefs,

- Occupational history, and

- Performance patterns.

The 2nd section gathers information about the client's perceptions of barriers and supports in their physical and social environments. The 3rd section in the template evaluates the client's perceptions of cultural, personal, temporal, and virtual contexts as they relate to meaningful occupation. The template concludes with a goal-setting section to guide the practitioner in identifying occupational performance limitations that are of a high priority to the client and in determining desired results.

The *AOTA Occupational Profile Template* is intended for use in establishing a detailed occupational profile and client-centered goals across settings and populations. No psychometric data are available (AOTA, 2014).

Canadian Occupational Performance Measure

The Canadian Occupational Performance Measure (COPM) is a semistructured interview tool used to guide collaborative discussion regarding clients' perceptions of occupational performance (Carswell et al., 2004). Using the COPM, the therapist interviews the client to identify performance problems in the areas of

- Self-care (personal care, functional mobility, community management),

- Productivity (paid or unpaid work, household management, play and school), and

- Leisure (quiet recreation, active recreation, socialization).

The client then rates the importance of each identified performance problem on a scale from 1 to 10. For the 5 most important goals, the client uses a 10-point scale to rate their current performance level and current satisfaction level. To score the measure, the practitioner then divides the total performance or satisfaction score by the number of problems to obtain an average performance or satisfaction score, respectively.

The COPM is a useful tool for determining a client's occupational profile, for goal setting, and for use as a client-centered outcome measure. The measure has been applied extensively in populations of patients with stroke or traumatic brain injury (Jenkinson et al., 2007; Phipps & Richardson, 2007; Yang et al., 2017). Use of the COPM has also been reported with clients with chronic pain, arthritis, cerebral palsy, and developmental coordination disorder, but the measure may be used with clients with any condition (Carpenter et al., 2001; Kjeken et al., 2005; Novak et al., 2009; Taylor et al., 2007). Test–retest reliability, interrater reliability, and internal consistency of the measure are acceptable (Cup et al., 2003). The minimal clinically important difference for COPM scores is 2 points.

Occupational Performance History Interview

The Occupational Performance History Interview (OPHI–II) is a semistructured interview (Kielhofner et al., 2001) that is rooted in the Model of Human Occupation (Kielhofner & Henry, 1988; Kielhofner et al., 1989). The current version of this instrument consists of an interview, rating scales for use with information obtained during the interview, and a method for recording qualitative data from the interview (Kielhofner & Henry, 1988). The interview evaluates

- Activity and occupational choices,

- Critical life events,

- Daily routines,

- Occupational roles, and

- Occupational behavior settings.

After the interview, the therapist completes

- The Occupational Competence scale as a quantitative measure of the extent to which the client is able to continue a satisfying and productive occupational performance pattern;

- The Occupational Identity scale as a measure of the extent to which the client has developed a positive occupational identity; and

- The Occupational Behavior Settings scale as a measure of the support of the home, work, and leisure environments for occupational performance.

The recording of qualitative data from the interview focuses on the overall course of the client's life story and themes found in the story (Kielhofner et al., 2001). The OPHI may be used with any population as long as the clients have sufficient cognitive capacity to engage in the interview process. The OPHI has demonstrated acceptable levels of reliability and validity (Henry et al., 1994; Kielhofner et al., 1991, 2001; Lynch & Bridle, 1993).

Activity Card Sort

The Activity Card Sort (ACS) evaluates a client's daily life participation through the use of photos of activities placed on cards or a tablet (Baum & Edwards, 2008). Activities are sorted by the client according to the categories of "never done," "do less than in the past," "do more than in the past," "do the same amount as in the past," and "given up." These categories may be in reference to a time point, such as an illness, injury, or simply aging.

The activity cards include instrumental activities, low-demand leisure activities, high-demand leisure activities, and social activities. The ACS provides insight into the person's family and community activities and their level of participation. The measure helps the practitioner to determine why clients may be doing something less or have given it up and to identify activities families can use to engage their loved one (Fox et al., 2017). The OPHI also records and evaluates changes in participation over time and can serve as an outcome measure in clinic and research settings (Bailey et al., 2009; Baum, 1995; Edwards et al., 2006; Eriksson et al., 2013; Hartman-Maeir et al., 2007; Perlmutter et al., 2010). Furthermore, the ACS may be used as a basis for goal setting.

Since the original ACS was developed by Baum and Edwards in 1993 for use with older adults, there have been many culture- and population-specific adaptations of the measure. The ACS has demonstrated excellent reliability and validity (Baum & Edwards, 2001; Chan et al., 2006; Hamed & Holm, 2013; Katz et al., 2003; Laver-Fawcett et al., 2016; Lyons et al., 2010; Orellano et al., 2012; Poerbodipoero et al., 2016). Research has provided support for the ACS as an accepted measure of activity engagement and participation (Tse et al., 2013).

Essential Information From the Occupational Profile

The first domain of the C–FE is referred to as the occupational narrative. This is synonymous with what is described in this chapter as the occupational profile. In the process of obtaining an occupational history, by using formal measures and informal interviews, the occupational therapist builds an occupational profile that forms the foundation for assessment and treatment.

The information from the occupational profile provides the therapist with information related to the client's level of engagement in specific occupations, but, indirectly, it also provides the occupational therapist with additional information that is essential for treatment planning. The following are some examples of additional information that practitioners can obtain from the occupational profile.

Saliency

In geography, a *salience* is something that stands out from a contour. In neuroscience, the word *saliency* is used to describe items in an array to which the individual allocates cognitive resources (i.e., the most personally important information in the environment). Building on these definitions, in the context of interpretation of an occupational profile, **saliency** denotes the quality of being the most noticeable or important.

An occupational profile is essential in helping the occupational therapist understand which occupations are the most salient to the client or care partner. As the practitioner is developing an occupational profile and, ultimately, establishing goals with a client, a knowledge of the client's previous level of occupational performance is, of course, important, but the saliency of the occupations to the individual is also central to the occupational profile.

The most salient occupations should be prioritized whenever possible, not only in the selection of performance-based tests (PBTs) that the test taker can appreciate as relevant to their life circumstances but also in the structure of treatment sessions. Saliency is the first priority in this regard; however, it needs to be balanced with the client's current level of functioning, practical considerations related to the treatment setting, and the ultimate goals of treatment.

For example, the most salient task to the client may not currently be an appropriate therapeutic goal for several reasons, including but not limited to the following:

- The task might present no or very limited challenge to the client.

- The task might not be addressable in the current treatment setting (e.g., driving, in an acute care setting).

In these cases, the occupational therapy practitioner should have a conversation with the client, their care partner, or both to acknowledge the importance of the activity to the client but discuss why it might not be the most appropriate, to help build rapport.

Habitual vs. Novel Tasks

Although saliency helps the occupational therapist understand which occupations are most important to the client, an occupational profile can also provide important information about a client's familiarity and experience with occupations. Familiarity and experience with occupations can generally be described in 2 categories: habitual and novel. **Habitual tasks** are the occupations that the client has the most experience with. They tend to be very routinized, often occur in the same context with minimal or no changes in task demands, and do not require sustained conscious attention. An example of occupations that are often habitual is basic ADLs.

Novel tasks either are less familiar to the client or often occur in dynamic environments with changing task demands. Therefore, they often require a greater degree of vigilance and high-level cognitive processing. A common example of a task that is typically considered novel is managing household finances. Although components of paying bills and managing finances may be habitual to a client, the dynamic nature of the task (e.g., changes in which bills need to be paid, fluctuations in income, long-term budgeting) makes it more novel.

Although ADLs and finance management are typical examples, it is important to note that there is great variability in what clients consider habitual or novel for most occupations. For example, **Bob** lives alone in an apartment, does not finance anything on credit, does not have savings or investments, gets money orders to pay rent and utilities, and has had the same typical expenses for many years. In Bob's case, paying bills is very much a habitual task.

In contrast, **Mark** works a commission-based job with income that varies from month to month. He has varying expenses that come due at different times, helps support other family members whose needs change monthly, and has a portfolio of investments that he contributes to as he is able. In Mark's case, paying bills may be a much more novel task.

It is important to understand, however, that tasks that are novel can be modified to be more habitual, and tasks that were once habitual may become more novel after an injury or illness. ADLs are habitual until an individual has a stroke and cannot use 1 side of their body. After an illness or injury, cooking may be very novel until the kitchen is modified, the types of food cooked are simplified, and the individual starts using a meal service to do meal planning.

Why is this information important in an occupational profile that addresses functional cognition? First, the neuroanatomical correlates and cognitive demands for how people accomplish habitual and novel tasks are different. Novel tasks

- Require much more complex and integrated brain activation (executive function),
- Are more conscious processes, and
- Are much more susceptible to even mild changes in cognitive capacity.

Habitual tasks, in contrast,

- Rely more on limited subcortical and cerebellar structures,
- Require less conscious thought, and
- Are often not as impaired among people with mild to moderate cognitive limitations (Camina & Güell, 2017).

Therefore, understanding the mechanism of injury or disease etiology, the prognosis, and which neuroanatomical structures and networks are affected not only will help explain changes in the occupational profile but also will help with treatment planning.

Second, practitioners need to know the degree to which a task is habitual or novel to interpret performance on a PBT of functional cognition. Consider Bob from the previous example of paying bills. Bill paying has posed limited demands on Bob, and he pays the same bills in the same way week after week. A complex bill-paying activity that requires monthly budgeting, writing checks, and using an online bill-pay system, however, would be very novel. One might expect that Bob would find this assessment very challenging, but it would likely not be a very salient activity for him, because he would recognize bill paying as a relatively insignificant and nondemanding part of his life.

In contrast, for Mark, this same bill-paying PBT might be much more salient. Given his far more extensive experience in complex budgeting and bill paying, however, one also might expect him to accomplish the assessment with less difficulty than Bob. Without the context from the occupational profile, Bob might be inappropriately identified as having a profound change in functional cognition, or vice versa for Mark.

Third, occupational therapy practitioners need to know the degree to which a task is habitual or novel for treatment planning. For example, imagine that Mark has a progressive neurocognitive disorder (e.g., Alzheimer's disease, dementia). The practitioner knows that habitual tasks are typically spared longer than the ability to accomplish novel tasks, and individuals can learn new habitual tasks using behavioral methods (Kawai et al., 2002). It therefore might be more appropriate to use more task-based approaches (e.g., task simplification, environmental modification, behavioral training) rather than trying to help Mark learn strategies to maintain his independence. The practitioner needs the occupational profile, with an understanding of the likely course of illness progression, to determine the appropriate approach to support Mark's independence as long as possible with paying bills. Without knowledge from the occupational profile, there is no way to appropriately set goals for treatment.

Motivation

Knowing what is most important to the client (i.e., saliency) and their level of familiarity with their occupations (habitual vs. novel) forms the basis of understanding what is motivating to the client. *Motivation* is the individual's willingness to engage in an activity. This is not a new concept for occupational therapists, but it is important to discuss related to addressing functional cognition.

Rehabilitation for functional–cognitive loss, or even rehabilitation in general, involves helping clients learn new ways to do familiar activities. This can be frustrating and challenging, and it can cause a lot of mental distress for the client. Educational psychology, a field focused on understanding teaching and learning, has much to offer rehabilitation when it comes to how to support learning. In educational psychology, motivation has been understood and studied for almost 100 years (Leeper, 1935).

Motivation is responsible for determining how an individual engages in goal-directed behavior, how energy is allocated to a task, and even how the individual engages and uses the available cognitive-processing ability (Ormrod et al., 2008). Marshaling the client's motivation is a core component of every intervention approach discussed in this text, and knowing what motivates a client comes from the occupational profile.

Care Support Involvement

People with cognitive impairments may have difficulty differentiating between current activity participation and competency and the participation and competency that were present for them at one time but are no longer current. Particularly individuals with awareness problems and those who are experiencing limitations in their short-term memory may have difficulty placing their engagement in an activity in a current context. If such problems are present, the individuals will need the assistance of a family member or knowledgeable friend to confirm the narrative of the occupational history they have reported.

A recent meta-analysis of the correlation between an implicit test and self-reported measures suggests that the low correlation may be due to motivational biases, lack of introspective representation, or difficulty with information retrieval from memory (Hofmann et al., 2005). Particularly after an incident such as a stroke or injury, a person may remember only what they could do before the event when being asked to self-describe their capacity. Thus, the clinician may have to give them a specific context in which to answer the questions. In this instance, it would be helpful to have the perspective of a care partner to help obtain an occupational history and build an occupational profile. The occupational therapy practitioner should bear in mind, however, that the care partner's report is also not without bias and may at times misrepresent how much and how often support is provided (Wadley et al., 2003).

Conclusion and Next Steps

This chapter has reviewed the importance of an occupational profile in understanding what is salient and familiar to the client as well as methods to develop an occupational profile. The occupational profile, in turn, drives the selection of a performance-based assessment to evaluate functional–cognitive status. On the basis of the information obtained in the occupational profile, the performance-based assessment, and pertinent information related to the client's overall functional status (e.g., prognosis, strengths and deficits), the occupational therapist can work with the client and care partner to establish goals for treatment. The therapist then uses the occupational profile to select treatment activities, regardless of which intervention approach is chosen.

The next chapters in this text discuss specific performance-based assessments that can be used in practice, along with the clients they are most appropriate for. The common thread through all of this content is the tie-back to the occupational profile and the importance of the specific activity to the client in selection and use of that assessment.

References

American Occupational Therapy Association. (2014). Occupational therapy practice framework: Domain and process (3rd ed.). *American Journal of Occupational Therapy, 68*(Suppl. 1), S1–S48. https://doi.org/10.5014/ajot.2014.682006

American Occupational Therapy Association. (2017). AOTA's occupational profile template. *American Journal of Occupational Therapy, 71*(Suppl. 2), 7112420030. https://doi.org/10.5014/ajot.2017.716S12

Bailey, R., Kaskutas, V., Fox, I., Baum, C. M., & Mackinnon, S. E. (2009). Effect of upper extremity nerve damage on activity participation, pain, depression, and quality of life. *Journal of Hand Surgery, 34*, 1682–1688. https://doi.org/10.1016/j.jhsa.2009.07.002

Baum, C. M. (1995). The contribution of occupation to function in persons with Alzheimer's disease. *Journal of Occupational Science, 2*, 59–67. https://doi.org/10.1080/14427591.1995.9686396

Baum, C. M., & Edwards, D. (2001). *The Washington University Activity Card Sort*. St. Louis: PenUltima Press.

Baum, C. M., & Edwards, D. F. (2008). *Activity Card Sort* (2nd ed.). Bethesda, MD: American Occupational Therapy Association.

Camina, E., & Güell, F. (2017). The neuroanatomical, neurophysiological and psychological basis of memory: Current models and their origins. *Frontiers in Pharmacology, 8*, 438. https://doi.org/10.3389/fphar.2017.00438

Carpenter, L., Baker, G. A., & Tyldesley, B. (2001). The use of the Canadian Occupational Performance Measure as an outcome of a pain management program. *Canadian Journal of Occupational Therapy, 68*, 16–22. https://doi.org/10.1177/000841740106800102

Carswell, A., McColl, M. A., Baptiste, S., Law, M., Polatajko, H., & Pollock, N. (2004). The Canadian Occupational Performance Measure: A research and clinical literature review. *Canadian Journal of Occupational Therapy, 71*, 210–222. https://doi.org/10.1177/000841740407100406

Chan, V. W., Chung, J. C., & Packer, T. L. (2006). Validity and reliability of the Activity Card Sort–Hong Kong version. *OTJR: Occupation, Participation and Health, 26*, 152–158. https://doi.org/10.1177/153944920602600405

Cup, E. H. C., Scholte op Reimer, W. J. M., Thijssen, M. C., & Van Kuyk-Minis, M. A. H. (2003). Reliability and validity of the Canadian Occupational Performance Measure in stroke patients. *Clinical Rehabilitation, 17*, 402–409. https://doi.org/10.1191/0269215503cr635oa

Edwards, D. F., Hahn, M., Baum, C., & Dromerick, A. W. (2006). The impact of mild stroke on meaningful activity and life satisfaction. *Journal of Stroke and Cerebrovascular Diseases, 15*, 151–157. https://doi.org/10.1016/j.jstrokecerebrovasdis.2006.04.001

Eriksson, G., Baum, M. C., Wolf, T. J., & Connor, L. T. (2013). Perceived participation after stroke: The influence of activity retention, reintegration, and perceived recovery. *American Journal of Occupational Therapy, 67*, e131–e138. https://doi.org/10.5014/ajot.2013.008292

Fox, K., Morrow-Howell, N., Herbers, S., Battista, P., & Baum, C. M. (2017). Activity disengagement: Understanding challenges and opportunities for reengagement. *Occupational Therapy International, 2017*, 1983414. https://doi.org/10.1155/2017/1983414

Hamed, R., & Holm, M. B. (2013). Psychometric properties of the Arab Heritage Activity Card Sort. *Occupational Therapy International, 20*, 23–34. https://doi.org/10.1002/oti.1335

Hartman-Maeir, A., Soroker, N., Ring, H., Avni, N., & Katz, N. (2007). Activities, participation and satisfaction one-year post stroke. *Disability and Rehabilitation, 29*, 559–566. https://doi.org/10.1080/09638280600924996

Henry, A., Tohen, M., Coster, W., & Tickle-Degnen, L. (1994, July). *Predicting psychosocial functioning and symptomatic recovery of adolescents and young adults following a first psychotic episode.* Paper presented at the joint annual conference of the American Occupational Therapy Association and the Canadian Association of Occupational Therapists, Boston.

Hofmann, W., Gawronski, B., Gschwendner, T., Le, H., & Schmitt, M. (2005). A meta-analysis on the correlation between the Implicit Association Test and explicit self-report measures. *Personality and*

Social Psychology Bulletin, 31, 1369–1385. https://doi.org/10.1177/0146167205275613

Jenkinson, N., Ownsworth, T., & Shum, D. (2007). Utility of the Canadian Occupational Performance Measure in community-based brain injury rehabilitation. *Brain Injury, 21,* 1283–1294. https://doi.org/10.1080/02699050701739531

Katz, N., Karpin, H., Lak, A., Furman, T., & Hartman-Maeir, A. (2003). Participation in occupational performance: Reliability and validity of the Activity Card Sort. *OTJR: Occupation, Participation and Health, 23,* 10–17. https://doi.org/10.1177/153944920302300102

Kawai, H., Kawamura, M., Mochizuki, S., Yamanaka, K., Arakaki, H., Tanaka, K., & Kawachi, J. (2002). Longitudinal study of procedural memory in patients with Alzheimer-type dementia. *No To Shinkei, 54,* 307–311.

Kielhofner, G., & Henry, A. D. (1988). Development and investigation of the Occupational Performance History Interview. *American Journal of Occupational Therapy, 42,* 489–498. https://doi.org/10.5014/ajot.42.8.489

Kielhofner, G., Henry, A. D., & Walens, D. (1989). *A user's guide to the Occupational Performance History Interview.* Bethesda, MD: American Occupational Therapy Association.

Kielhofner, G., Henry, A. D., Walens, D., & Rogers, E. S. (1991). A generalizability study of the Occupational Performance History Interview. *OTJR: Occupation, Participation and Health, 11,* 292–306. https://doi.org/10.1177/153944929101100503

Kielhofner, G., Mallinson, T., Forsyth, K., & Lai, J.-S. (2001). Psychometric properties of the second version of the Occupational Performance History Interview (OPHI–II). *American Journal of Occupational Therapy, 55,* 260–267. https://doi.org/10.5014/ajot.55.3.260

Kjeken, I., Dagfinrud, H., Slatkowsky-Christensen, B., Mowinckel, P., Uhlig, T., Kvien, T. K., & Finset, A. (2005). Activity limitations and participation restrictions in women with hand osteoarthritis: Patients' descriptions and associations between dimensions of functioning. *Annals of the Rheumatic Diseases, 64,* 1633–1638. https://doi.org/10.1136/ard.2004.034900

Laver-Fawcett, A., Brain, L., Brodie, C., Cardy, L., & Manaton, L. (2016). The face validity and clinical utility of the Activity Card Sort–United Kingdom (ACS–UK). *British Journal of Occupational Therapy, 79,* 492–504. https://doi.org/10.1177/0308022616629167

Leeper, R. (1935). The role of motivation in learning: A study of the phenomenon of differential motivational control of the utilization of habits. *Pedagogical Seminary and Journal of Genetic Psychology, 46,* 3–40. https://doi.org/10.1080/08856559.1935.10533143

Lynch, K. B., & Bridle, M. J. (1993). Construct validity of the Occupational Performance History Interview. *OTJR: Occupation, Participation and Health, 13,* 231–240. https://doi.org/10.1177/153944929301300402

Lyons, K. D., Li, Z., Tosteson, T. D., Meehan, K., & Ahles, T. A. (2010). Consistency and construct validity of the Activity Card Sort (modified) in measuring activity resumption after stem cell transplantation. *American Journal of Occupational Therapy, 64,* 562–569. https://doi.org/10.5014/ajot.2010.09033

Novak, I., Cusick, A., & Lannin, N. (2009). Occupational therapy home programs for cerebral palsy: Double-blind, randomized, controlled trial. *Pediatrics, 124,* e606–e614. https://doi.org/10.1542/peds.2009-0288

Orellano, E. M., Ito, M., Dorne, R., Irizarry, D., & Dávila, R. (2012). Occupational participation of older adults: Reliability and validity of the Activity Card Sort–Puerto Rican version. *OTJR: Occupation, Participation and Health, 32,* 266–272. https://doi.org/10.3928/15394492-20110708-01

Ormrod, J. E., Anderman, E. M., & Anderman, L. (2008). *Educational psychology: Developing learners.* London: Pearson.

Perlmutter, M. S., Bhorade, A., Gordon, M., Hollingsworth, H. H., & Baum, M. C. (2010). Cognitive, visual, auditory, and emotional factors that affect participation in older adults. *American Journal of Occupational Therapy, 64,* 570–579. https://doi.org/10.5014/ajot.2010.09089

Phipps, S., & Richardson, P. (2007). Occupational therapy outcomes for clients with traumatic brain injury and stroke using the Canadian Occupational Performance Measure. *American Journal of Occupational Therapy, 61,* 328–334. https://doi.org/10.5014/ajot.61.3.328

Poerbodipoero, S. J., Sturkenboom, I. H., Van Hartingsveldt, M. J., Nijhuis-van der Sanden, M. W., & Graff, M. J. (2016). The construct validity of the Dutch version of the Activity Card Sort. *Disability and Rehabilitation, 38,* 1943–1951. https://doi.org/10.3109/09638288.2015.1107779

Taylor, S., Fayed, N., & Mandich, A. (2007). CO–OP intervention for young children with developmental coordination disorder. *OTJR: Occupation, Participation and Health, 27,* 124–130. https://doi.org/10.1177/153944920702700402

Tse, T., Douglas, J., Lentin, P., & Carey, L. (2013). Measuring participation after stroke: A review of frequently used tools. *Archives of Physical Medicine and Rehabilitation, 94,* 177–192. https://doi.org/10.1016/j.apmr.2012.09.002

Wadley, V. G., Harrell, L. E., & Marson, D. C. (2003). Self- and informant report of financial abilities in patients with Alzheimer's disease: Reliable and valid? *Journal of the American Geriatrics Society, 51,* 1621–1626. https://doi.org/10.1046/j.1532-5415.2003.51514.x

Yang, S.-Y., Lin, C.-Y., Lee, Y.-C., & Chang, J.-H. (2017). The Canadian Occupational Performance Measure for patients with stroke: A systematic review. *Journal of Physical Therapy Science, 29,* 548–555. https://doi.org/10.1589/jpts.29.548

6

Baseline Cognitive Screening Tools

DOROTHY FARRAR EDWARDS, PhD; MUHAMMAD O. AL-HEIZAN, MS, OT; AND GORDON MUIR GILES, PhD, OTR/L, FAOTA

LEARNING OBJECTIVES

After completing this chapter, readers should be able to

- Distinguish between screening and diagnostic measures,
- Identify the characteristics of reliable and valid screening measures,
- Compare performance-based screening measures of functional cognition with neuropsychological screening measures, and
- Describe screening measures of functional cognition.

KEY TERMS AND CONCEPTS

- Diagnostic tests • Gold standard • Negative predictive value • Positive predictive value
- Receiver-operating characteristic curve analysis • Screening measures • Selective screening
- Sensitivity • Specificity

Introduction

The assessment process provides the foundation of occupational therapy practice. The assessment of an individual's functional status, competencies, and difficulties is essential for the planning and documenting of interventions (Dunn, 2005). Screening measures provide critical information for the identification and subsequent treatment or management of occupational performance deficits (Katz et al., 2011).

In general terms, the assessment process can be characterized as falling into 2 stages: screening tests, followed by more comprehensive diagnostic assessment. *Screening measures* are used when the presence of a condition is unknown, to assess the likelihood that a person has a particular problem or condition.

Diagnostic tests are used with people who have specific indications of a possible condition, problem, or illness. Thus, diagnostic tests are used to confirm the presence and extent of a problem on the basis of

- A reported history,

- Symptoms,

- Signs, or

- Positive screening-test results.

The goal of a diagnostic assessment is to identify the presence and often the extent of the problem or condition.

Neuropsychological diagnostic tests are reviewed briefly in Chapter 16, and Chapters 7–15 examine in detail tests that are considered diagnostic for functional cognition. A comparison of the characteristics of screening and diagnostic tests is presented in Exhibit 6.1. Both types of assessment are important for occupational therapy practice; however, it is important to use the most appropriate type of measure for the clinical situation and the needs of the individual being evaluated.

The focus of this chapter is on screening tests for the types of cognitive problems that may compromise ADL and IADL functioning. The most well-established screening tests come from neuropsychology, but also reviewed are some newer occupational therapy screening tests that use pseudo-functional tasks to evaluate functional cognition.

EXHIBIT 6.1. Characteristics of Screening and Diagnostic Tests

CHARACTERISTICS OF A SCREENING TEST	CHARACTERISTICS OF A DIAGNOSTIC TEST
The cutoff for a positive result is extremely sensitive and may result in numerous false positives.	The cutoff for a positive result is precisely defined, with stress being laid on diagnostic precision and accuracy.
The cost is usually low, because the accuracy is lower.	The cost is higher, because of the required accuracy.
The test results determine the level of risk and whether a diagnostic test is required.	The test provides a definitive diagnosis.
The test is usually brief.	The test is often more complex and time consuming.
The test is used with individuals who may be asymptomatic or who may be at risk for the condition or problem.	The test is used to confirm a problem or condition.

Screening as Part of Occupational Therapy Evaluation

When the occupational therapy practitioner is developing the client's occupational profile, it is often appropriate to ask questions of the client regarding

- Concerns related to occupational engagement,

- The client's status in a particular area, and

- Barriers perceived by the client.

In instances when the frequency of deficit in an area is low in a population (i.e., when there is a low base rate and when the diagnosis and circumstances of the patient suggest that a problem in an area is unlikely), screening may be limited to asking a question of the client or, when appropriate, of a knowledgeable informant about the client's functioning.

However, in many instances that are reviewed in this text, the client's self-report is an inadequate approach to screening. Hospitalized clients, particularly those with diagnoses associated with impaired functional cognition (e.g., stroke) and those older than 65, may be at increased risk for impaired functional cognition and may be unaware of their impairments, so the use of screening tests is indicated. Individuals admitted to acute or postacute settings are known to be at risk for postdischarge IADL impairment. Impaired functional cognition has been implicated as a significant source of IADL deficits, so the use of screening tests is indicated. It is also important to emphasize that whenever a screening test is indicated, the use of subjective, nonstandardized evaluations will not provide the quality of information needed for effective treatment planning and evaluation (Edwards et al., 2006; Korner-Bitensky et al., 2011), and a screening test with known reliability, validity, sensitivity, and specificity should be used.

The superiority of standardized assessment over the subjective evaluations of treating clinicians was illustrated in a study that compared the information obtained from a brief screening battery with a comprehensive chart review for 53 patients admitted to an acute hospital stroke unit. The formal screening detected significantly more impairments than were noted in the patients' charts at discharge. Thirty-five percent of the patients had 3 or more undetected impairments (Edwards et al., 2006).

Characteristics of Screening Tests

Screening tests are used in clinical practice to assess the likelihood that a person has a particular health problem or medical condition. The rationale is that if a problem or disease is identified early (before the manifestation of symptoms), then earlier treatment or intervention may lead to prevention of the condition, improved survival or function, and enhanced quality of life. Much of what we know about screening tests is derived from epidemiological studies that focused on population-based efforts to detect communicable diseases and to prevent chronic conditions (Wilson & Jungner, 1968).

In 1957, the Commission on Chronic Illness defined screening as "the presumptive identification of unrecognized disease or defect by the application of tests, examinations, or other procedures which can be applied rapidly" (p. 3). In this report, the commission further concluded that a screening test is not intended to be diagnostic. They advised that "persons with positive or suspicious findings must be referred to their physicians for diagnosis and treatment" (p. 45).

Screening tests may be offered to asymptomatic people who may have early disease or disease precursors, and test results are used to guide whether a diagnostic test should be offered. Diagnostic tests are offered to people who have a specific indication of possible illness (a history, symptom, sign, or positive screening-test result) to determine whether they have the disease in question.

Wilson and Jungner (1968) defined 3 types of screening:

1. Selective screening

2. Mass public health screening

3. Surveillance.

In this chapter we focus on *selective screening*—assessments used to evaluate individuals who are thought to be of high risk for the underlying problem when compared with the population at large. For example, hospital patients, both inpatients and outpatients, constitute a particularly high-risk population, and screening is likely to identify more individuals with potential impairment of functional cognition as compared with the patient population as a whole.

Screening tests are used to identify problems that otherwise might have been missed as well as to avoid unnecessarily subjecting patients to unneeded, more expensive, or invasive testing. The Care Tool required by the Improving Medicare Post-Acute Care Transformation Act (2014; Pub. L. 113–185) is an example of selective screening, because only Medicare patients are evaluated rather than all hospitalized adults.

Screening tests are evaluated on the basis of 2 separate but related perspectives. The first is the statistical examination of the test itself. Practitioners use very specific statistical criteria to evaluate the reliability and validity of screening measures. These include standard reliability and validity statistics and the determination of the sensitivity and specificity of the tests. These statistical criteria are discussed in the next section, on establishing the validity of screening tests.

Second, the clinical yield, or value of the results, is also an important determinant of the utility of a screening measure. Here the focus is not just on the statistical characteristics of a particular test but also on the ability of the test to quickly identify problems or the risk for problems before they become so serious that they require more intensive diagnostic testing and clinical intervention.

For example, the Centers for Medicare and Medicaid Services (CMS) have emphasized the importance of standardized screening as part of their aim to better meet the preventive care needs of older Americans. Medicare is placing an increased emphasis on preventive care services for older adults. With the passage of the Patient Protection and Affordable Care Act (2010; Pub. L. 111–148), newly revised guidelines for screening and preventive services have been issued by the U.S. Preventive Services Task Force and the Centers for Disease Control and Prevention. These population-specific guidelines place increased emphasis on identifying the risk of decreased functional status and multiple risk factor reduction, as opposed to more conventional, disease-focused guidelines, which are less suitable for maintaining physical function and quality of life.

In this case, CMS determined that there is a need for better evidence-based screening measures of physical performance, cognitive function, and ADL and IADL capacity appropriate for administration by primary care providers (Nicholas & Hall, 2011). Screening tests are not used for treatment planning, because many do not provide the types of information that are necessary for treatment planning. Rather, they are used to identify individuals in need of further evaluation and possible treatment.

Establishing the Validity of Screening Tests: Sensitivity, Specificity, and Positive and Negative Predictive Values

In the simplest approach to the use of screening tests, there are only 2 possible outcomes: *positive* (which suggests that the problem or condition is present) or *negative* (which suggests that the problem or condition is not present; Greenhalgh, 1997). Ideally, the screening test shows a positive result only if the condition is present and a negative result only if the condition is not present. Unfortunately, very few screening tests are this accurate, and most tests have both false-positive and false-negative outcomes. These possibilities are illustrated in Table 6.1.

Generally, screening tests are benchmarked, or compared with well-established diagnostic tests, often referred to as the *gold standard.* According to Greenhalgh (1997), the gold standard is a well-validated diagnostic test that is seen as definitive. The gold standard may not be perfect—in other words, there may be classification errors (false positives or false negatives)—but the test is considered the best test available under reasonable conditions.

A practitioner evaluates the possible outcomes shown in Table 6.1 and assesses the validity of the test by determining the sensitivity and specificity of the screening test compared with the gold standard. These are the most important characteristics to look for when considering adopting a screening test. The practitioner determines the validity of the test by examining sensitivity and specificity.

Sensitivity is the capacity of the test to correctly identify individuals with the condition or problem of interest. A highly sensitive test rarely misses individuals with the problem. Another way of looking at sensitivity is that there are very few false negatives. In other words, the test does not misclassify people with the problem as healthy or unimpaired when they in fact do have the condition (Maxim et al., 2014).

Specificity, in contrast, is the test's capacity to correctly identify individuals without the problem or condition as negative. Highly specific tests have very few false-positive findings: They do not identify people as having the condition when in fact they do not have the condition. Ideally, a screening test has high levels of sensitivity and specificity. Sensitivity and specificity values can range from 0% to 100%. The closer the value is to 100%, the greater is the likelihood that the screening test identifies both true positive and true negative classifications.

TABLE 6.1. Possible Screening Test Outcomes

POSITIVE OR NEGATIVE	PERSON HAS CONDITION	PERSON DOES NOT HAVE CONDITION	TOTAL
Positive	Correct result (true positive)	False positive	Total positive results
Negative	False negative	Correct result (true negative)	Total negative results
Subtotal	Total with the condition	Total without the condition	Total number screened

TABLE 6.2. Calculation of Sensitivity, Specificity, and Positive and Negative Predictive Values

TEST RESULT	CONDITION PRESENT	CONDITION ABSENT
Test positive	True positive (A)	False positive (B)
Test negative	False negative (C)	True negative (D)
Sensitivity or specificity	Sensitivity = A/(A + C)	Specificity = D/(B + D)
Predictive value	Positive predictive value = A/(A + B)	Negative predictive value = D/(C + D)

Often, 2 other related statistics are calculated. The first is *positive predictive value* (PPV). PPV is the percentage of individuals with a positive test who actually have the problem. This tells the practitioner how well the test is working. If the PPV value is high (as close to 100 as possible), then the PPV suggests that the screening test is doing as well as the gold standard.

Similarly, the *negative predictive value* (NPV) is the percentage of individuals with a negative test who do not have the problem. NPV tells the practitioner how many test negatives are true negatives. If this number is high (it should be close to 100), then it suggests that this new test is doing as well as the gold standard.

It is important to remember that the PPV and NPV are directly related to the prevalence of the condition in the population (the base rate). If all other factors remain constant, the PPV increases with increasing prevalence, and the NPV decreases with increasing prevalence (Parikh et al., 2008). The formulas used to calculate sensitivity, specificity, PPV, and NPV are presented in Table 6.2.

Criteria for Selection of a Screening Test

The circumstances surrounding the selection of a screening test determine the relative importance of sensitivity and specificity, because most screening tests are not equally sensitive and specific. In other words, it is important to carefully consider the practical and clinical consequences of a false-positive or a false-negative finding. In the case of a false negative (poor sensitivity), a person with the condition is incorrectly classified as not having the condition on the basis of the screening test.

In medical situations, a false negative can have significant consequences in the form of delayed diagnosis or incorrect or ineffective treatments. From an occupational therapy perspective, the impact of a false negative test may also be significant.

For example, a person with mild cognitive impairment may seem to be fully independent in complex IADLs, such as medication management or financial management, on the basis of a score within normal range on a cognitive screening test, such as the Mini-Mental State Examination (Folstein et al., 1975) or the Montreal Cognitive Assessment (Nasreddine et al., 2005).

However, there is growing evidence that these scales are not sensitive to subtle functional–cognitive impairment (Giles et al., 2017). The result of a false negative in this situation is that a client may be sent home after hospitalization without receiving the occupational therapy services that would support greater independence at home. In this situation, it is important to consider the sensitivity of the screening tool.

There are also consequences associated with false positives (poor specificity). False positives occur when a test is sensitive but not specific. A person who is misclassified as having a condition or problem on the basis of a screening test may be asked to undergo more intensive diagnostic testing or treatment procedures. Thus, they are exposed to unnecessary testing procedures and possibly emotional risks.

In addition to the personal consequences, false positives can place undue burden on practitioners by directing the use of limited or scarce clinical resources to individuals not in need of further evaluation or treatment. Low or poor specificity in a functional cognition screening tool may result in an overclassification of individuals as having impaired functional cognition, when in fact they are fully capable of optimal performance of essential IADLs.

One way that screening test developers address concerns about balancing sensitivity and specificity is through the use of a more sophisticated analysis technique called a *receiver-operating characteristic (ROC) curve analysis.* In the ROC analysis, the test developer can determine the cut score that optimizes the classification of true positives and true negatives on the screening test, as compared with the gold standard.

This analysis computes sensitivity, specificity, PPV, and NPV for a series of different screening-test cutoff scores. The area-under-the-curve statistic, also computed as part of overall ROC analysis, provides an additional indicator of validity because it measures the performance of a test over its whole range. The larger the area is, the better the performance is (Zweig & Campbell, 1993).

This method is more precise than the approach presented in Table 6.2. The best approach to selecting a screening measure is to carefully evaluate its reliability and validity and then decide, on the basis of the intended use of the test, on the optimal combination of sensitivity and specificity needed to fit the characteristics of the population to be screened and the prevalence and significance of the condition to be evaluated. Table 6.3 presents considerations for selecting a screening measure.

Approaches to Screening Functional Cognition

Functional cognition is an emerging area of occupational therapy practice. Although several assessments are described in this book, less attention has been paid to the development and validation of occupational therapy screening measures designed to identify individuals at risk for impaired functional cognition. Appendices 6.A–6.C include a selection of screening tools designed to identify individuals in need of more comprehensive assessment.

Ideally, the use of valid screening tools will help to identify individuals who are at risk for not qualifying for occupational therapy services despite the presence of deficits in functional cognition. The use of screening assessments will decrease the likelihood that individuals with functional–cognitive deficits are discharged without the occupational therapy services they need to support occupational performance in community or postacute settings. We have included descriptions of cognitive, performance, and self- and informant-report measures that can be used to identify potential deficits in functional cognition. These measures are briefly reviewed in Appendices 6.A–6.C. Two videos present the administration and scoring of the Menu Task, one showing perfect performance on the task (Video 6.1) and the other showing performance with errors (Video 6.2).

TABLE 6.3. Practical Considerations for Selecting a Screening Test

QUESTION	CONSIDERATIONS
Is this screening test relevant to my practice?	• Will it identify a treatable problem? • Will my clients consent to it? • Can it replace a less reliable or less valid measure?
Has the test been compared with a true gold standard?	• Has it been compared with anything at all? • There may be no gold standard for this area of practice. If not, how has the screening test been validated?
Was the validation sample appropriate given the conditions I wish to better identify?	• Very few screening measures are validated in truly representative populations. • Did the validation sample include individuals with mild and severe conditions, treated and untreated individuals, and persons with similar but potentially confusing conditions?
Is the test reproducible?	• Has test–retest or interrater reliability been established?
Has a sensible "normal range" been identified?	• If the test results in numerical rather than dichotomous (yes–no) scores, how were the abnormal values identified?

Source. "How to Read a Paper: Papers That Report Diagnostic or Screening Tests," by T. Greenhalgh, 1997, *BMJ, 315*, pp. 540–543.

Appendix 6.A. Cognitive Screening Measures

INSTRUMENT AND REFERENCE(S)	DESCRIPTION	PSYCHOMETRICS	STRENGTHS AND WEAKNESSES
Brief Interview for Mental Status (BIMS; Saliba et al., 2012)	The BIMS is a cognitive screen that includes items that measure temporal orientation, recall, and short-term memory. The BIMS is part of the federally mandated Minimum Data Set. It was designed to help identify older adults in nursing homes with cognitive deficits. The scores on the BIMS range from 0 to 15; scores of 13–15 are considered unimpaired cognitive function. The average time to complete the BIMS is 3.2 minutes.	The BIMS had high correlations with the Modified Mini-Mental State Examination (Folstein et al., 1975; $r =$ .90, $p <$ .0001). The area-under-the-curve (AUC) statistic for identifying any impairment was .93 for the BIMS. A total score below 13 had a sensitivity of .83 and a specificity of .91. The AUC for identifying moderate to severe impairment was .96 for the BIMS. A total score below 8 had a sensitivity of .83 and a specificity of .92 for identifying severe impairment.	*Strengths* • Easy to administer and score. • Suitable for more severe cognitive impairment. *Weaknesses* • May be inappropriate for patients with mild to moderate cognitive impairments. • Has not been adequately validated with populations outside nursing homes.

(Continued)

APPENDIX 6.A. Cognitive Screening Measures *(Cont.)*

INSTRUMENT AND REFERENCE(S)	DESCRIPTION	PSYCHOMETRICS	STRENGTHS AND WEAKNESSES
Mini-Mental State Examination (MMSE; Feliciano et al., 2013; Folstein et al., 1975)	The MMSE was developed as a brief screening tool to provide a quantitative evaluation of cognitive impairment and to record cognitive changes over time. The MMSE has 11 items that measure 5 areas of cognitive function: orientation, registration, attention and calculation, recall, and language. The total score on the MMSE is 30, with scores below 24 indicating impairment. The administration time of the MMSE is approximately 10 minutes.	The MMSE has norms based on age and education for reference (Crum et al., 1993). The reliability and validity of the MMSE have been extensively examined. The MMSE has low reported levels of sensitivity, particularly among individuals with mild cognitive impairment (MCI; Tombaugh & McIntyre, 1992). In a systematic review, the MMSE had a sensitivity of .88 and a specificity of .86 for dementia, with a score cutoff of 23–25 indicating significant impairment (Norris et al., 2016).	*Strengths* • Quick and easy to use. • Available in different languages. *Weaknesses* • May not be appropriate for patients who are hearing or visually impaired, are intubated, have low English literacy, or have other communication disorders. • Demonstrates marked ceiling effects among younger typical individuals and marked floor effects among individuals with moderate to severe impairment.
St. Louis University Mental Status Examination (SLUMS; Tariq et al. 2006)	The SLUMS is used to identify people with dementia or mild neurocognitive impairment (MNCI). The SLUMS has 11 items that cover orientation, memory, attention, and executive functions (EFs). The maximum score is 30 points. Cutoff scores for dementia or MNCI are based on education level. The SLUMS takes approximately 7 minutes to complete.	The SLUMS has normative data for comparison (Feliciano et al., 2013) as well as cutoff scores based on age and education for determining dementia or MNCI (Tariq et al., 2006). The SLUMS demonstrated criterion-related validity with the MMSE (*r* = .75). The SLUMS was able to significantly predict mortality and institutionalization of individuals with dementia (Cruz-Oliver et al., 2012). The cutoff scores for dementia and MNCI had sensitivities that ranged from .92 to 1.00 and specificities that ranged from .76 to 1.00 (Tariq et al., 2006).	*Strengths* • May be more sensitive than other cognitive measures in detecting MNCI. • Has items assessing logical memory and size differentiation, unlike other cognitive screens. *Weaknesses* • Has not been used with a wide range of clinical populations. • No information is available regarding the reliability of the measure.
Montreal Cognitive Assessment (MoCA; Nasreddine et al., 2005)	The MoCA was designed as a rapid screening instrument for the detection of MCI. The MoCA assesses the following cognitive domains: attention and concentration, EFs, memory, language, visuoconstructional skills, conceptual thinking, calculations, and orientation. Total score on the MoCA is 30 points, with a cutoff score of 26 indicating impairment. The MoCA takes approximately 10–15 minutes to complete.	The MoCA had excellent internal consistency (.83) and test–retest reliability (*r* =.92). The MoCA had high correlations with the MMSE (*r* = .87) (Nasreddine et al., 2005). At a cutoff score of 26, the MoCA had a 90% sensitivity in identifying clients with MCI and a 100% sensitivity in identifying clients with Alzheimer's disease. It had a specificity of 87%. The sensitivity of the MoCA in detecting MCI has been reported to be high in several other studies.	*Strengths* • Available in various languages. • Has strong psychometric properties. • Simple to score. *Weaknesses* • Has not been examined for ceiling or floor effects. • Is not suitable for individuals with language or visual impairments.

(Continued)

APPENDIX 6.A. Cognitive Screening Measures *(Cont.)*

INSTRUMENT AND REFERENCE(S)	DESCRIPTION	PSYCHOMETRICS	STRENGTHS AND WEAKNESSES
Trail Making Test (TMT; Reitan, 1932)	The TMT consists of Parts A and B. In Part A, clients are asked to connect numbered circles scattered across a page. In Part B, they are asked to connect circles with alternating numbers and letters scattered across a page. The TMT can be administered in paper-and-pencil, computerized, or smartphone versions. Part A and Part B are scored separately. The score for each task is the number of seconds required to complete the task. Timing should start as soon as the instruction is given to begin. Administration time is between approximately 5 and 10 minutes.	O'Donnell et al. (1994) reported the face validity of the TMT in a sample of 117 community-dwelling patients. The results suggest that the TMT is a complex test that involves aspects of attention. In addition, the same study examined the convergent validity of the TMT and 4 other neuropsychological tests: Category Test (Mack & Carlson, 1978), Wisconsin Card Sorting Test (Meier, 1974), Paced Auditory Serial-Addition Task (Gronwall, 1977), and Visual Search and Attention Test (Trenerry et al., 1990). O'Donnell et al.'s findings suggest adequate correlations between the TMT and the other measures (R^2 = .38, .31, .44, and .30, respectively), on the basis of Pearson product–moment correlations. Matarazzo et al. (1974) examined the test–retest reliability for Part A and Part B of the TMT (R^2 = .78 and .67, respectively) among participants with diffuse cerebrovascular disease. Interrater reliability has been found to be high for both Part A (r = .94) and Part B (r = .90; Fals-Stewart, 1992).	*Strengths* • Relatively easy to administer. • Short in duration. *Weaknesses* • Could be skewed to more-educated individuals. • The instructions could be confusing for some individuals. • Cannot be administered to illiterate clients, non-English speakers, or individuals with hand impairments.

Appendix 6.B. Performance Measures

INSTRUMENT AND REFERENCE(S)	DESCRIPTION	PSYCHOMETRICS	STRENGTHS AND WEAKNESSES
Menu Task (MT; Edwards et al., 2019)	The MT is a brief performance-based screening measure of functional cognition that involves a selection of menu items following a set of rules and restrictions. It is based on the Multiple Errands Test–Revised (Morrison et al., 2013). The MT has a maximum score of 12 points. The average administration time of the MT is 183 seconds.	The MT has moderate internal consistency (α = .70) and excellent interrater reliability (intraclass correlation coefficient = 1). The MT had higher correlations with the Montreal Cognitive Assessment (MoCA) and Trail Making Test Part B, which supports construct validity. MT scores were significantly lower for groups impaired on the Brief Interview for Mental Status and MoCA than for groups not impaired on those measures, which supports predictive validity. The MT scores were predictive of self-reported IADL impairments. Furthermore, measures of executive function significantly predicted MT scores, which demonstrates construct validity (Al-Heizan et al., 2018). A cutoff score of 6 had an area-under-the-curve (AUC) statistic of .78, a sensitivity of .80, and a specificity of .65.	*Strengths* • Designed for the purpose of detecting functional–cognitive deficits. • Follows performance-based testing principles of functional cognition. *Weaknesses* • Has not yet been examined in a clinical setting. • May have ceiling effects.
Allen Cognitive Level Screen–5 (ACLS–5; Allen et al., 2007)	The ACLS–5 is a leather-lacing standardized screening test of functional cognition designed to provide a quick estimate of cognitive abilities within Cognitive Levels 3, 4, and 5 on the Allen Scale of levels and modes of performance. This is a 26-point scale ranging from 1.0 (low) to 6.0 (high). The Large ACLS–5 (LACLS–5) is intended for use with individuals who have impaired vision or hand function. It takes approximately 15–30 minutes to complete.	The ACLS–5 has high interrater reliability, with 100% correspondence on the Allen Scale. The LACLS–5 had moderate correlations and functional independence rating (r = .55; Scanlan & Still, 2013). Cairns et al. (2013) found high correlations between the LACLS–5 and the Medication Adherence Rating Scale (r = .71). The LACLS–5 had a sensitivity of .86 and specificity of .81 in distinguishing between cognitively typical individuals and individuals with dementia (Wesson et al., 2017).	*Strength* • Standardized screen with comparisons with Allen Cognitive Scale levels. *Weakness* • Additional studies are needed to examine the psychometrics of the ACLS–5 and LACLS–5.

(Continued)

APPENDIX 6.B. Performance Measures *(Cont.)*

INSTRUMENT AND REFERENCE(S)	DESCRIPTION	PSYCHOMETRICS	STRENGTHS AND WEAKNESSES
Medi-Cog (Anderson et al., 2008)	The Medi-Cog is a combination of the Mini-Cog and the Medication Transfer Screen (MTS). The Mini-Cog is a widely used 2-part rapid screening measure that incorporates a 3-word recall test of memory and a clock-drawing test. It takes 2–3 minutes to administer. The MTS is a paper-and-pencil skills screen of medication management. Participants must read 4 prescription instructions, correctly decipher each instruction by writing the number of pills in appropriate compartments on a "virtual pillbox" that is printed on a paper, and answer a question about the pill count. Possible scores range from 0 to 10: 5 points from the Mini-Cog, and 5 points from the MTS. The average time to complete the Medi-Cog is 6.9 minutes.	The Medi-Cog had moderate correlations with the Mini-Mental State Examination ($r = .50$). The Medi-Cog had a sensitivity of 80% and a specificity of 61% in identifying 70% accuracy in pillbox assessment. In addition, the sensitivity was 72% and specificity was 61% for identifying 80% accuracy in pillbox assessment.	*Strength* • Designed specifically for screening for medication management problems. *Weakness* • No information regarding the reliability of the measure.
Performance Assessment of Self-Care Skills (PASS) Medication Management task (PMMT; Holm & Rogers, 2008)	The PASS is a performance-based test designed to document functional status. The full PASS consists of 26 core tasks divided into 4 domains, including cognitive IADLs. The PMMT is categorized as 1 of the cognitive IADL tasks on the PASS. The PASS has independence, safety, and adequacy measures (performance process and quality). Clients are presented with 2 pill bottles and a printed 4 × 7–cell medication organizer and are asked to follow the instructions on the pill bottle labels to lay out medications. Scoring is based on need for cueing or assistance.	The PASS has been found to have high interrater reliability on measures of independence (96%), safety (97%), and adequacy (88%), as well as high validity among these measures (Holm & Rogers, 2008). The PASS has content validity that was based primarily on the content of validated tools, such as the IADL Scale developed by Lawton and Brody (1969). Construct validity of the PASS was established with factor analysis and a Rasch analysis (Chisholm, 2005). The Cognitive IADL tasks of the PASS were able to distinguish between individuals with mild cognitive impairment and those with typical cognition, with an AUC statistic of .81, sensitivity of 75%, and specificity of 73% (Rodakowski et al., 2014).	*Strengths* • Clinically relevant tool that guides intervention. • Strong ecological validity. *Weakness* • More research is needed on the utility of the PMMT in clinical settings.

Appendix 6.C. Self-Report and Informant-Report Measures

INSTRUMENT AND REFERENCE(S)	DESCRIPTION	PSYCHOMETRICS	STRENGTHS AND WEAKNESSES
Functional Behavior Profile (FBP; Baum & Edwards, 2000; Baum et al., 1993)	The FBP is a clinical assessment used to guide placement and discharge decisions after stroke. The FBP can also be used in an interview with a caregiver at home or in an outpatient setting. The measure has 27 items; responses range from 0 to 4. Total score on the FBP is 108. Administration time is 10–20 minutes.	The FBP had good internal consistency (.86; Baum & Edwards, 2000). FBP was based on the comprehensive occupational therapy evaluation, which supports content validity. The FBP had high correlation with the Katz Index of Independence in Activities of Daily Living (r = .85) and the Blessed Dementia Scale (r = .83; Baum et al., 1993). The FBP had a sensitivity of .75 and a specificity of .68 in identifying individuals with stroke who needed supervision (Baum & Edwards, 2000; Baum et al., 1993).	*Strengths* • Quick and easy to use. • Strong reliability. *Weakness* • Has not been examined in different clinical populations.
Behavior Rating Inventory of Executive Function–Adult Version (BRIEF–A; Roth et al., 2005)	The BRIEF–A is a 75-item self-report of executive functioning (EF) across a range of situations. It provides information based on 2 indexes—the Behavioral Regulation Index (BRI) and the Metacognition Index (MI)—and 9 subscales. The BRI measures inhibition, shifting, emotional control, and self-monitoring. The MI measures initiation, working memory, planning and organization, organization of materials, and task monitoring. The BRIEF–A takes about 10–15 minutes to complete.	The BRIEF–A has been standardized and validated for ages 18–90. The MI and BRI indexes have a reported high internal consistency (α = .93–.96). The BRIEF–A had moderate to strong correlations with measures of EF (r = .63–.74), which demonstrates construct validity. Significant differences were found between healthy individuals and patients with traumatic brain injury on both BRIEF–A indexes, which supports concurrent validity.	*Strengths* • A reasonably brief measure of EF difficulties. • Does not require formal training to administer or score. • Covers various aspects of EF. *Weaknesses* • Validation based on U.S sample only. • Scoring has to be done by hand unless the computer scoring program is used. • Self-report may not be accurate.
Alzheimer's Disease Cooperative Study—ADL Inventory Scale (ADCS; Galasko et al., 1997)	The ADCS is a self- or informant-report measure used to describe actions or behaviors of individuals during ADL and IADL performances as they are perceived. The ADCS is composed of 23 items that each assesses a specific ADL or IADL. Items consist of performance descriptors with assigned numeric values, and each item may range from 0 to 7 points. The test administrator scores the measure by adding the points of each item to obtain a score out of a maximum of 78 points. A score of 78 indicates a high level of self-reported ADL or IADL performance.	The applicability of ADCS items was determined by performance rates of 90% or higher among control participants or participants with Alzheimer's disease and by whether patients with a wide range of dementia severities attempted to perform the ADL (Galasko et al., 1997). Items with moderate to very good agreement fell into the .4–.75 range, indicating test–retest reliability (Galasko et al., 1997). Finally, correlations between levels of performance for each item on the ADCS and dementia severity, as indexed by a gold-standard screening tool, the Mini-Mental State Examination, were shown to be statistically significant (p < .001; Galasko et al., 1997). Informant and proxy ratings have been found to be highly correlated on the ADCS (Howland et al., 2017).	*Strength* • Easy to use and interpret. *Weaknesses* • May contain ambiguous questions for the reporter. • More studies are needed to support the psychometric properties.

(Continued)

APPENDIX 6.C. Self-Report and Informant-Report Measures *(Cont.)*

INSTRUMENT AND REFERENCE(S)	DESCRIPTION	PSYCHOMETRICS	STRENGTHS AND WEAKNESSES
Lawton IADL Scale (Lawton & Brody, 1969)	The Lawton IADL Scale was developed to assess the more complex ADLs necessary for living in the community. It contains 8 items, with a summary score from 0 (low function) to 8 (high function). Administration time is 10–15 minutes.	Interrater reliability on the measure was .85. Researchers tested the validity of the Lawton IADL Scale by determining the correlation of the Lawton IADL with 4 scales that measured domains of functional status: the Physical Classification (6-point rating of physical health), Mental Status Questionnaire (10-point test of orientation and memory), Behavior and Adjustment Rating Scales (4- to 6-point measure of intellectual, personal, behavioral and social adjustment), and the Physical Self-Maintenance Scale (6-item test of ADLs). A total of 180 research participants participated in the study; however, few received all 5 evaluations. Moderate to high correlations were obtained.	*Strengths* • Easy to administer. • Widely used in both research and clinical practice. *Weaknesses* • May overestimate or underestimate ability. • May not be sensitive to small, incremental changes in function.

References

Al-Heizan, M. O., Giles, G. M., Wolf, T. J., & Edwards, D. F. (2018). The construct validity of a new screening measure of functional cognitive ability: The Menu Task. *Neuropsychological Rehabilitation*, 1–12. https://doi.org/10.1080/09602011.2018.1531767

Allen, C. K., Austin, S. L., David, S. K., Earhart, C. A., McCraith, D. B., & Riska-Williams, L. (2007). *Manual for the Allen Cognitive Level Screen–5 (ACLS–5) and Large Allen Cognitive Level Screen–5 (LACLS–5)*. Camarillo, CA: ACLS & LACLS Committee.

Anderson, K., Jue, S., & Madaras-Kelly, K. (2008). Identifying patients at risk for medication mismanagement: Using cognitive screens to predict a patient's accuracy in filling a pillbox. *Consultant Pharmacist, 6*, 459–472. https://doi.org/info:doi/10.4140/TCP.n.2008.459

Baum, M. C., & Edwards, D. F. (2000). Documenting productive behaviors: Using the Functional Behavior Profile to plan discharge following stroke. *Journal of Gerontological Nursing, 26*, 34–43. https://doi.org/10.3928/0098-9134-20000401-07

Baum, C., Edwards, D. F., & Morrow-Howell, N. (1993). Identification and measurement of productive behaviors in senile dementia of the Alzheimer type. *Gerontologist, 33*, 403–408. https://doi.org/10.1093/geront/33.3.403

Cairns, A., Hill, C., Dark, F., McPhail, S., & Gray, M. (2013). The Large Allen Cognitive Level Screen as an indicator for medication adherence among adults accessing community mental health services. *British Journal of Occupational Therapy, 76*, 137–143. https://doi.org/10.4276/030802213X13627524435180

Chisholm, D. (2005). *Disability in older adults with depression*. Doctoral dissertation, University of Pittsburgh, Pittsburgh. Retrieved from http://d-scholarship.pitt.edu/9697/

Commission on Chronic Illness. (1957). *Chronic illness in the United States, Volume 1: Prevention of chronic illness*. Cambridge, MA: Harvard University Press.

Crum, R. M., Anthony, J. C., Bassett, S. S., & Folstein, M. F. (1993). Population-based norms for the Mini-Mental State Examination by age and educational level. *JAMA, 269*, 2386–2391. https://doi.org/10.1001/jama.1993.03500180078038

Cruz-Oliver, D. M., Malmstrom, T. K., Allen, C. M., Tumosa, N., & Morley, J. E. (2012). The Veterans Affairs Saint Louis University Mental Status Exam (SLUMS Exam) and the Mini-Mental Status Exam as predictors of mortality and institutionalization. *Journal of Nutrition, Health and Aging, 16*, 636–641. https://doi.org/10.1007/s12603-012-0098-9

Dunn, W. (2005). Measurement issues and practices. In D. W. Law & C. M. Baum (Eds.), *Measuring occupational performance: Supporting best practice in occupational therapy* (2nd ed., pp. 22–29). Thorofare, NJ: Slack.

Edwards, D. F., Hahn, M. G., Baum, C. M., Perlmutter, M. S., Sheedy, C., & Dromerick, A. W. (2006). Screening patients with stroke for rehabilitation needs: Validation of the post-stroke rehabilitation guidelines. *Neurorehabilitation and Neural Repair, 20*, 42–48. https://doi.org/10.1177/1545968305283038

Edwards, D. F., Wolf, T. J., Marks, T., Alter, S., Larkin, V., Padesky, B. L., . . . Giles, G. M. (2019). Reliability and validity of a functional cognition screening tool to identify the need for occupational therapy. *American Journal of Occupational Therapy, 73*, 7302205050. https://doi.org/10.5014/ajot.2019.028753

Fals-Stewart, W. (1992). An interrater reliability study of the Trail Making Test (Parts A and B). *Perceptual and Motor Skills, 74*, 39–42. https://doi.org/10.2466/pms.1992.74.1.39

Feliciano, L., Horning, S. M., Klebe, K. J., Anderson, S. L., Cornwell, R. E., & Davis, H. P. (2013). Utility of the SLUMS as a cognitive screening tool among a nonveteran sample of older adults. *American Journal of Geriatric Psychiatry, 21*, 623–630. https://doi.org/10.1016/j.jagp.2013.01.024

Folstein, M. F., Folstein, S. E., & McHugh, P. R. (1975). "Mini-Mental State": A practical method for grading the cognitive state of patients for the clinician. *Journal of Psychiatric Research, 12(3)*, 189–198. https://doi.org/10.1016/0022-3956(75)90026-6

Galasko, D., Bennett, D., Sano, M., Ernesto, C., Thomas, R., Grundman, M., & Ferris, S. (1997). An inventory to assess activities of daily living for clinical trials in Alzheimer's disease. *Alzheimer Disease and Associated Disorders, 11*(Suppl. 2), S33–S39. https://doi.org/10.1097/00002093-199700112-00005

Giles, G. M., Edwards, D. F., Morrison, M. T., Baum, C., & Wolf, T. J. (2017). Screening for functional cognition in postacute care and the Improving Medicare Post-Acute Care Transformation (IMPACT) Act of 2014. *American Journal of Occupational Therapy, 71,* 7105090010. https://doi.org/10.5014/ajot.2017.715001

Greenhalgh, T. (1997). How to read a paper: Papers that report diagnostic or screening tests. *BMJ, 315,* 540–543. https://doi.org/10.1136/bmj.315.7107.540

Gronwall, D. M. (1977). Paced Auditory Serial-Addition Task: A measure of recovery from concussion. *Perceptual and Motor Skills, 44,* 367–373.

Holm, M. B., & Rogers, J. C. (2008). The Performance Assessment of Self-Care Skills (PASS). In B. Hemphill-Pearson (Ed.), *Assessments in occupational therapy mental health* (2nd ed., pp. 101–112). Thorofare, NJ: Slack.

Howland, M., Allan, K. C., Carlton, C. E., Tatsuoka, C., Smyth, K. A., & Sajatovic, M. (2017). Patient-rated versus proxy-rated cognitive and functional measures in older adults. *Patient Related Outcome Measures, 8,* 33–42. https://doi.org/10.2147/PROM.S126919

Improving Medicare Post-Acute Care Transformation Act of 2014, Pub. L. 113–185, 42 U.S.C. § 1305 et seq.

Katz, N., Baum, C., & Maeir, A. (2011). Introduction to cognitive intervention and cognitive functional evaluation. In N. Katz (Ed.), *Cognition, occupation, and participation across the life span: Neuroscience, neurorehabilitation, and models of intervention in occupational therapy* (3rd ed., pp. 3–13). Bethesda, MD: AOTA Press.

Korner-Bitensky, N., Barrett-Bernstein, S., Bibas, G., & Poulin, V. (2011). National survey of Canadian occupational therapists' assessment and treatment of cognitive impairment post-stroke. *Australian Occupational Therapy Journal, 58,* 241–250. https://doi.org/10.1111/j.1440-1630.2011.00943.x

Lawton, M. P., & Brody, E. M. (1969). Assessment of older people: Self-maintaining and instrumental activities of daily living. *Gerontologist, 9,* 179–186. https://doi.org/10.1093/geront/9.3_Part_1.179

Mack, J. L., & Carlson, N. J. (1978). Conceptual deficits and aging: The Category Test. *Perceptual and Motor Skills, 46*(1), 123–128.

Matarazzo, J. D., Wiens, A. N., Matarazzo, R. G., & Goldstein, S. G. (1974). Psychometric and clinical test–retest reliability of the Halstead Impairment Index in a sample of healthy, young, normal men. *Journal of Nervous and Mental Disease, 158,* 37–49. https://doi.org/10.1097/00005053-197401000-00006

Maxim, L. D., Niebo, R., & Utell, M. J. (2014). Screening tests: A review with examples. *Inhalation Toxicology, 26,* 811–828. https://doi.org/10.3109/08958378.2014.955932

Meier, M. J. (1974). Some challenges for clinical neuropsychology. In R. M. Reitan & L. A. Davison (Eds.), *Clinical neuropsychology: Current status and applications.* Washington, DC: V. H. Winston.

Morrison, M. T., Giles, G. M., Ryan, J. D., Baum, C. M., Dromerick, A. W., Polatajko, H. J., & Edwards, D. F. (2013). Multiple Errands Test–Revised (MET–R): A performance-based measure of executive function in people with mild cerebrovascular accident. *American Journal of Occupational Therapy, 67,* 460–468. https://doi.org/10.5014/ajot.2013.007880

Nasreddine, Z. S., Phillips, N. A., Bédirian, V., Charbonneau, S., Whitehead, V., Collin, I., . . . Chertkow, H. (2005). The Montreal Cognitive Assessment, MoCA: A brief screening tool for mild cognitive impairment. *Journal of the American Geriatrics Society, 53,* 695–699. https://doi.org/10.1111/j.1532-5415.2005.53221.x

Nicholas, J. A., & Hall, W. J. (2011). Screening and preventive services for older adults. *Mount Sinai Journal of Medicine, 78,* 498–508. https://doi.org/10.1002/msj.20275

Norris, D., Clark, M. S., & Shipley, S. (2016). The Mental Status Examination. *American Family Physician, 94,* 635–641.

O'Donnell, J. P., Macgregor, L. A., Dabrowski, J. J., Oestreicher, J. M., & Romero, J. J. (1994). Construct validity of neuropsychological tests of conceptual and attentional abilities. *Journal of Clinical Psychology, 50,* 596–600. https://doi.org/10.1002/1097-4679(199407)50:4<596::AID-JCLP2270500416>3.0.CO;2-S

Parikh, R., Mathai, A., Parikh, S., Chandra Sekhar, G., & Thomas, R. (2008). Understanding and using sensitivity, specificity and predictive values. *Indian Journal of Ophthalmology, 56,* 45–50. https://doi.org/10.4103/0301-4738.37595

Patient Protection and Affordable Care Act, Pub. L. 111–148, 42 U.S.C. §§ 18001–18121 (2010).

Reitan, R. M. (1932). *Trail Making Test: Manual for administration and scoring.* Tucson, AZ: Reitan Neuropsychology Laboratory.

Rodakowski, J., Skidmore, E. R., Reynolds, C. F., III, Dew, M. A., Butters, M. A., Holm, M. B., . . . Rogers, J. C. (2014). Can performance on daily activities discriminate between older adults with normal cognitive function and those with mild cognitive impairment? *Journal of the American Geriatrics Society, 62,* 1347–1352. https://doi.org/10.1111/jgs.12878

Roth, R. M., Isquith, P. K., & Gioia, G. A. (2005). *Behavior Rating Inventory of Executive Function: Adult version: Examiner's manual.* Lutz, FL: Psychological Assessment Resources.

Saliba, D., Buchanan, J., Edelen, M. O., Streim, J., Ouslander, J., Berlowitz, D., & Chodosh, J. (2012). MDS 3.0: Brief Interview for Mental Status. *Journal of the American Medical Directors Association, 13,* 611–617. https://doi.org/10.1016/j.jamda.2012.06.004

Scanlan, J. N., & Still, M. (2013). Functional profile of mental health consumers assessed by occupational therapists: Level of independence and associations with functional cognition. *Psychiatry Research, 208,* 29–32. https://doi.org/10.1016/j.psychres.2013.02.032

Tariq, S. H., Tumosa, N., Chibnall, J. T., Perry, M. H., III, & Morley, J. E. (2006). Comparison of the Saint Louis University Mental Status Examination and the Mini-Mental State Examination for detecting dementia and mild neurocognitive disorder—A pilot study. *American Journal of Geriatric Psychiatry, 14,* 900–910. https://doi.org/10.1097/01.JGP.0000221510.33817.86

Tombaugh, T. N., & McIntyre, N. J. (1992). The Mini-Mental State Examination: A comprehensive review. *Journal of the American Geriatrics Society, 40,* 922–935. https://doi.org/10.1111/j.1532-5415.1992.tb01992.x

Trenerry, M. R., Crosson, B., DeBoe, J., & Leber, W. R. (1990). *Visual Search and Attention Test.* Odessa, FL: Psychological Assessment Resources.

Wesson, J., Clemson, L., Crawford, J. D., Kochan, N. A., Brodaty, H., & Reppermund, S. (2017). Measurement of functional cognition and complex everyday activities in older adults with mild cognitive impairment and mild dementia: Validity of the Large Allen's Cognitive Level Screen. *American Journal of Geriatric Psychiatry, 25,* 471–482. https://doi.org/10.1016/j.jagp.2016.11.021

Wilson, J. M. G., & Jungner, G. (1968). *Principles and practice of screening for disease.* Geneva: World Health Organization.

Zweig, M. H., & Campbell, G. (1993). Receiver-operating characteristic (ROC) plots: A fundamental evaluation tool in clinical medicine. *Clinical Chemistry, 39,* 561–577.

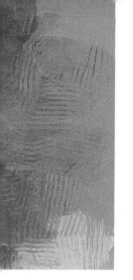

 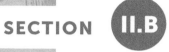
Assessment

Functional Cognition in the Community and IADLs:
Performance-Based Assessment Tools

7

The Executive Function Performance Test

CAROLYN M. BAUM, PhD, OTR/L, FAOTA; DOROTHY FARRAR EDWARDS, PhD;
ANNA E. BOONE, MSOT, PhD, OTR/L; AND TIMOTHY J. WOLF, OTD, PhD, OTR/L, FAOTA

LEARNING OBJECTIVES

After completing this chapter, readers should be able to

- Explain the purpose and the properties of the Executive Function Performance Test,
- Discuss the role of functional task performance in the evaluation of cognitive processes,
- Understand how to support performance with the level of cueing that meets the client's needs,
- Describe an approach to teach a family how to support the client's successful performance, and
- Understand how to describe the client's current level of function in documentation.

KEY TERMS AND CONCEPTS

- Completion • Executive Function Performance Test • Executive functions • Initiation • Judgment and safety
- Organization • Sequencing

Introduction

The occupational therapist's lens addresses the complex interactions of biological, psychological, and social capacities of those they serve. Furthermore, it focuses on the importance of the fit among the person, the task, and the environment to support the person's occupational performance. Before researchers learned of the role of cognition in everyday performance, activity analysis primarily concentrated on the movement and strength necessary to perform functional tasks.

In the 1980s, practitioners recognized that cognitive skills also play a critical role in occupational performance. This new understanding required the development of performance-based measures to analyze an individual's capacity to perform cognitively demanding tasks. The *Executive Function Performance Test* (EFPT) is such a measure (Baum et al., 2008).

Executive functions (EFs) are an interrelated set of cognitive abilities that organize and direct complex, goal-directed activities (Toglia & Katz, 2018). The cognitive components of EF include working memory, attention, inhibitory control, and initiation.

People need these EFs to

- Support adaptive behaviors,
- Generate problem-solving strategies,
- Maintain and update goals,
- Monitor the consequences of actions, and
- Apply prior knowledge to anticipate future events (Miyake & Shah, 1999).

From a performance-based perspective, people need EFs to make plans, initiate actions, and modify activities as they experience problems or as information from the environment changes (Fitzpatrick & Baum, 2012).

Chen and colleagues (2006) suggested that EFs are central to the learning, relearning, and retraining necessary for successful rehabilitation of individuals with impaired functional cognition. Implementation of effective occupational therapy interventions addressing these deficits is based on comprehensive assessment of the client's capacity to perform complex life activities. The EFPT provides the information the practitioner needs to guide rehabilitation interventions and family education designed to support the client's occupational performance in context. Use of the EFPT helps to determine the client's ability to live independently, the level and frequency of cues they need for independence, and specific EF components supporting or inhibiting performance.

The EFPT was developed to provide a performance-based, standardized assessment of cognitive function (Baum & Edwards, 1993). EFs traditionally have been measured by standard neuropsychological evaluations, but the functional cognition necessary to perform in daily life is often missed, because neuropsychological tests are administered in a simplified, structured, and supportive environment (Lezak et al., 2004; Prigatano, 1999). Neuropsychological tests gather information about specific aspects of cognition, such as memory, attention, or planning. The EFPT

- Assesses the person's ability to initiate, organize, and sequence actions;

- Measures the person's ability to use judgment and complete a task; and

- Records how cognition functions support the person's performance of daily activities.

The EFPT does not examine what individuals cannot do. Rather, it identifies what they can do and how much assistance they need in accomplishing those actions.

There are several ecologically valid, performance-based IADL assessments that measure the capacity of a person to perform a structured everyday life activity, some of which are discussed in this text. Although these measures reveal problems in cognitive and processing skills, most do not record the person's capabilities when they are provided with progressive levels of support, although such information is necessary to developing a treatment plan. The EFPT (Baum & Wolf, 2013; Baum et al., 2008) was developed to identify supports needed to help those with executive dysfunction perform daily tasks, and it fills a gap that many other currently available assessments do not address.

Performance-based tests yield specific understanding of the impact that a cognitive problem is having on the tasks that are central to daily life. A screening tool such as the Montreal Cognitive Assessment (MoCA; Nasreddine et al., 2005) can indicate whether a client is experiencing severe cognitive difficulties, but performance-based tests provide a more direct evaluation of functional–cognitive deficits for clients who score as cognitively intact or show only mild impairment on the MoCA (Nasreddine et al., 2005; Toglia et al., 2017).

EFPT Structure

By using a cueing system as part of the assessment process, practitioners can capture a wider range of abilities among people previously assumed to be untestable because of poor performance on standard neurocognitive measures. The EFPT cueing system is standardized and relates to the degree of cognitive impairment affecting task performance. The cueing system gives the test administrator a straightforward assessment of the assistance the individual requires to perform tasks; thus, it is a clinically useful test that can be used in practice and research.

The initial version of the EFPT examines the execution of 4 basic tasks that are essential for self-maintenance and independent living:

1. Simple cooking

2. Telephone use

3. Medication management

4. Bill payment (Baum et al., 2008).

The tasks included in the EFPT were selected because they represent complex activities needed for independence in community settings (i.e., cooking, making a phone call, taking medication, paying a bill).

An alternate version (aEFPT) has been developed with slight modifications to the task demands of the original 4 tasks (i.e., cooking pasta instead of oatmeal, calling a physician's office instead of a grocery store, sorting medications instead of taking medications, ordering items from a catalogue instead of paying 2 bills; Hahn et al., 2014). Rand and colleagues (2018) also developed alternate, Internet-based forms of the Bill Pay and Telephone Use tasks. A more complex version of the EFPT, the EFPT–Enhanced, is currently undergoing psychometric evaluation among persons with stroke and with cancer-related cognitive impairment.

The EFPT assesses an individual's ability to complete 5 executive components within each subtask (see Exhibit 7.1). Using the definitions in Exhibit 7.1, the test administrator can record the EFs that are involved in each task by identifying the level of guidance (cueing) the person needs to perform the task. The levels of assistance are scored as follows:

- No cue required (0)

- Indirect verbal guidance (1)

- Gestural guidance (2)

- Direct verbal assistance (3)

- Physical assistance (4)

- The test administrator does the step for the person (5).

These levels of cues make it possible to record the degree of assistance required by even someone with severe cognitive impairment, yet the measure is sensitive enough to identify an individual who requires only minimal cues. Knowledge of what cueing support the client needs to function safely and how cognitive components are integrated in functional performance informs treatment planning and family education related to maintaining client engagement (Baum & Edwards, 2003; see Exhibit 7.2).

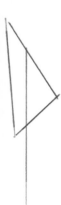

EXHIBIT 7.1. Executive Function Components Assessed in Each Subtask of the EFPT

EXECUTIVE FUNCTION COMPONENT	DEFINITION
Initiation	The start of motor activity that begins a task.
Organization	The physical arrangement of the environment, tools, and materials to facilitate efficient and effective performance of the steps required to complete the task. The individual correctly retrieves and uses the items that are necessary for the task.
Sequencing	The coordination and proper ordering of the steps that compose the task. A proper allotment of attention to each step is required. The individual carries out the steps in an appropriate order, attends to each step appropriately, and can switch attention from 1 step to the next.
Judgment and safety	The use of reason and decision-making capabilities to intentionally avoid physically, emotionally, or financially dangerous or problematic situations. The individual exhibits an awareness of danger by actively avoiding or preventing the creation of a dangerous or problematic situation.
Completion	The inhibition of motor performance, driven by the knowledge that the task is finished. The person does not perseverate and instead terminates task performance by indicating verbally or by physically moving away from the area of the last step.

Note. EFPT = Executive Function Performance Test.
Source. Adapted from *Executive Function Performance Test Manual,* by C. M. Baum and T. J. Wolf, 2013, St. Louis: Washington University in St. Louis. In the public domain.

EXHIBIT 7.2. Cueing Principles for the EFPT

- The test administrator delivers the cues necessary to help the test taker avoid errors and complete the tasks. Even individuals with severe cognitive loss who require multiple step-by-step cues or physical assistance may complete the EFPT.
- During performance difficulty, the test administrator must wait to give the test taker time to process before giving a cue, but they must also time the cues to prevent the test taker from making an error.
- Unless the participant is in danger (e.g., putting a hot pad on the burner, touching the burner to see whether it is on), the test administrator does not intervene until the test taker shows they are not processing to move to the next step.
- The test administrator gives 2 cues of each kind before progressing to the next cueing level.
- If the test taker is still unable to perform a step in a task after gestural and verbal assistance, the test administrator should do the step for the test taker, who should then be cued back to the next step in the task sequence.
- If the test taker needs direct verbal cues in 1 aspect of the observation (organization, sequencing, judgment, and safety), the test administrator should provide the verbal cues to finish the task without starting back through the level sequence each time.
- Test administrators will often find themselves accidentally combining different levels of cues. The score for degree of assistance must reflect the highest level of cueing used to facilitate task completion.
- The test administrator should not initiate conversations during the test, and "cheerleading" is to be avoided (i.e., do not give positive or negative feedback).

Note. EFPT = Executive Function Performance Test.
Source. Adapted from *Executive Function Performance Test Manual,* by C. M. Baum and T. J. Wolf, 2013, St. Louis: Washington University in St. Louis. In the public domain.

Psychometric Properties

The EFPT has been translated into Hebrew, Swedish, French, Italian, and Spanish. It has been validated for people with a variety of conditions affecting cognitive performance (e.g., stroke, multiple sclerosis [MS], schizophrenia, traumatic brain injury [TBI]). The EFPT has demonstrated good discriminant validity between healthy adults and persons with mild cognitive impairment from stroke (Baum et al., 2008), MS (Kalmar et al., 2008), and TBI (Baum et al., 2017). The EFPT has also been found to discriminate between groups of people with mild and moder-

ate impairment in stroke (Baum et al., 2008), MS (Kalmar et al., 2008), schizophrenia (Katz et al., 2007), and TBI (Baum et al., 2017).

Test–retest reliability has not been established because of the learning effect inherent in performance-based tests of cognition. Good to excellent interrater reliability has been demonstrated among patients with stroke for

- The overall EFPT (intraclass correlation [ICC] = .91),
- Cooking (ICC = .94),
- Bill Pay (ICC = .89),

- Medication Management (ICC = .94), and

- Telephone Use (ICC = .79).

Adequate internal consistency of the measure has been evaluated among persons with stroke (Cronbach's α = .77–.94) and among persons with schizophrenia (Cronbach's α = .88).

The EFPT has moderate correlations with neurological tests known to be measures of EF, including the Delis–Kaplan Executive Function System's Trail Making subtest (Delis et al., 2001), the Wisconsin Card Sorting Test (Heaton et al., 1993), and the National Institutes of Health Toolbox's Fluid Cognition and Crystalized Cognition composite scores (Weintraub et al., 2014). Excellent correlations exist with the Assessment of Motor and Process Skills (Cederfeldt et al., 2015; Fisher & Jones, 2010). Correlation coefficients between the EFPT and the total Behavioral Assessment of the Dysexecutive Syndrome profile revealed moderate to high correlations (Katz et al., 2007). Predictive validity was determined in a sample of persons with TBI, with the EFPT total task score predicting self-reported independence (Baum et al., 2017; Wilson et al., 1996).

Psychometric testing with the aEFPT has revealed the tasks to be reliable, with no significant differences demonstrated in performance on the EFPT tasks compared with the aEFPT tasks. Furthermore, performance on the aEFPT demonstrated moderate to high correlations with neuropsychological cognitive assessments (Hahn et al., 2014). Reliability of the form has also been demonstrated with Internet-based versions of the Bill Pay task and Telephone Use task (Rand et al., 2018).

Target Population

Functional–cognitive changes occur frequently in chronic neurologic and metabolic diseases, including Alzheimer's disease (Baum & Edwards, 1993); Parkinson's disease (Cahn et al., 1998; Klepac et al., 2008); MS (Birnboim & Miller, 2004); TBI (Goverover & Hinojosa, 2002); stroke (Baum et al., 2008); spinal cord injury (Hanks et al., 1999); and psychiatric disorders, in particular schizophrenia (Katz et al., 2007; Rempfer et al., 2003) and depression (Brown et al., 2014). More recently, deficits in functional cognition have been recognized as secondary consequences of cancer treatment (Nieuwenhuijsen et al., 2009) as well as in diabetes (Gaspar et al., 2016), chronic obstructive pulmonary disease (Dodd et al., 2010), and kidney disease (Zammit et al., 2015).

Functional–cognitive issues also require attention among people with autism; children with known sensory-processing problems; people with eating disorders (Dohle et al., 2018); and adults with behavioral conditions, including substance abuse (Perry, 2016; Rezapour et al., 2015). The EFPT may be applied in any of these populations or others in which there are suspected functional–cognitive deficits. The EFPT is particularly useful for those with mild to moderate cognitive deficits, which might not be adequately detected with often-used neuropsychological quick-screen measures (Toglia et al., 2017).

Administration

Practitioners should consult the EFPT test manual for test administration guidelines and a list of required supplies. The manual includes the forms, the labels to personalize the tasks, and the script for the administration of the EFPT. The EFPT itself and the training manual are free and available online (http://www.ot.wustl.edu/about/resources/executive-function-performance-test-efpt-308). The materials include all of the assessment forms and a scoring sheet that can be placed in the individual's medical record. Some hospital systems have asked that the scoring sheet be included in their electronic medical record; this is possible because the tool is in the public domain.

The EFPT tasks can be administered in a clinic's life skills area or in a home. Three of the tasks—Bill Pay, Medication Management, and Telephone Use—can be administered in a hospital room. In the absence of a kitchen, practitioners can administer the test using a portable burner and water from a pitcher. All of the items to administer the assessment are placed in a box and can be used at the point of testing.

The training manual includes all of the test materials, such as the script, labels, and bills; however, the test administrator will need to purchase items necessary for the tasks and the distractors. The items are listed and can be purchased at any grocery or general merchandise store for less than $50. The instructions to administer the test are listed in Exhibit 7.3, but readers should review the test manual for details regarding cueing. Video 7.1 provides an example of the instructions for the cooking subtest as well as an example of the cueing provided to the participant.

Scoring

The individual task sheets and the final scoring sheets are in the test manual located online. For each task, the test administrator calculates the highest level of cueing in the 5 domains:

1. **Initiation** (i.e., the start of motor activity that begins a task)

2. **Organization** (i.e., the physical arrangement of the environment, tools, and materials to facilitate efficient and effective performance of the steps required to complete the task)

3. **Sequencing** (i.e., the coordination and proper ordering of the steps that compose the task)

4. **Judgment and safety** (i.e., the use of reason and decision-making capabilities to intentionally avoid physically, emotionally, or financially dangerous or problematic situations)

5. **Completion** (i.e., the inhibition of motor performance driven by the knowledge that the task is finished).

EXHIBIT 7.3. Step-by-Step Instructions for Administering the EFPT

1. Begin the EFPT with the script and all of the pretest questions (see the EFPT manual).
2. Leave all of the items necessary for all of the tasks in the box on a table (the "materials table"). Put it on a lower table or stool if the person sits in a wheelchair. (Bills and other mail should be mixed together in a sealable plastic bag. The account book or checkbook should have checks included inside. All other items are loose in the box.)
3. Ask the person to begin the task (use the script available in the EFPT manual).
4. Offer assistance only after the participant has made a good attempt to process the actions necessary to carry out the step. Use the cueing guidelines.
5. Complete the cueing chart and behavior assessment chart for each task.
6. Time each of the tasks, and write down in minutes and seconds the time the test taker spends on each task on the task sheet.
7. Complete the score sheet with the information from each task sheet.

Note. EFPT = Executive Function Performance Test.
Source. Adapted from *Executive Function Performance Test Manual*, by C. M. Baum and T. J. Wolf, 2013, St. Louis: Washington University in St. Louis. In the public domain.

The administrator then sums these values to create a score for each subtask. They may calculate EF domain scores (e.g., initiation) by summing each of the domain components across tasks (e.g., all initiation components).

Documentation

Table 7.1 shows EFPT scoring for an example client, on the basis of the test material available online. A short summary of the client's test results is given. The occupational therapy practitioner could report this information at a case conference and include it in the client's record to document the cognitive problems the client is having in performing tasks and the level of cueing needed.

TABLE 7.1. Example EFPT Scoring Representation

MEASURED ITEM	CONTROL	CLIENT
Task		
Cooking	4.03	7
Bill Pay	0.38	5
Medication Management	1.82	4
Telephone Use	0.92	14
Cognitive construct		
Initiation	0.50	8
Organization	0.47	10
Sequencing	1.63	18
Judgment and safety	0.61	18
Completion	0.60	1

Note. EFPT = Executive Function Performance Test.

In this example, the report would include that the client was administered the EFPT, a standardized functional–cognitive assessment, and that the client required verbal cues in initiating, organizing, sequencing, and being safe in performing tasks. The client's occupational performance indicates that they may pose a safety risk. The occupational therapy practitioner could use an example from the EFPT to illustrate this. The client required a direct verbal cue to turn off the stove, required a direct verbal cue to avoid paying a bill when there were insufficient funds in the account, and had to be cued to take their medication rather than another person's.

The report should indicate the level of assistance the client is likely to require (e.g., the client requires a caregiver who can provide direct cues to help with instrumental tasks). If the client is independent or requires only limited help with organization, that can also be reported. The report might also include a statement regarding the client's efficiency in the tasks. Finally, through comparison with the client's predictions of performance or recall of performance, the practitioner may draw conclusions regarding self-awareness.

Interpretation and Intervention Considerations

The EFPT provides information regarding the functional–cognitive capabilities of the client. If clients are responding to cues in the assessment, they will likely respond best to strategy-based intervention methods. For example, Cognitive Orientation to daily Occupational Performance involves application of a global problem strategy, generation of domain-specific strategies, and use of guided discovery methods (Dawson et al., 2017). If the client consistently requires physical assistance, a skill- or habit-training approach, such as the Neurofunctional Approach, may be indicated (Clark-Wilson et al., 2014).

In both situations, the family will need to learn strategies to support the client in full engagement outside of the therapy environment. After the family observes the level of cueing provided by the occupational therapist, it is essential that the therapist give them the opportunity to be successful in providing cues to support the client's performance in the supervised environment. Families are more effective in providing support at home if they have successful experiences (Kinney & Stephens, 1989; Lawton et al., 1991).

If the client has problems initiating a task, the family must know that the client will need a cue to get them started on a task. If the client has trouble with organization, the family may have to lay out clothes or organize a work area where all the tools are located so the client can do a task. If the client has trouble performing an activity in the correct sequence, it is important for the family to know what that means and what the client requires in terms of supervision. If safety is a problem, the family needs to provide a sufficient level of supervision. If the client has trouble ending an activity at the appropriate stage, the family needs to understand perseveration and how to assist the client in ending an activity.

References

Baum, C. M., Connor, L. T., Morrison, T., Hahn, M., Dromerick, A. W., & Edwards, D. F. (2008). Reliability, validity, and clinical utility of the Executive Function Performance Test: A measure of executive function in a sample of people with stroke. *American Journal of Occupational Therapy, 62*, 446–455. https://doi.org/10.5014/ajot.62.4.446

Baum, C., & Edwards, D. F. (1993). Cognitive performance in senile dementia of the Alzheimer's type: The Kitchen Task Assessment. *American Journal of Occupational Therapy, 47*, 431–436. https://doi.org/10.5014/ajot.47.5.431

Baum, C. M., & Edwards, D. F. (2003). What persons with Alzheimer's disease can do: A tool for communication about everyday activities. *Alzheimer's Care Quarterly, 4*, 108–118.

Baum, C. M., & Wolf, T. J. (2013). *Executive Function Performance Test manual.* St. Louis: Washington University in St. Louis.

Baum, C. M., Wolf, T. J., Wong, A. W. K., Chen, C. H., Walker, K., Young, A. C., . . . Heinemann, A. W. (2017). Validation and clinical utility of the Executive Function Performance Test in persons with traumatic brain injury. *Neuropsychological Rehabilitation, 27*, 603–617. https://doi.org/10.1080/09602011.2016.1176934

Birnboim, S., & Miller, A. (2004). Cognitive strategies application of multiple sclerosis patients. *Multiple Sclerosis Journal, 10*, 67–73. https://doi.org/10.1191/1352458504ms980oa

Brown, P. J., Sneed, J. R., Rutherford, B. R., Devanand, D. P., & Roose, S. P. (2014). The nuances of cognition and depression in older adults: The need for a comprehensive assessment. *International Journal of Geriatric Psychiatry, 29*, 506–514. https://doi.org/10.1002/gps.4033

Cahn, D. A., Sullivan, E. V., Shear, P. K., Pfefferbaum, A., Heit, G., & Silverberg, G. (1998). Differential contributions of cognitive and motor component processes to physical and instrumental activities of daily living in Parkinson's disease. *Archives of Clinical Neuropsychology, 13*, 575–583. https://doi.org/10.1093/arclin/13.7.575

Cederfeldt, M., Carlsson, G., Dahlin-Ivanoff, S., & Gosman-Hedstrom, G. (2015). Inter-rater reliability and face validity of the Executive Function Performance Test (EFPT). *British Journal of Occupational Therapy, 78*, 563–569. https://doi.org/10.1177/0308022615575744

Chen, A. J. W., Abrams, G. M., & D'Esposito, M. (2006). Functional reintegration of prefrontal neural networks for enhancing recovery after brain injury. *Journal of Head Trauma Rehabilitation, 21*, 107–118. https://doi.org/10.1097/00001199-200603000-00004

Clark-Wilson, J., Giles, G. M., & Baxter, D. M. (2014). Revisiting the Neurofunctional Approach: Conceptualizing the core components for the rehabilitation of everyday living skills. *Brain Injury, 28*, 1646–1656. https://doi.org/10.3109/02699052.2014.946449

Dawson, D. R., McEwen, S. E., & Polatajko, H. J. (Eds.) (2017). *Cognitive Orientation to daily Occupational Performance in Occupational Therapy: Using the CO–OP Approach™ to enable participation across the lifespan.* Bethesda, MD: AOTA Press.

Delis, D. C., Kaplan, E., & Kramer, J. H. (2001). *Delis–Kaplan Executive Function System.* San Antonio: Psychological Corporation.

Dodd, J. W., Getov, S. V., & Jones, P. W. (2010). Cognitive function in COPD. *European Respiratory Journal, 35*, 913–922. https://doi.org/10.1183/09031936.00125109

Dohle, S., Diel, K., & Hofmann, W. (2018). Executive functions and the self-regulation of eating behavior: A review. *Appetite, 124*, 4–9. https://doi.org/10.1016/j.appet.2017.05.041

Fisher, A. G., & Jones, K. B. (2010). *Assessment of Motor and Process Skills: Vol. 1: Development, standardization, and administration manual* (7th ed.). Ft. Collins, CO: Three Star Press.

Fitzpatrick, S., & Baum, C. M. (2012). Executive functions. In L. M. Carey (Ed.), *Stroke rehabilitation: Insights from neuroscience and imaging* (pp. 208–221). New York: Oxford University Press. https://doi.org/10.1093/med/9780199797882.003.0015

Gaspar, J. M., Baptista, F. I., Macedo, M. P., & Ambrósio, A. F. (2016). Inside the diabetic brain: Role of different players involved in cognitive decline. *ACS Chemical Neuroscience, 7*, 131–142. https://doi.org/10.1021/acschemneuro.5b00240

Goverover, Y., & Hinojosa, J. (2002). Categorization and deductive reasoning: Predictors of instrumental activities of daily living performance in adults with brain injury. *American Journal of Occupational Therapy, 56*, 509–516. https://doi.org/10.5014/ajot.56.5.509

Hahn, B., Baum, C., Moore, J., Ehrlich-Jones, L., Spoeri, S., Doherty, M., & Wolf, T. J. (2014). Development of additional tasks for the Executive Function Performance Test. *American Journal of Occupational Therapy, 68*, e241–e246. https://doi.org/10.5014/ajot.2014.008565

Hanks, R. A., Rapport, L. J., Millis, S. R., & Deshpande, S. A. (1999). Measures of executive functioning as predictors of functional ability and social integration in a rehabilitation sample. *Archives of Physical Medicine and Rehabilitation, 80*, 1030–1037. https://doi.org/10.1016/S0003-9993(99)90056-4

Heaton, R. K., Chelune, G. J., Talley, J. L., Kay, G. G., & Curtiss, G. (1993). *Wisconsin Card Sorting Test (WCST): Manual: Revised and expanded.* Lutz, FL: Psychological Assessment Resources.

Kalmar, J. H., Gaudino, E. A., Moore, N. B., Halper, J., & Deluca, J. (2008). The relationship between cognitive deficits and everyday functional activities in multiple sclerosis. *Neuropsychology, 22*, 442–449. https://doi.org/10.1037/0894-4105.22.4.442

Katz, N., Tadmor, I., Felzen, B., & Hartman-Maeir, A. (2007). Validity of the Executive Function Performance Test in individuals with schizophrenia. *OTJR: Occupation, Participation and Health, 27*, 44–51. https://doi.org/10.1177/153944920702700202

Kinney, J. M., & Stephens, M. A. P. (1989). Hassles and uplifts of giving care to a family member with dementia. *Psychology and Aging, 4*, 402–408. https://doi.org/10.1037/0882-7974.4.4.402

Klepac, N., Trkulja, V., Relja, M., & Babić, T. (2008). Is quality of life in non-demented Parkinson's disease patients related to cognitive performance? A clinic-based cross-sectional study. *European Journal of Neurology, 15*, 128–133. https://doi.org/10.1111/j.1468-1331.2007.02011.x

Lawton, M. P., Brody, E. M., & Saperstein, A. R. (1991). *Respite for caregivers of Alzheimer patients: Research and practice.* New York: Springer.

Lezak, M. D., Howieson, D. B., Loring, D. W., Hannay, H. J., & Fischer, J. S. (2004). *Neuropsychological assessment.* New York: Oxford University Press.

Miyake, A., & Shah, P. (Eds.). (1999). *Models of working memory: Mechanisms of active maintenance and executive control.* Cambridge, England: Cambridge University Press.

Nasreddine, Z. S., Phillips, N. A., Bédirian, V., Charbonneau, S., Whitehead, V., Collin, I., . . . Chertkow, H. (2005). The Montreal Cognitive Assessment, MoCA: A brief screening tool for mild cognitive impairment. *Journal of the American Geriatrics Society, 53,* 695–699. https://doi.org/10.1111/j.1532-5415.2005.53221.x

Nieuwenhuijsen, K., De Boer, A., Spelten, E., Sprangers, M. A., & Verbeek, J. H. (2009). The role of neuropsychological functioning in cancer survivors' return to work one year after diagnosis. *Social and Behavioral Dimensions of Cancer, 18,* 589–597. https://doi.org/10.1002/pon.1439

Perry, C. J. (2016). Cognitive decline and recovery in alcohol abuse. *Journal of Molecular Neuroscience, 60,* 383–389. https://doi.org/10.1007/s12031-016-0798-4

Prigatano, G. P. (1999). *Principles of neuropsychological rehabilitation.* New York: Oxford University Press.

Rand, D., Ben-Haim, K. L., Malka, R., & Portnoy, S. (2018). Development of Internet-based tasks for the Executive Function Performance Test. *American Journal of Occupational Therapy, 72,* 7202205060. https://doi.org/10.5014/ajot.2018.023598

Rempfer, M. V., Hamera, E. K., Brown, C. E., & Cromwell, R. L. (2003). The relations between cognition and the independent living skill of shopping in people with schizophrenia. *Psychiatry Research, 117,* 103–112. https://doi.org/10.1016/S0165-1781(02)00318-9

Rezapour, T., Hatami, J., Farhoudian, A., Sofuoglu, M., Noroozi, A., Daneshmand, R., . . . Ekhtiari, H. (2015). NEuro COgnitive REhabilitation for Disease of Addiction (NECOREDA) program: From development to trial. *Basic and Clinical Neuroscience, 6,* 291–298.

Toglia, J., Askin, G., Gerber, L. M., Taub, M. C., Mastrogiovanni, A. R., & O'Dell, M. W. (2017). Association between 2 measures of cognitive instrumental activities of daily living and their relation to the Montreal Cognitive Assessment in persons with stroke. *Archives of Physical Medicine and Rehabilitation, 98,* 2280–2287. https://doi.org/10.1016/j.apmr.2017.04.007

Toglia, J., & Katz, N. (2018). Executive functioning: Prevention and health promotion for at-risk populations and those with chronic disease. In N. Katz & J. Toglia (Eds.), *Cognition, occupation, and participation across the lifespan: Neuroscience, neurorehabilitation, and models of intervention in occupational therapy* (4th ed., pp. 129–140). Bethesda, MD: AOTA Press.

Weintraub, S., Dikmen, S. S., Heaton, R. K., Tulsky, D. S., Zelazo, P. D., Slotkin, J., . . . Gershon, R. (2014). The Cognition Battery of the NIH Toolbox for Assessment of Neurological and Behavioral Function: Validation in an adult sample. *Journal of the International Neuropsychological Society, 20,* 567–578. https://doi.org/10.1017/S1355617714000320

Wilson, B. A., Alderman, N., Burgess, P. W., Emslie, H., & Evans, J. (1996). *Behavioural Assessment of the Dysexecutive Syndrome.* Suffolk, England: Thames Valley Test Company.

Zammit, A. R., Katz, M. J., Lai, J. Y., Zimmerman, M. E., Bitzer, M., & Lipton, R. B. (2015). Association between renal function and cognitive ability domains in the Einstein Aging Study: A cross-sectional analysis. *Journals of Gerontology, Series A: Biomedical Sciences and Medical Sciences, 70,* 764–770. https://doi.org/10.1093/gerona/glu185

Weekly Calendar Planning Activity

ALEXIS LUSSIER, MS, OTR/L; MEGHAN DOHERTY, OTD, OTR/L;
AND JOAN TOGLIA, PhD, OTR/L, FAOTA

LEARNING OBJECTIVES

After completing this chapter, readers should be able to

- Describe the background, purpose, and aims of the Weekly Calendar Planning Activity (WCPA) to assess executive function;
- Describe the administration, utility, and clinical applications of the WCPA;
- Identify quantitative and qualitative information obtained from the WCPA; and
- Discuss how the results of the WCPA can be used to guide treatment planning.

KEY TERMS AND CONCEPTS

- Cognitive strategy • Executive function • Instrumental activity of daily living • Self-awareness
- Weekly Calendar Planning Activity

Introduction

The **Weekly Calendar Planning Activity** (WCPA) is a performance-based measure of functional cognition (Toglia, 2015a). This tabletop assessment asks the test taker to perform an **instrumental activity of daily living** (IADL) task. *IADLs* are "activities that support daily life within the home and community and that often require more complex interactions than those used in ADLs" (American Occupational Therapy Association, 2014, p. S43).

The WCPA requires the test taker to enter a 10- to 18-item list of fixed and flexible appointments into a blank weekly schedule while adhering to rules, monitoring time, and reconciling conflicting task demands. During the task, demands are placed on the test taker's **executive function** (EF) processes, which can be described as "an inter-related set of abilities responsible for directing and coordinating cognitive control and goal directed actions" (Toglia & Katz, 2018, p. 129).

Specific EF demands placed on the test taker during this activity include

- Planning,
- Organization,
- Inhibition,
- Working memory, and
- Flexibility.

Additionally, successful adherence to a provided set of rules engages prospective memory, mental tracking, and problem solving.

The test administrator or occupational therapist observes the client's use of **cognitive strategy**, which can be defined as "a mental plan of action that helps a person to learn, problem solve, and perform" (Toglia et al., 2012, p. 227). The activity part of the assessment is followed by a semistructured interview,

EXHIBIT 8.1. WCPA Levels of Difficulty

LEVEL 1 (least difficult)	LEVEL 2	LEVEL 3 (most difficult)
• Organized checklist of appointments • Cue to checklist is provided • Preplanning is not required	• Unorganized list of appointments • No cue provided • Preplanning and reorganization required	• Paragraph of appointments • Irrelevant information included • Requires sorting out relevant information and preplanning
Appointments and errands to be scheduled: Adult/Older Adult (Level 1, Version A) ☐ Dentist on Thursday at 3:00 p.m. (1 hour) ☐ Lunch with a friend on Tuesday from 1:00–2:00 p.m. ☐ Haircut on Monday from 11:00 a.m.–12:00 p.m. ☐ Volunteer at People to People on Friday from 9:00–10:30 a.m. ☐ Movies with friends on Thursday from 7:00–11:00 p.m. ☐ Walk neighbor's dog on Thursday morning before 11:00 a.m. (half hour)	**Appointments and errands to be scheduled: Adult/Older Adult (Level 2, Version A)** Dentist on Thursday at 3:00 p.m. (1 hour) One-hour visit with cousin who is only available on Thursday between 2:30 and 4:00 p.m. or on Monday or Tuesday between 1:00 and 2:30 p.m. Carpool: One morning at 9:00 a.m. and 1 afternoon at 3:00 p.m. (45 minutes) Phone conference before 2:00 p.m. on Tuesday (half-hour) Doctor appointment Monday or Friday afternoon at 2:00 p.m. (90 minutes)	**Appointments and errands to be scheduled: Adult/Older Adult (Level 3, Version A)** You have a dentist appointment on Thursday at 3:00 p.m. for an hour. Also, you need to call to renew your prescription and pick up the medication. You take your medication 3 times a day (8:00 a.m., noon, and 9:00 p.m.) and will be out of medication after taking your last pill on Tuesday at noon. Make time to go to the pharmacy; it is open 9 a.m. to 3 p.m. daily and will take a half-hour You have plans to go out with your friends to the movies on Thursday from 7:00 to 11:00 p.m. You have a nice pair of pants to wear.

Note. WCPA = Weekly Calendar Planning Activity.
Source. From *Weekly Calendar Planning Activity Part I: Introduction and Overview* [video file], by J. Toglia and A. Lussier, November 29, 2017. Retrieved from https://youtu.be/rJ4Czn17y0M. Copyright © 2018 by J. Toglia. Used with permission.

which provides valuable insight into a client's perception of their performance and level of ***self-awareness,*** or ability to self-monitor performance as well as recognize and correct errors (Zlotnik & Toglia, 2018).

The WCPA has good clinical utility, because it is easily portable and can be used consistently in any setting (Toglia, 2015a). The assessment includes 3 levels of difficulty, which can accommodate varying levels of ability (see Exhibit 8.1). The Level 2 version of the WCPA has a shortened 10-item list (WCPA–10) that is useful in clinical settings where there are time constraints.

Background and Theory

EF

It is well understood that EF processes are instrumental to successful participation in ADLs (Adamit et al., 2015; Miyake & Friedman, 2012; Toglia, Lahav, et al., 2017; Zelazo et al., 2016). EFs support a person's ability to engage in goal-oriented actions required for independent occupational participation and community engagement. Habitual activities and everyday routines are accomplished automatically and procedurally, placing minimal demands on EF (Norman

& Shallice, 1986; Wood & Rünger, 2016). It is therefore necessary to examine and understand EF control in the context of novel, nonroutine, and complex multistep activities (Burgess et al., 2006).

During performance of the WCPA, subtle deficits in EF are highlighted through error pattern analysis and observations of performance, including strategy use. The addition of rules, conflicting task demands, and unfamiliar appointments creates novelty and places increased demands on the test taker while they are entering appointments into a daily calendar (Toglia & White, 2019).

The WCPA is theoretically based on the Dynamic Interactional Model of cognition and is frequently used with the Multicontext Approach (Toglia, 2018; see Chapter 20). The model focuses on the relationships among personal context, self-awareness, and strategy use in combination with activity demands and the environment to understand functional cognition. It emphasizes the idea that one can best understand cognitive dysfunction by analyzing the pattern of errors, process strategies, and self-monitoring or awareness that are reflected during performance, rather than identifying specific deficits.

Development of the Tool

The WCPA has been studied with populations ranging from healthy adolescents ages 12 or older to community-dwelling older adults up to age 94 (Stephens & Berryhill, 2016; Toglia, 2015a). It has also been examined in a variety of clinical populations, including at-risk youth (Weiner et al., 2012) and youth with epilepsy (Zlotnik et al., 2018).

Normative data on healthy controls are included in the WCPA manual (ages 16 to 94) as well as in published studies (ages 12 to 88). These data provide a foundation for interpretation of WCPA performance (Toglia, 2015a). This is important because "typical" performance is not always clear in cognitively demanding functional activities, without a means of normative comparison (Bottari & Dawson, 2011; Toglia, Askin, et al., 2017).

The WCPA manual includes raw-score-to-percentile conversions according to version used and specific age groups (Toglia, 2015a). Normative data collection on the WCPA–10 for young and older adults is currently in progress. Table 8.1 presents a summary of the WCPA versions and age ranges for which normative data are available. Psychometric properties that have been published thus far are reported in Table 8.2 and include discriminant validity, convergent validity, and interrater reliability.

In addition to the studies presented in Table 8.2, several pilot studies have been completed recently. For example, Kizony et al. (2018) reported discrimination between age-matched healthy controls and people with stroke in Israel. Recently, Toglia et al. (2018) also reported that the short version of the WCPA (WCPA–10) discriminated between adults with acquired brain injury and age-matched healthy controls. Additionally, Goverover et al. (2019) completed a study that found that the WCPA discriminated between people with multiple sclerosis (MS) and cognitive impairment and healthy controls or people with MS and no cognitive impairment.

The WCPA has been published in Swedish by the Swedish Association of Occupational Therapists (Toglia, 2017) and in Dutch (Toglia, 2015b) and has been translated into Arabic and Hebrew (Amer et al., 2016; Grinblatt et al., 2012). Scores demonstrate stability across cultures in adults, except for strategy use and time for completion. Test administrators should mindfully interpret these latter aspects of performance with individuals from varying cultural backgrounds (Toglia, Lahav, et al., 2017).

Target Population

EF deficits typically can be seen in a wide variety of clinical populations (see Exhibit 8.2). The WCPA may detect subtle, as well as overt, EF difficulties and can be used with a variety of diagnoses, including neurological and chronic illnesses as well as developmental and mental health disorders. The WCPA is appropriate for individuals who are generally independent in basic and routine ADLs but show greater difficulty in complex IADL tasks (Toglia, 2015a). Individuals for whom this assessment is suitable are oriented, demonstrate the ability to sustain attention for 10 minutes, and can comprehend written sentences (Toglia, 2015a).

It is beneficial if the test has face validity with the client—that is, if their occupational profile shows they are familiar with using a calendar, planner, or smartphone to schedule appointments. The WCPA is not appropriate for individuals who cannot read or write or those with low vision who have not yet established magnification options. The test has 3 versions for use with

- Middle and high school students (ages 12 to 18),
- Youth (ages 16 to 21), and
- Adults and older adults (ages 18 to 94).

Normative scores for these populations are available for comparison.

The Montreal Cognitive Assessment (MoCA; Nasreddine et al., 2005) is frequently used as a cognitive screening tool to identify adults with mild cognitive impairment, and occupational therapists can consider it for use before giving the WCPA. Toglia, Askin, et al. (2017) found that IADL performance could not be reliably predicted among people with MoCA scores of 20 and above. Therefore, these individuals would benefit from further assessment with the WCPA or other performance-based IADL assessments. Although screening tools such as the MoCA

TABLE 8.1. Summary of WCPA Versions and Age Ranges, With Normative Data

WCPA VERSION	AGE RANGE	*N*	SOURCE(S)
Level 2 (United States)	16–94	435	(Toglia, 2015a)
Level 2, Hebrew version (Israel)	18–88	433	(Toglia, Lahav, et al., 2017)
Youth Level 2, Version A	16–21	49	(Toglia, 2015a; Toglia & Berg, 2013)
Middle School and High School Level 2, Version A (Hebrew version)	12–18	109	(Zlotnik & Toglia, 2018)
Level 3, Version A	18–87	175	(Toglia, 2015a)
Student	20–34	157	(Lahav et al., 2018)

Note. WCPA = Weekly Calendar Planning Activity.

TABLE 8.2. Psychometric Properties of the WCPA

POPULATION	PSYCHOMETRIC PROPERTIES	RESULTS
At-risk youth (Weiner et al., 2012)	High interrater reliability for total accuracy scores	ICC = .99
Community and at-risk youth (Toglia & Berg, 2013)	Discriminant validity between typical and at-risk youth on various performance measures	The community group entered a greater number of appointments, had greater accuracy, made fewer errors, and used more strategies as compared with the at-risk group.
College students with and without ADHD (Lahav et al., 2018)	Moderate to high test–retest reliabilities for performance measures	ICCs = .60–.85
	Interrater reliability	r_s = .937–.989
	Discriminant validity between ADHD and control group on various performance measures	College students without ADHD had fewer missing appointments, used less time, entered more appointments, followed more rules, and used more strategies than college students with ADHD.
Typical adolescents and those with epilepsy (Zlotnik et al., 2018)	Discriminant validity between group with epilepsy and typical control group on various performance measures	Typical adolescents had higher efficiency scores and more accurate appointments and strategies used as compared with the epilepsy group.
Adult age and cultural differences in Israel and the United States (Toglia, Lahav, et al., 2017)	Discriminant validity between older and younger groups on various performance measures	Significant differences were found between adults younger and older than age 65 years, in both countries, on the majority of WCPA variables, with the exception of time.
Healthy controls and teenagers with ABI (Doherty et al., 2017)	Discriminant validity between participants with ABI and controls on various performance measures	ABI group had longer total time and used fewer strategies as compared with control group.
	Convergent validity with moderate to fair correlations across all measures	
WCPA in MS: top-down assessment of EFs (Goverover et al., 2019)	Discriminant validity among participants with MS and cognitive impairments, those with MS without cognitive impairments, and healthy controls	Significant between-group differences on the WCPA number of correct appointments entered, number of rules followed, and total number of errors committed were found between MS participants and other groups.
	Concurrent validity with a standardized measure of EF and a functional–cognitive measure	WCPA accuracy, number of strategies used, and number of rules followed were associated with better performance on another functional–cognitive test.
		Significant associations were found between a neuropsychological measure of EF and the WCPA number of accurate appointments entered and number of rules followed.

Note. ABI = acquired brain injury; ADHD = attention deficit hyperactivity disorder; EF(s) = executive function(s); ICC(s) = intraclass correlation(s); MS = multiple sclerosis; WCPA = Weekly Calendar Planning Activity.

can be helpful in determining appropriateness of the WCPA, a comprehensive occupational profile and evaluation are most valuable to determine whether the WCPA is appropriate.

Administration

Training and Preparation

In preparation for administration of the WCPA, the examiner should read and understand the WCPA manual (Toglia, 2015a) to become familiar with instructions and procedures. They should read the examples of after-task interview scripts and

probes that are included in the manual and become familiar with the range of strategies typically used. Additional resources for review include the WCPA narrated presentations and training videos that can be found on https://www.multicontext.net.

After reviewing these materials, the prospective test administrator is encouraged to practice before clinical use, including role-playing and administering the measure to healthy individuals, colleagues, and people from various age groups to enhance their knowledge and gain proficiency with the procedures. Finally, the test administrator must select the appropriate level of difficulty and version of the calendar, considering the participant's age and level of function. All of the calendar versions

EXHIBIT 8.2. Clinical Populations With Possible EF Deficits

NEUROLOGICAL INJURY OR ILLNESS	CHRONIC ILLNESS	DEVELOPMENTAL DISORDERS	MENTAL HEALTH DISORDERS	OTHER
• Stroke • TBI • Brain tumor • MS • Mild cognitive impairment • Parkinson's disease	• Cancer • Renal or cardiac disease • COPD • Lupus • Rheumatoid arthritis • Diabetes	• Autism • Learning disabilities • ADHD • Cerebral palsy • Pediatric TBI or brain tumors	• Schizophrenia • Susbtance abuse • Bipolar disorder • Depression	• Youth or adults with concussion • PTSD • At-risk youth • Youth with epilepsy • Community-dwelling older adults

Note. ADHD = attention deficit hyperactivity disorder; COPD = chronic obstructive pulmonary disease; EF = executive function; MS = multiple sclerosis; PTSD = posttraumatic stress disorder; TBI = traumatic brain injury.
Source. From *Weekly Calendar Planning Activity Part I: Introduction and Overview* [video file], by J. Toglia and A. Lussier, November 29, 2017. Retrieved from https://youtu.be/rJ4Czn17y0M. Copyright © 2018 by J. Toglia. Used with permission.

and forms for administration are included in the appendix of the test manual as well as on a flash drive that accompanies the manual (see Exhibit 8.3).

The WCPA manual is available from AOTA Press. In addition, Toglia and Lussier (2017) created a video illustrating WCPA administration procedures. The video shows a sample of correct administration procedures of the WCPA, including setup and oral instructions, procedures during the task performance, and the after-task interview.

Before the Task

Once all the appropriate forms and items are gathered (highlighters, pens, small clock or watch if needed), they must be placed directly in front of the client as illustrated in the WCPA manual and as shown in Video 8.1. Test materials include an abbreviated sheet of instructions and rules, which remains in front of the test taker for the duration of the task. The assessment should be set up in a well-lit and clutter-free environment, without nontest-relevant distractions.

Scripted instructions are provided orally. The test taker should be asked to restate directions and be provided with an

opportunity to ask questions. It is essential that the test administrator feel that the client understands the 5 rules:

1. Leave the specified day free.

2. Do not cross out appointments once they are entered.

3. Inform the examiner when it is a specified time.

4. Do not respond to distracting questions from the examiner.

5. Inform the examiner when finished.

Once they have explained and reviewed the instructions and rules, the examiner states, "Let's begin," and starts a timer.

If there are concerns about the client's memory, comprehension, or understanding of the directions and rules before they begin the task, the examiner can ask the client specific questions using the sample calendar sheet, such as, "Show me how you would indicate an appointment for 45 minutes." The client can also be asked to fully teach back the directions to ensure understanding so that the test can proceed. These adaptations were not used or necessary with healthy controls during normative studies and could potentially facilitate performance. Therefore,

EXHIBIT 8.3. Forms and Materials Needed for WCPA Administration

FORMS NEEDED	
EXAMINER	**CLIENT**
• Examiner directions for all levels • Adult background form (optional) • WCPA recording form • After-task interview and rating scale • Calendar scoring worksheet • Observation form (optional)	• WCPA instruction sheet • Appointments and errands to be scheduled (list or paragraph) • Blank weekly calendar • Weekly calendar sample
ADDITIONAL MATERIALS NEEDED	
EXAMINER	**CLIENT**
• Stopwatch	• Pens • 2 different color highlighters • 1 or 2 pieces of blank scrap paper • Watch or clock in clear sight

Source. From *Weekly Calendar Planning Activity (WCPA): A Performance Test of Executive Function*, by J. Toglia, 2015, Bethesda, MD: AOTA Press. Copyright © 2015 by the American Occupational Therapy Association. Used with permission.

they should be avoided unless required, because more structured procedures for directions could also mask subtle EF deficits.

During the Task

Immediately after the client begins the task, the test administrator observes how they go about entering appointments into the calendar and managing conflicts. During the task, the test administrator asks the test taker 3 distracting questions at specific time intervals (i.e., at 2, 5, and 10 minutes), which the test taker previously has been instructed to ignore. The test administrator records the test taker's ability to cope with these task interruptions and brief distractions.

The test administrator also observes and records multiple components of performance during the task, including

- Planning time (seconds),

- Total time (minutes),

- Rule adherence,

- Type and number of strategies used, and

- Spontaneous self-recognition of errors.

Other performance observations are also recorded, such as frequency with which the test taker refers to the instruction sheet and calendar error management. The WCPA calendar includes purposeful errors (i.e., Saturday–Sunday reversal, appointments that extend past calendar time, and change in the evening time from 15-minute to half-hour time slots). These components provide important qualitative information as to how the test taker copes with the unexpected (Toglia, 2015a).

The WCPA scoring worksheet includes a self-recognition column that the examiner uses during performance to indicate the test taker's acknowledgment of an error or attempt to fix a mistake. The test administrator is encouraged to use the optional observation form to record entry order of appointments and any other observations, comments, or errors specific to each appointment. This provides greater detail about the test taker's performance and the process and methods used and is also helpful during scoring and analysis.

After the Task

Once the test taker indicates that they are finished, the test administrator and test taker immediately engage in a semistructured after-task interview. The interview is an important component of the WCPA and provides an opportunity for the test administrator to obtain any clarification needed or to verify observations made during the task. It also provides key information on the test taker's

- Perceptions of task challenges,

- Methods or strategies used,

- Ability to generate alternative strategies, and

- Overall perceptions of the activity and their performance.

To conclude, the test taker completes a 4-question self-rating form and is asked to self-estimate the time needed to complete the task and performance accuracy. This information, in comparison with actual performance, provides an indication of the test taker's self-awareness.

Scoring

Each version of the WCPA includes a scoring worksheet to assist the test administrator in evaluating performance. The first step in scoring involves identifying appointments entered as well as those that are missing. Next, the examiner generally identifies whether each appointment entered is correct or incorrect. Other scores include the number of rules adhered to, number of strategies used, planning time, and total time needed for task completion.

The test administrator has the option of obtaining a detailed error analysis by categorizing each error according to 4 specified error codes:

1. Repetition

2. Location

3. Time

4. Incomplete.

Examples of these errors include repeating an appointment entry, placing an appointment in the wrong location or on the wrong day, allotting an incorrect amount of time, or inaccurately entering an appointment name, respectively. This detailed method of scoring provides greater insight into the underlying impairments that might have contributed to difficulty with the assessment, can guide clinical decision making, and provides implications for treatment.

The test administrator can calculate an optional efficiency score to help understand the relationship between accuracy and speed when the test taker performs this task. Normative data and percentiles exist for comparison in the WCPA manual for the 17-item versions for ages 16 to 94. The test administrator can create a visual representation of performance with a visual performance profile or error analysis summary visual profile to provide an overview of strengths and weaknesses and error patterns.

Documentation

Documentation of performance on the WCPA should focus on the test taker's objective performance during the test as well as on how their performance might affect their IADLs. Documentation should begin with a general statement about the client's performance and observed error patterns. Next, the occupational therapist can include any difficulties the client encountered with physically completing the task, assistance given, and any environmental factors that might have influenced the results.

Examples of environmental factors include clinic or room atmosphere, interruptions, or self-generated distractions of the client (e.g., using their smartphone, initiating conversations).

Next, the occupational therapist can use 1 or more WCPA forms to include a visual performance profile, error analysis profile, or normative comparison to summarize the client's objective performance. Main scores to include are

- Total time (minutes),

- Planning time (seconds),

- Total number of strategies used,

- Total number of appointments entered and whether any were missing,

- Total number of correct appointments,

- Total number of errors,

- Total number of rules followed, and

- Efficiency score.

The next level of detail for documentation includes review of strategies used and errors made. Strategy use can be defined by total number, frequency, consistency, and type. Total strategy use can be compared with normative data for adults. Errors can be defined by total number, frequency of each of the 4 types of errors, and whether the client demonstrated self-recognition of any errors made. Total errors can also be compared with normative data. If an efficiency score was calculated, it should be included in documentation.

Next, the test administrator should document the self-awareness of the test taker. This includes a general statement of partial or full recognition of difficulties or challenges encountered during the test. Next, the administrator should detail the experience during the task. For example, did the test taker show self-recognition of errors at the time they were made? The test administrator could include a more subjective reflection on the test taker's behavior during the task—for example, any verbal statements of difficulty or frustration or any facial expressions that might reveal the feelings of the test taker during the task.

Finally, the test administrator summarizes the findings from the after-task interview. How well did the test taker estimate their performance? Could the test taker describe the process or strategies used? Do the test taker's self-ratings match those of the test administrator?

Interpretation and Intervention Considerations

Interpretation of WCPA performance translates directly to 3 important areas of consideration for treatment:

1. Error pattern analysis

2. Strategy use

3. Self-awareness.

By observing task performance and discussing it after the activity, the occupational therapist gleans valuable information to apply when structuring daily therapy sessions and when selecting an appropriate cognitive intervention approach. Synthesizing the various aspects of task performance is crucial to interpret the client's capabilities.

Errors

Analysis of the number and types of errors committed during the WCPA (i.e., omissions, repetition, location, time, or incomplete) can aid the occupational therapist in identifying error patterns that might be present in other cognitively challenging daily life activities. For example, if a person tended to omit or miss information during the WCPA, it is important to determine whether this same error pattern emerges during other complex activities.

It is important to note whether the person spontaneously self-recognizes errors or self-corrects errors during the task as well as acknowledges difficulties after the activity. Awareness of performance errors suggests that the person may be a good candidate for intervention that focuses on helping them to develop strategies to prevent or effectively manage performance errors.

Because lists are an inherent part of many daily activities, multiple errors on the WCPA also suggest that the person needs assistance in managing lists. Treatment can focus on either adapting and simplifying lists or helping the person effectively use strategies to manage use of lists and prevent errors across different situations.

Following Rules

The 5 rules given during the task add complexity by increasing cognitive load and further stress the test taker's ability to keep track of information, inhibit distracting or irrelevant information, and multitask. The person needs to keep the rules in mind as they carry out the task. Most healthy people are able to follow at least 4 rules (Toglia, 2015a).

Rules that are broken are analyzed in combination with error patterns and strategy use. The client's ability to adhere to rules can be used in the design of future treatment sessions. If the person shows an inability to handle the level of complexity of the WCPA, the occupational therapist may need to downgrade the demands for initial treatment. The client may not be ready for multitasking in simulated daily activities.

Strategies

Analysis of strategy use includes information obtained both from the after-task interview and from observations of strategy use during the task. Some strategies cannot be observed but are described by the person during the after-task interview, such as manipulating information using working memory or recognizing that the list includes both fixed and flexible appointments and setting priorities. The number, type, frequency, and effectiveness of strategies used are considered as well as the person's ability to generate alternative strategies.

Typical adults use an average of 4 strategies to complete the WCPA (Toglia, 2018). Using too many strategies (e.g., 9 to 10) can negatively affect performance by increasing time, effort, or confusion. Similarly, using too few strategies can also negatively affect performance (Toglia, 2015a).

Strategies that healthy controls were commonly observed to use during the WCPA are grouped into 4 major categories on the basis of how they support performance on the WCPA:

1. Enhance attention to features (e.g., crossing off, using finger, highlighting)

2. Keep track (e.g., using verbal rehearsal, crossing off items)

3. Simplify or organize information (e.g., rearranging materials, using a written plan)

4. Self-monitor performance (e.g., self-checking, pausing and rereading).

Typically, healthy controls used strategies from 3 or all 4 of these categories. The most effective strategy for completing the WCPA successfully involves entering fixed appointments first (Toglia, 2015a).

Clinical observations of strategy use include lack of initiation of strategies, ineffective or inefficient use of strategies, inability to adjust strategies or task methods when they do not work, restricted range of strategies, inconsistent strategy use, and poor strategy selection. For example, a test taker might highlight, use their finger, and underline key words (attention to features). However, none of these strategies is effective if the test taker is having difficulty keeping track of information or organizing information. The strategy selected needs to match the cognitive performance errors.

Another test taker might fail to initiate strategies and might not use any methods to help keep track of appointments they entered (e.g., crossing off). As a result, some appointments are missed, and others are entered twice. Strategy use is interpreted in relation to performance and in combination with other WCPA measures to provide a foundation for treatment.

Self-Awareness

The test administrator observes self-awareness both through watching a client's performance and from probing during the after-task interview. Self-awareness is not all or none. Often, a person has mixed insight about their strengths and weaknesses. Some test takers also may have only a vague sense of their cognitive issues, which the occupational therapist could glean from a general statement such as, "My memory isn't as good" or "That test was hard."

During the WCPA, the test administrator should watch for instances of the test taker self-correcting their work. This might be an indicator of self-recognition of specific errors after they have been committed on the calendar or of other self-talk, such as test takers catching themselves before making an error. Facial expressions, statements of the difficulty of the task, frustration, or signs that the test taker is upset at the challenge may also indicate self-awareness of challenges during the task.

After the test taker finishes the task, the test administrator asks them both quantitative and qualitative questions to estimate their performance. Test takers are asked to self-reflect on their process of task completion, strategies they used, and anything they could have done differently. They are asked to estimate their performance time and accuracy and to use quantitative ratings of

1. Efficiency,

2. Task difficulty,

3. Task completion, and

4. Their management of multiple components of the test.

Test administrators rate these 4 items on the basis of their observation and compare their responses with the responses of the test taker. A match indicates better self-awareness of strengths and weaknesses (Toglia, 2015a).

Emotional Stability–Instability

A test taker might have emotional reactions to the challenge presented by the WCPA. Management of emotions in the face of challenge is part of good functional cognition. Demonstrations of frustration, anxiety, or other behavior during the WCPA might be observed in terms of facial expressions or through negative statements verbalized by the test taker. If these types of behaviors are demonstrated, the occupational therapist can address them in follow-up treatment sessions by improving the test taker's awareness of their emotional reactions and by teaching them to implement strategies to modulate anxiety, frustration, or anger.

Synthesizing the Results of the WCPA

Interpretation of the WCPA involves combining and synthesizing information on error patterns, strategy use, and self-awareness obtained through objective scores or ratings, observations, and the test taker's own perceptions of their performance. Interpretation of only 1 score or area (e.g., number of errors) should be avoided, because it can be misleading (Toglia, 2015a). Combinations of scores and qualitative information across different areas (performance, strategies, awareness) yield different WCPA performance patterns.

Two test takers might have the same score on the WCPA and exhibit the same error pattern; however, the implications for treatment might be different when the therapist interprets all aspects of performance together. For example, a test taker might spend several minutes planning but still miss several items on the list. They might forget rules and fail to use strategies to help keep track of information. After the task, however, they might demonstrate good awareness of performance challenges. In this situation, treatment might focus on helping the person anticipate task challenges (before the task), self-monitor performance, and develop effective methods to keep track of information during performance.

Similarly, another test taker might quickly jump into the task without planning, miss items on the list, break several rules (e.g., answer all distracting questions, cross out appointments), jump impulsively from 1 part of the list to another, fail to use strategies, and overestimate performance. In this case, treatment might first focus on helping the person to recognize the need to plan ahead and use a slower, more organized approach. As awareness emerges, treatment might then progress to helping the person develop strategies to pace actions and restrain impulsive responses.

These 2 examples illustrate the importance of examining all aspects of the WCPA simultaneously when interpreting performance. They also demonstrate that even when 2 test takers have the same accuracy score and make the same type of error (omissions), differences among other aspects of the WCPA performance profile can result in different implications for treatment. The WCPA manual discusses the wide range and variety of WCPA performance patterns that can be observed and reviews implications for treatment.

Other Considerations for WCPA Interpretation

There is no scaled scoring available for the WCPA; however, normative scores for the 17-item version are available for ages 16 to 21 (Youth Version, Level 2) and ages 18 to 94 (Adult Version, Levels 2 and 3) and can be found in the WCPA manual (Toglia, 2015a). Zlotnik and Toglia (2018) published normative data for the middle school–high school version from a study of Israeli teens ages 12 to 18. Information from the WCPA performance profile is very valuable for communicating with an interdisciplinary health care team as well as with a client's family. The WCPA should not be used for treatment and is intended for assessment only.

Treatment Planning

The first step to selecting a cognitive treatment approach is determining a client's level of awareness of their deficits (Haskins et al., 2012). The WCPA provides ample information about a test taker's self-awareness during an IADL task requiring EF. A mismatch between self-ratings and the occupational therapist's observations after test performance or a poor description of the process and strategies the test taker used might indicate that they would benefit from a treatment approach that focuses on improving awareness, facilitating error pattern recognition, and increasing strategy use, such as the Multicontext Approach (Toglia, 2018). If a client demonstrates errors on the WCPA but can verbalize recognition of these errors during and after the task, they might have enough self-awareness to respond to a metacognitive strategy training intervention, such as either the Cognitive Orientation to daily Occupational Performance approach (Skidmore et al., 2017) or the Multicontext Approach.

If a client exhibits defensive denial or shows lack of awareness as well as significantly impaired short-term memory, a task-specific approach that focuses on improving functional performance of selected tasks, such as the Neurofunctional Approach (Clark-Wilson et al., 2014; Giles, 2018), may be most appropriate for the client with profound functional impairments. This client might not be able to complete the WCPA. Poor performance on the WCPA might also indicate that additional testing is warranted with a less complex test, such as the Executive Function Performance Test (Baum et al., 2008). Alternatively, the client might need tests of memory or attention.

Case Example 8.1 presents a comprehensive summary of performance, scoring, documentation, and interpretation of the WCPA with an adult neurological client.

CASE EXAMPLE 8.1. Darius: Adult Neurological Client

Darius is a 48-year-old African-American factory supervisor who is married and has 2 children. He lives in an apartment in New York City with elevator access. Before he experienced a right cerebral vascular accident, Darius was independent in all activities and consistently used schedules to manage his employees and keep track of his children's sports events.

Darius is currently independent with all self-care activities; however, he requires assistance from his wife for IADLs such as managing his finances and keeping track of his appointments. When questioned, Darius did not spontaneously report any difficulties or changes in cognitive status. His goals include returning to work, getting back to regularly practicing sports with his children, and attending their games. Darius is attending outpatient occupational therapy twice weekly.

The **occupational therapist** administered the WCPA (Level 2, Version A) as 1 component of Darius's occupational therapy assessment, which also included examination of other routines and habits, interests, and goals. The OT chose this measure to provide information on Darius's ability to cope with a cognitively challenging everyday

(Continued)

CASE EXAMPLE 8.1. Darius: Adult Neurological Client *(Cont.)*

EXHIBIT 8.4. Darius's WCPA Calendar

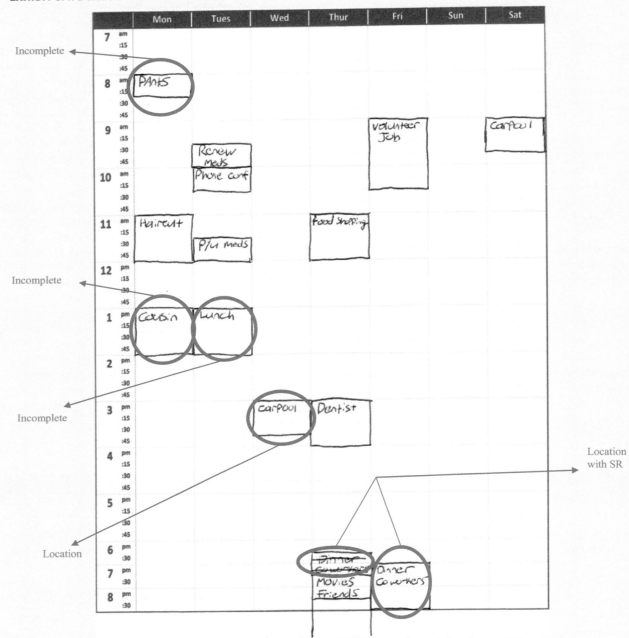

Note. SR = self-recognition of errors.
Source. From *Weekly Calendar Planning Activity (WCPA): A Performance Test of Executive Function*, by J. Toglia, 2015, Bethesda, MD: AOTA Press. Copyright © 2015 by the American Occupational Therapy Association. Used with permission.

(Continued)

CASE EXAMPLE 8.1. Darius: Adult Neurological Client *(Cont.)*

activity, including the ability to plan, recognize potential conflicts, make performance adjustments, simultaneously keep track of information, restrain impulsive responses, self-monitor performance, and use efficient strategies or methods (Toglia, 2015a).

Darius demonstrated difficulty with planning ahead, keeping track of appointments and rules, and managing the information presented during the task. This report presents a summary of results in the areas of performance, strategy use, and awareness. Exhibit 8.4 depicts Darius's completed calendar, with errors highlighted. Exhibit 8.5 depicts the scoring worksheet for Darius's calendar performance.

EXHIBIT 8.5. Darius's Calendar Scoring Worksheet (WCPA Adult/Older Adult Level 2, Version A)

ENTERED	MISSING	ERROR	ACCURATE	SR	APPOINTMENTS
✓			✓		Mon.: Haircut from 11:00 a.m.–12:00 p.m.
✓		I			Mon. or Tues.: Visit with cousin between 1:00 and 2:00 p.m. or 1:30 and 2:30 p.m. or on Thurs. between 2:30 and 3:30 p.m. or 3:00 and 4:00 p.m.
✓			✓		Mon. anytime or Tues. a.m.: Call to renew prescription
✓		I			Tues.: Lunch with friend from 1:00–2:00 p.m.
✓			✓		Tues.: Phone conference before 2:00 p.m. (30 min)
✓			✓		Mon. or Tues.: Medication picked up between 9:00 a.m. and 3:00 p.m. (30 min). Must have previously called to renew prescription.
	✓				Thurs.: Walk neighbor's dog before 11:00 a.m. (30 min)
✓			✓		Thurs.: Dentist at 3:00 p.m. (1 hr)
✓			✓		Thurs.: Movies with friends from 7:00–11:00 p.m.
✓			✓		Fri.: Volunteer job from 9:00–10:30 a.m. (90 min)
✓		L		✓	Thurs. or Fri.: Dinner, coworkers, starting between 6:30 and 8:00 p.m. (2 hr)
✓		I			Mon. or Fri.: Pick up dry cleaning between 8:00 a.m. and 4:00 p.m. (30 min)
	✓				Fri., Sat., or Sun. morning: Exercise at the gym (45 min)
	✓				Doctor: Mon. or Fri. afternoon at 2:00 p.m. (90 min)
✓			✓		Food shopping before Fri. (1 hr)
✓			✓		Carpool: One morning at 9:00 a.m. (45 min)
✓		L			Carpool: One afternoon at 3:00 p.m. (45 min)
14	3	5	9	1	**Total all columns** The number of appointments in the missing + error + accurate columns should equal 17.

Note. I = incomplete error; L = location error; SR = self-recognition of errors.
Source. From *Weekly Calendar Planning Activity (WCPA): A Performance Test of Executive Function*, by J. Toglia, 2015, Bethesda, MD: AOTA Press. Copyright © 2015 by the American Occupational Therapy Association. Used with permission.

(Continued)

CASE EXAMPLE 8.1. Darius: Adult Neurological Client *(Cont.)*

Performance Analysis

The results summarized in Exhibit 8.6 demonstrate a pattern of significantly below-average performance in appointments entered (14 of 17), accuracy (9 of 14), and rules followed (2 of 5). Darius performed below average in strategy usage (3) and used significantly less time to plan (8 seconds) and complete the task (7 minutes) than more than 90% of people in his age group. Darius's efficiency can be considered average. He rushed through the task and used few strategies (3) to help manage the information (checking off appointments, rearranging materials, using a finger).

Darius also demonstrated impulsive and disinhibited tendencies; he missed 3 appointments, entered appointments incompletely, and could not effectively manage conflicting task demands. Darius entered a flexible appointment on Thursday before noticing a fixed appointment that needed to be entered there (demonstrating a lack of preplanning). He crossed out the appointment (a rule break) and moved it to Friday. Darius made 3 incomplete errors by not entering the entire or complete appointment into the calendar (e.g., "cousin" instead of "visit with cousin") as stated in the directions. Darius also made 2 location errors by placing items in the wrong location, day, or time slot (see Exhibits 8.4 and 8.5).

EXHIBIT 8.6. Darius's Visual Performance Profile

PERCENTILE	ENTERED APPT.	ACCURATE APPT.	RULES FOLLOWED	STRATEGIES USED	PLANNING TIME	TOTAL TIME	EFFICIENCY	PERCENTILE
>95								>95
>75					✓ (8 sec)	✓ (7 min)		>75
70								70
60								60
50								50
40								40
30							✓ (87.5)	30
25								25
20								20
10				✓ (3)				10
<5	✓ (14 of 17)	✓ (9 of 14)	✓ (2 of 5)					<5
PERCENTILE	ENTERED APPT.	ACCURATE APPT.	RULES FOLLOWED	STRATEGIES USED	PLANNING TIME	TOTAL TIME	EFFICIENCY	PERCENTILE

Note. Appt. = appointment.
Source. From *Weekly Calendar Planning Activity (WCPA): A Performance Test of Executive Function*, by J. Toglia, 2015, Bethesda, MD: AOTA Press. Copyright © 2015 by the American Occupational Therapy Association. Used with permission.

(Continued)

CASE EXAMPLE 8.1. Darius: Adult Neurological Client *(Cont.)*

Strategy Use

Strategy Frequency

Darius used only 3 strategies throughout the activity, and he used them inconsistently and ineffectively. He switched between 2 strategies, which led to confusion and omissions.

Task Methods and Strategies

Darius consistently checked off appointments; however, he occasionally checked them off before putting them in the calendar, and he switched between checking off and crossing out appointments. This led to confusion: Darius thought he had entered 3 appointments that he did not enter. He also rearranged the materials, covering up the instruction sheet without realizing. Darius approached the task by going 1 by 1 down the appointment list. This is an inefficient task method and ultimately led to conflicts and rule breaks.

Strategy Generation

In the after-task interview, Darius did not list any additional strategies and was unable to identify anything he would do differently if he were to complete the task again.

Self-Monitoring and Awareness

During the Task

During the activity, Darius spontaneously identified 1 conflict. He crossed out the appointment (rule break) and rescheduled it, which indicates awareness of the rule break and self-recognition of 1 error. Darius did not seem to recognize any other errors.

After-Task Self-Perceptions

Darius stated that the task was not challenging for him and reported that he would not do anything differently if he were to perform it again. He rated himself positively and stated that the task was easy for him. Darius also underestimated the time he used, and he overstated his accuracy by 7 appointments.

Performance Summary and Treatment Recommendations

In summary, Darius demonstrated difficulty in managing information and efficiently navigating this multistep activity. His performance was characterized by a tendency to miss needed information. The majority of errors included appointments that were either missed entirely or incomplete.

Failure to plan ahead and a tendency to rush through the task in a haphazard manner contributed to Darius's difficulties. He initiated and used strategies, but his inability to pace performance or self-monitor compromised his effective use of strategies. Darius demonstrated limitations in awareness, in that he did not consistently self-recognize errors or acknowledge challenges during or after the task, and he overestimated performance.

(Continued)

CASE EXAMPLE 8.1. Darius: Adult Neurological Client *(Cont.)*

Occupational therapy treatment that is directed at helping to optimize Darius's use of strategies is recommended. As a first step, this involves helping Darius recognize and monitor performance challenges. The OT can use guided questions and structured methods of self-evaluation to help Darius discover performance errors himself in the context of functional–cognitive activities. As his awareness improves, treatment can focus on increasing the effectiveness and efficiency of his strategy use across different activities, as is described in Chapter 20 on the Multicontext Approach. See Exhibit 8.7 for a short sample documentation and summary of Darius's performance.

EXHIBIT 8.7. Short Sample Documentation of Darius's WCPA Performance

Darius completed the WCPA, a performance-based test of EF, and demonstrated difficulty with planning ahead, keeping track of appointments and rules, and managing the information presented during the task. Darius
- Planned for 8 seconds before beginning the task,
- Took 7 minutes to complete the test,
- Entered 14/17 appointments (with 9/14 accurate),
- Followed 2/5 rules, and
- Made inconsistent use of 3 strategies: checking off appointments entered, rearranging materials, and using a finger.

Darius made 5 errors of varying types; he completed the task quickly but had low accuracy because he rushed through the task. Darius completed the assessment with an efficiency score in the 30th percentile (average). He showed poor awareness of his deficits during and after the task, overestimating his performance and stating that the task was not challenging. Darius initiated and used strategies; however, strategy use was often ineffective. His performance on the WCPA indicates that Darius is likely to encounter significant difficulty in performing requirements of his job (managing schedules) as well as other cognitively challenging IADLs, such as grocery shopping from a list, following a recipe, or following directions to place pills in an organizer.

Conclusion

The WCPA is a valuable performance-based measure of functional cognition (Toglia, 2015a). It is portable, it is applicable to many clients of different ages and different diagnoses, and it can be administered quickly in a variety of settings. The occupational therapist can glean valuable information regarding the client's cognitive strategy use, errors, planning, and problem solving to aid in treatment planning and improve IADL participation.

In addition, the after-task interview provides valuable insight into a client's level of self-awareness. Determining performance patterns on the WCPA allows the occupational therapist to determine how deficits of functional cognition affect participation to improve occupational performance and support a return to productive roles.

References

Adamit, T., Maeir, A., Ben Assayag, E., Bornstein, N. M., Korczyn, A. D., & Katz, N. (2015). Impact of first-ever mild stroke on participation at 3 and 6 month post-event: The TABASCO study. *Disability and Rehabilitation, 37,* 667–673. https://doi.org/10.3109/09638288.2014.923523

Amer, N., Marom, B., & Kizony, R. (2016, July). *Construct validity of the Weekly Calendar Planning Activity in Arabic speaking people with stroke.* Poster presentation at the 13th conference of the Neuropsychological Rehabilitation Special Interest Group of the World Federation for Neurorehabilitation, Glasgow, Scotland.

American Occupational Therapy Association. (2014). Occupational therapy practice framework: Domain and process (3rd ed.). *American Journal of Occupational Therapy, 68*(Suppl. 1), S1–S48. https://doi.org/10.5014/ajot.2014.682006

Baum, C. M., Connor, L. T., Morrison, T., Hahn, M., Dromerick, A. W., & Edwards, D. F. (2008). Reliability, validity, and clinical utility of the Executive Function Performance Test: A measure of executive function in a sample of people with stroke. *American Journal of Occupational Therapy, 62,* 446–455. https://doi.org/10.5014/ajot.62.4.446

Bottari, C., & Dawson, D. R. (2011). Executive functions and real-world performance: How good are we at distinguishing people with acquired brain injury from healthy controls? *OTJR: Occupation, Participation and Health, 31*(Suppl.), S61–S68. https://doi.org/10.3928/15394492-20101108-10

Burgess, P. W., Alderman, N., Forbes, C., Costello, A., Coates, L. M., Dawson, D. R., . . . Channon, S. (2006). The case for the development and use of "ecologically valid" measures of executive function in experimental and clinical neuropsychology. *Journal of the International Neuropsychological Society, 12,* 194–209. https://doi.org/10.1017/S1355617706060310

Clark-Wilson, J., Giles, G. M., & Baxter, D. M. (2014). Revisiting the Neurofunctional Approach: Conceptualizing the core components for the rehabilitation of everyday living skills. *Brain Injury, 28,* 1646–1656. https://doi.org/10.3109/02699052.2014.946449

Doherty, M., Dodd, J., & Berg, C. (2017). Validation of the Weekly Calendar Planning Activity with teenagers with acquired brain injury. *Archives of Physical Medicine and Rehabilitation, 98,* e130. https://doi.org/10.1016/j.apmr.2017.08.423

Giles, G. M. (2018). Neurofunctional Approach to rehabilitation after brain injury. In N. Katz & J. Toglia (Eds.), *Cognition, occupation, and participation across the lifespan: Neuroscience, neurorehabilitation, and models of intervention in occupational therapy* (4th ed., pp. 419–442). Bethesda, MD: AOTA Press.

Goverover, Y., Toglia, J., & DeLuca, J. (2019). The Weekly Calendar Planning Activity in multiple sclerosis: A top-down assessment of executive functions. *Neuropsychological Rehabilitation.* Online publication. https://doi.org/10.1080/09602011.2019.1584573

Grinblatt, N., Offek, H., Gebert, M., Kizony, R., & Tau-Cohen, S. (2012). Establishing the reliability and validity of the Weekly Calendar Planning Assessment in a healthy population in Israel. *Israeli Journal of Occupational Therapy, 21,* H67–H87.

Haskins, E. C., Cicerone, K. D., & Trexler, L. E. (2012). *Cognitive rehabilitation manual: Translating evidence-based recommendations into practice.* Reston, VA: ACRM Publishing.

Kizony, R., Marom, B., & Osman, S. (2018, October). *Executive functions of people with stroke: Validity of an ecologically valid assessment.* Poster presentation at the 11th World Stroke Congress, Montreal.

Lahav, O., Ben-Simon, A., Inbar-Weiss, N., & Katz, N. (2018). Weekly Calendar Planning Activity for university students: Comparison of individuals with and without ADHD by gender. *Journal of Attention Disorders, 22,* 368–378. https://doi.org/10.1177/1087054714564621

Miyake, A., & Friedman, N. P. (2012). The nature and organization of individual differences in executive functions: Four general conclusions. *Current Directions in Psychological Science, 21,* 8–14. https://doi.org/10.1177/0963721411429458

Nasreddine, Z. S., Phillips, N. A., Bédirian, V., Charbonneau, S., Whitehead, V., Collin, I., . . . Chertkow, H. (2005). The Montreal Cognitive Assessment, MoCA: A brief screening tool for mild cognitive impairment. *Journal of the American Geriatrics Society, 53,* 695–699. https://doi.org/10.1111/j.1532-5415.2005.53221.x

Norman, D. A., & Shallice, T. (1986). Attention to action: Willed and automatic control of behavior. In R. J. Davidson, G. E. Schwartz, & D. Shapiro (Eds.), *Consciousness and self-regulation: Advances in research and theory* (pp. 1–18). New York: Plenum. https://doi.org/10.1007/978-1-4757-0629-1_1

Skidmore, E., McEwen, S., Green, D., Van den Houten, J., Dawson, D., & Polatajko, H. (2017). Essential elements and key features. In D. R. Dawson, S. E. McEwen, & H. Polatajko (Eds.), *Cognitive Orientation to daily Occupational Performance in occupational therapy: Using the CO–OP Approach™ to enable participation across the lifespan* (pp. 11–20). Bethesda, MD: AOTA Press.

Stephens, J. A., & Berryhill, M. E. (2016). Older adults improve on everyday tasks after working memory training and neurostimulation. *Brain Stimulation, 9,* 553–559. https://doi.org/10.1016/j.brs.2016.04.001

Toglia, J. (2015a). *Weekly Calendar Planning Activity (WCPA): A performance test of executive function.* Bethesda, MD: AOTA Press.

Toglia, J. (2015b). *Weekly Calendar Planning Activity (WCPA): Assessment van het executief functioneren*—Nederlandse versie [Weekly Calendar Planning Activity (WCPA: Assessment of executive function—Netherlands version] (E. T. Van Schouwen, Trans.). Enkhuizen, The Netherlands: Hersenwerk.

Toglia, J. (2017). *Veckoplanering i kalender. Aktivitetsbaserat test av exekutiva funktioner (WCPA–SE)* [Weekly Calendar Planning Activity: Activity-based test of executive functions (WCPA–SE)]. Nacka: Swedish Association of Occupational Therapists.

Toglia, J. (2018). The Dynamic Interactional Model and the Multicontext Approach. In N. Katz & J. Toglia (Eds.), *Cognition, occupation, and participation across the lifespan: Neuroscience, neurorehabilitation,*

and models of intervention in occupational therapy (4th ed., pp. 355–385). Bethesda, MD: AOTA Press.

Toglia, J., Askin, G., Gerber, L. M., Taub, M. C., Mastrogiovanni, A. R., & O'Dell, M. W. (2017). Association between 2 measures of cognitive instrumental activities of daily living and their relation to the Montreal Cognitive Assessment in persons with stroke. *Archives of Physical Medicine and Rehabilitation, 98,* 2280–2287. https://doi.org/10.1016/j.apmr.2017.04.007

Toglia, J., & Berg, C. (2013). Performance-based measure of executive function: Comparison of community and at-risk youth. *American Journal of Occupational Therapy, 67,* 515–523. https://doi.org/10.5014/ajot.2013.008482

Toglia, J., & Katz, N. (2018). Executive function: Prevention and health promotion for at-risk populations and those with chronic disease. In N. Katz & J. Toglia (Eds.), *Cognition, occupation, and participation across the lifespan: Neuroscience, neurorehabilitation, and models of intervention in occupational therapy* (4th ed., pp. 129–141). Bethesda, MD: AOTA Press.

Toglia, J., Lahav, O., Ari, E. B., & Kizony, R. (2017). Adult age and cultural differences in performance on the Weekly Calendar Planning Activity (WCPA). *American Journal of Occupational Therapy, 71,* 7105270010. https://doi.org/10.5014/ajot.2016.020073

Toglia, J., & Lussier, A. (2017, November 29). *Weekly Calendar Planning Activity Part I: Introduction and overview* [video file]. Retrieved from https://youtu.be/rJ4Czn17y0M

Toglia, J. P., Rodger, S. A., & Polatajko, H. J. (2012). Anatomy of cognitive strategies: A therapist's primer for enabling occupational performance. *Canadian Journal of Occupational Therapy, 79,* 225–236. https://doi.org/10.2182/cjot.2012.79.4.4

Toglia, J., Steinberg, C., & Mastrogiovanni, A. (2018, April). *The Weekly Calendar Planning Activity (WCPA): Analysis of performance in persons with acquired brain injury.* Short Course 360 presented at the AOTA Annual Conference & Expo, Salt Lake City.

Toglia, J., & White, S. (2019). Weekly Calendar Planning Activity. In B. J. Hemphill-Pearson & C. K. Urish (Eds.), *Assessments in occupational therapy mental health: An integrative approach* (3rd ed., pp. 219–238). Thorofare, NJ: Slack.

Weiner, N. W., Toglia, J., & Berg, C. (2012). Weekly Calendar Planning Activity (WCPA): A performance-based assessment of executive function piloted with at-risk adolescents. *American Journal of Occupational Therapy, 66,* 699–708. https://doi.org/10.5014/ajot.2012.004754

Wood, W., & Rünger, D. (2016). Psychology of habit. *Annual Review of Psychology, 67,* 289–314. https://doi.org/10.1146/annurev-psych-122414-033417

Zelazo, P. D., Blair, C. B., & Willoughby, M. T. (2016). *Executive function: Implications for education* (NCER 2017-2000). Washington, DC: National Center for Education Research.

Zlotnik, S., Schiff, A., Ravid, S., Shahar, E., & Toglia, J. (2018). A new approach for assessing executive functions in everyday life, among adolescents with genetic generalised epilepsies. *Neuropsychological Rehabilitation.* https://doi.org/10.1080/09602011.2018.1468272

Zlotnik, S., & Toglia, J. (2018). Measuring adolescent self-awareness and accuracy using a performance-based assessment and parental report. *Frontiers in Public Health, 6,* 15. https://doi.org/10.3389/fpubh.2018.00015

9

The Multiple Errands Test–Revised

DOROTHY FARRAR EDWARDS, PhD, AND
M. TRACY MORRISON, OTD, OTR/L

LEARNING OBJECTIVES

After completing this chapter, readers should be able to

- Understand the goal of assessing functional cognition in dynamic real-world settings,
- Describe how the key elements of the Multiple Errands Test–Revised (MET–R) assess aspects of functional cognition,
- Describe the development of the MET as a performance-based test of functional cognition, and
- Describe how to use the results from the MET to inform treatment goals and select therapeutic interventions.

KEY TERMS AND CONCEPTS

- Multiple Errands Test • Multiple Errands Test–Revised • Performance efficiency

Introduction

As noted in Chapter 1, "Understanding Functional Cognition," functional cognition is a global, "top-down" construct that incorporates executive function (EF) and other cognitive domains as well as performance skills, habits, and routines. Thus, EF skills are a critical component of functional cognition. The term *executive function* describes the effortful thinking necessary to perform complex activities, often of competing priority, in changing environments.

EFs enable humans to effectively and efficiently perform multiple activities across time and multiple contexts. These higher order mental processes are conceptualized as working memory, mental flexibility, and self-control abilities. EFs enable people to conduct their daily life by enacting goal-directed actions that reflect their personal preferences (Diamond, 2013).

From an occupational therapy perspective, functional cognition skills are best measured through performance-based evaluations and during the performance of complex daily activities. Individuals with strong EF skills demonstrate effi-

cient and effective occupational performance across varied activities, contexts, and task demands. Individuals with weak EF skills experience decreased occupational performance and quality of life.

However, the measurement of EFs has been particularly challenging for researchers and clinicians alike, because the behaviors associated with EFs are not readily observable during the predictable experiences found in clinical contexts (Morrison et al., 2013). Standardized neuropsychological tests, such as the Wisconsin Card Sorting Test (Berg, 1948), the Stroop Color and Word Test (Stroop, 1935), or self-rating scales (e.g., Behavior Rating Inventory of Executive Function; Gioia et al., 2000a, 2000b), provide information about executive abilities. However, these measures were not developed to predict how well an individual is able to manage the complexities of everyday life, and therefore they should be complemented with performance-based assessments that provide real-time information about the client's EF abilities (Roth et al., 2013).

Performance-based tests of EFs require that the test administrator observe and assess the test taker's performance in the completion of typically novel and complex multicomponent, multistep activities. Performance-based tests are intentionally designed to be less structured to create open-ended test scenarios that elicit the test taker's effortful and creative thinking skills. To successfully complete the tasks, the test taker must problem solve, plan, initiate, monitor, and flexibly adjust how they perform the tasks. Performance-based tests present challenges to the client through a dynamic interaction among complex task parameters, human EF, ability and motivation, and multiple environmental factors.

This chapter examines the Multiple Errands Test–Revised (Morrison et al., 2013), which is based on the **Multiple Errands Test** (MET), developed by Shallice and Burgess (1991). The MET is a performance-based assessment of EF conducted in dynamic, naturalistic social environments. It is designed to identify deficits not captured by standard neuropsychological measures and less demanding performance-based assessments of functional cognition.

Development

Shallice and Burgess (1991) developed the MET to assess action-dependent EF among 3 community-dwelling individuals with frontal lobe impairments. The MET was designed for use with individuals who test as average to above average on IQ and basic cognitive tests. The measure captures behavioral inefficiencies and difficulty completing complex tasks in dynamic natural settings.

According to Shallice and Burgess (1991), the MET is a scientific observational tool that illuminates the real-life functional deficits of individuals with frontal lobe damage. With the development of the MET, Shallice and Burgess launched a new area of research exploring the value of performance-based testing of EF. The MET captures EF deficits on complex, novel shopping and information-retrieval tasks under time pressure and with rule constraints (Burgess, 2000; Manchester et al., 2004; Shallice & Burgess, 1991).

The developers of the MET published simplified versions of the test (Alderman et al., 2003; Knight et al., 2002). However, the complex scoring systems used in both the original and the simplified versions limited the clinical utility of the assessment. The MET scoring system had low interrater reliability and did not produce a set of quantitative scores that could be easily used in research settings (Knight et al., 2002).

In response to this problem, Dawson and her colleagues (2009) incorporated all of the elements of the simplified version of the MET into the Baycrest version of the MET (B–MET) and added a standardized scoring procedure to the test. The B–MET has well-established reliability, validity, and clinical utility (Clark et al., 2012, 2017).

Morrison and her colleagues (2013) also addressed problems with the scoring of the MET in the creation of the **Multiple Errands Test–Revised** (MET-R). The MET-R, which is the focus of this chapter, provides a series of quantitative scores based on an objective scoring rubric. The MET–R also introduced an assessment of performance efficiency, which has been shown to be sensitive in distinguishing individuals with mild cognitive impairment (MCI) from healthy controls. Since the publication of the B–MET and the MET–R, many additional versions of the original MET have been described (Burns & Neville, 2016; Burns et al., 2018; Cipresso et al., 2014; Steverson et al., 2017; Valls-Serrano et al., 2018). Table 9.1 presents the historical development of the MET.

Reliability and Validity

The MET–R is a naturalistic functional–cognitive assessment developed as an occupational therapy interpretation of the MET for use in clinical practice. This test was validated on the campus of a public hospital. The MET–R is standardized, with quantitative scores that inform occupational therapy treatment planning (Morrison et al., 2013).

Interrater reliability of the MET–R was established with both observed and video-recorded test performances. Two independent raters (1 administering the test and another observing performance on the test) tested and observed 10 test takers

TABLE 9.1. Evolution of the Design and Scoring of the Multiple Errands Test

MET VERSION	TEST DESIGN
MET (Shallice & Burgess, 1991)	To identify behaviors and everyday life deficits associated with frontal lobe impairments
MET–Hospital Version (Knight et al., 2002)	To apply the MET to people who cannot be assessed in a public setting because of mobility limitations, behavioral problems, or mental health
MET–Simplified Version (Alderman et al., 2003)	To use with a range of people with neurological deficits who are routinely encountered in clinical settings
Baycrest MET (Dawson et al., 2009)	Hospital version based on the MET–Simplified; includes standardized scoring
MET–Revised (Morrison et al., 2013)	Hospital version based on the MET–Simplified; includes further standardized scoring and instructions as well as the performance efficiency score
Virtual MET (Cipresso et al., 2014)	To use with test takers who might be unable to walk around easily, to reduce test time, and to improve clinical utility

completing the MET–R. The researchers compared the raters' scores for all of the scored MET–R sections (i.e., tasks completed, total rule breaks, total locations, number of passes, and total time expended) using an intraclass correlation analysis. The intraclass correlation coefficients were 1 for all scored sections of the test for both direct observation and video-recorded comparisons.

The researchers explored the discriminant validity of MET–R by comparing the MET–R performance of 21 age-, education-, and gender-matched control participants with the performance of 25 individuals with mild stroke. Although the control group performed better than the participants with mild stroke on all test components, the test was sufficiently demanding that the control participants successfully completed an average of 15 of the 17 tasks, and some broke rules during testing. The performance scores of the participants with mild stroke were significantly lower than the scores for the control participants for the MET–R components, including

- Total tasks completed ($p < .001$),

- Rule breaks ($p < .001$), and

- Performance efficiency ($p < .002$).

The researchers established concurrent validity by comparing the MET–R task completion score with the total score on the Executive Function Performance Test (EFPT; Baum et al., 2008), an established performance-based assessment of EF (see Chapter 7). The correlation was .55. This moderate correlation was expected, given the differences in test administrator support, task demands, and level of structure in the testing environment.

Target Population

The MET–R was validated with a sample of individuals with mild stroke. Clinicians have used the MET–R to assess adults with MCI associated with a variety of neurocognitive conditions. Often these individuals perform well within the normal range on cognitive screening measures, such as the Montreal Cognitive Assessment (Nasreddine et al., 2005), the Mini-Mental State Examination (Folstein et al., 1975), the Brief Interview for Mental Status (Saliba et al., 2012), or the St. Louis University Mental Status Scale (Tariq et al., 2006). Individuals with MCI often perform well on more comprehensive neuropsychological measures of learning and memory.

A hierarchical approach to functional–cognitive assessment suggests that the MET–R is appropriate for use with individuals who are fully independent in ADLs but who are experiencing difficulty in performance of complex IADLs. A performance-based assessment protocol for people with mild to moderate impairment might include, in hierarchical order,

- An ADL measure (e.g., FIM®; Granger et al., 1993),

- An IADL measure (e.g., the EFPT), and

- A measure of higher order EF (e.g., the MET–R).

Patients who have ADL deficits will most likely be referred for rehabilitative services, during the course of which they likely will be assessed for cognitive function and EFs. ADL measures such as the FIM, however, may not be sensitive to subtle EF impairments. Therefore, further assessment is needed to predict the potential for functional–cognitive independence in community settings.

Administration

The MET–R was described by Morrison et al. (2013), and a MET–R manual describing test administration and scoring is presented in Video 9.1. The MET–R manual also provides the information needed for occupational therapists who wish to implement MET–R testing in their practice. Before administering the MET–R, the test administrator instructs the test taker to read the test instructions and rules. After this step, the test administrator tells test takers to take as much time as needed to review the instructions and to begin the test when they are ready. The test instructions are presented in Exhibit 9.1.

On initiating the test, test takers must carry out several unstructured tasks in novel and potentially highly stimulating environments. The tasks are simple everyday tasks, and the order in which they are executed is determined by the test taker. The unstructured format is an important difference between the MET–R and typical neuropsychological and tabletop tests.

The order in which test takers perform test components determines their performance efficiency, because the tasks must be grouped by location and meet the requirements stipulated in the test rules. Test takers who apply the strategy of sequentially executing the tasks often realize midway through the MET–R that they must change their strategy to complete the remaining tasks without accruing additional rule breaks. Test takers must also remember to complete a prospective task several minutes after beginning the test.

By design, the MET–R creates a high level of challenge, because it is conducted in a dynamic environment that requires walking and communicating with strangers. Additionally, the test takers must execute multiple tasks, manage money, calculate, and prospectively remember to complete all test items. Exhibit 9.2 presents the required tasks and their locations. The test taker is given a map to guide their performance (see Exhibit 9.3), and the administrator is given a map to record it (see Exhibit 9.4).

Scoring

The scoring system developed for the MET–R transitions from the interpretive methods used in the original version of the MET to a pragmatic and structured scoring system designed to improve the test's reliability and clinical utility (Morrison et al., 2013). Rather than interpret the quality of the test taker's behaviors, the test administrator gathers quantitative data that can be used to generate a series of quantitative scores, including the performance efficiency value. The scoring system uses scoring

EXHIBIT 9.1. MET–R: Task List

In this exercise you should complete the following in any order:
You should:
- **Collect something for the examiner from the Information Desk and do what is necessary.**
- **Buy 4 pieces of candy (This is 1 item).**
- **Buy a get well card.**
- **Buy a Coca-Cola.**
- **Telephone Bonnie Logsdon at 286-1619 and say where you are, who you are, and what time it is.**
- **Leave something to be mailed to Dr. Alex Dromerick with your examiner.**
- **You should also obtain the following information:**
- **What is the closing time of the uniform shop on a Thursday?** _____
- **What is the opening time of the gift shop on a Friday?**_____
- **What is the price of a bag of Pringles chips?**_____
- **Where is the chapel located?**_____

You should meet me at the fountain 10 minutes after you have started the task and tell me the time
You should tell me when you have completed the exercise.

While carrying out this exercise you must obey the following rules:
1. You must carry out all these tasks but may do so in any order.
2. You should spend no more than $4.50.
3. You should stay within the limits of the main floor of the hospital (i.e., the 1ˢᵗ floor).
4. You should not enter any of the hospital treatment areas or "staff only" areas.
5. You should buy no more than 2 items in the gift shop.
6. Take as little time to complete this exercise without rushing excessively.
7. You should not go back into an area you have already been in (e.g., the gift shop).
8. Do not speak to us unless this is part of the exercise.

Your examiner is: Dr. Tracy Morrison

Dr. Alex Dromerick
Dept. of Neurology
St. Louis, Mo. 63112

Source. Based on "Multiple Errands Test–Revised (MET–R): A Performance-Based Measure of Executive Function in People With Mild Cerebrovascular Accident," by M. T. Morrison et al., 2013, *American Journal of Occupational Therapy, 67,* pp. 460–468. Copyright © 2013 by the American Occupational Therapy Association. Used with permission.

EXHIBIT 9.2. MET–R: Tasks Shown by Location

INFORMATION DESK	GIFT SHOP	HALLWAY	VENDING AREA	PAY PHONE BOOTH
• Collect something for the examiner from the Information Desk • . . . and do what is necessary. • What is the closing time of the uniform shop on a Thursday? • Where is the chapel located?	• Buy 4 pieces of candy (this is 1 item). • What is the opening time of the gift shop on a Friday? • What is the price of a bag of Pringles chips? • Buy a get well card.	• You should tell me when you have completed the exercise. • You should meet me at the fountain 10 minutes after you have started the task • . . . and tell me the time. • Leave something to be mailed to Dr. Alex Dromerick with your examiner.	• Buy a Coca-Cola.	• Telephone Bonnie Logsdon at 286-1619 • . . . and say where you are, • . . . who you are, • . . . and what time it is.

Source. Based on "Multiple Errands Test–Revised (MET–R): A Performance-Based Measure of Executive Function in People With Mild Cerebrovascular Accident," by M. T. Morrison et al., 2013, *American Journal of Occupational Therapy, 67,* pp. 460–468. Copyright © 2013 by the American Occupational Therapy Association. Used with permission.

EXHIBIT 9.3. MET–R: Test Taker's Map

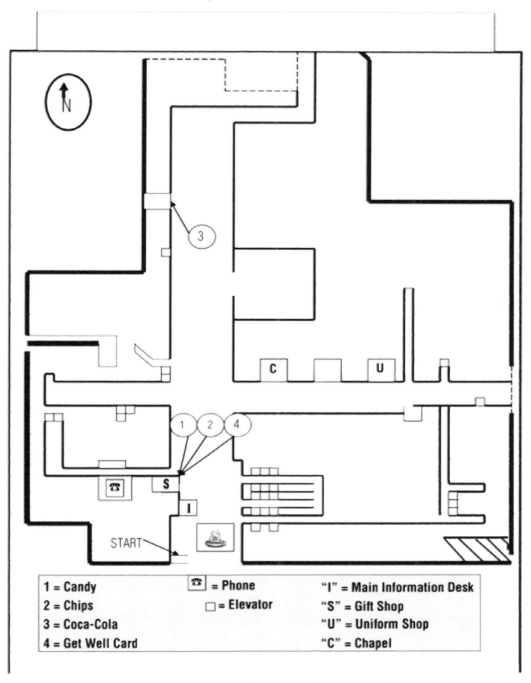

1 = Candy   ☎ = Phone   "I" = Main Information Desk
2 = Chips   ☐ = Elevator   "S" = Gift Shop
3 = Coca-Cola   "U" = Uniform Shop
4 = Get Well Card   "C" = Chapel

EXHIBIT 9.4. MET–R: Administrator's Observation of Performance Map

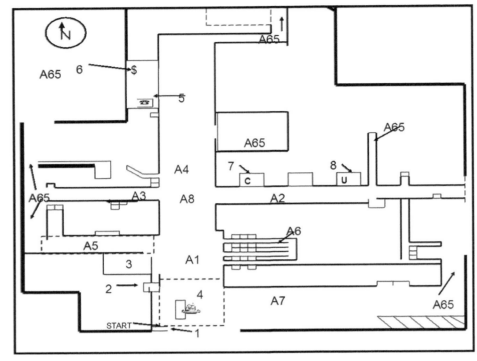

Source. Based on "Multiple Errands Test–Revised (MET–R): A Performance-Based Measure of Executive Function in People With Mild Cerebrovascular Accident," by M. T. Morrison et al., 2013, *American Journal of Occupational Therapy, 67*, pp. 460–468. Copyright © 2013 by the American Occupational Therapy Association. Used with permission.

methods commonly used in the cognitive neurosciences to objectify qualitative data for spatial learning and memory tasks that require environmental navigation (O'Keefe & Nadel, 1979).

During the test performance, the test administrator follows the participant and uses an observational rating form (see Exhibit 9.4) and a scoring form (see Exhibit 9.5). The MET–R includes the following scores:

- Total time to complete
- Total number of locations visited
- Total number of tasks completed
- Total number of passes
- Total number of rule breaks.

Table 9.2 presents the definitions of each of these scoring items.

Test scores can be further converted into a ratio to result in a performance efficiency score. The performance efficiency score assumes a normal distribution of 0 to 1, with a perfect score of 1.0. Performance efficiency is calculated through the following formula:

1. The first step is to calculate the optimal or ideal score, which is based on completing all tasks and visiting the least number of locations during the test. This value is called ***performance***

efficiency and is calculated with the following formula: performance efficiency = (total number of tasks; least number of locations) = ideal value as denominator.

2. The 2nd step involves including the ideal value as the denominator in the equation (actual number of tasks completed) / (actual number of locations) / ideal value as denominator.

Documentation

The scoring forms also record the test taker's demographic information, mood, and pretest assessment of the skills needed to complete the MET–R. As noted, a sample scored MET–R form is presented in Exhibit 9.5.

Interpretation and Intervention Considerations

The different MET–R component scores provide a comprehensive evaluation of the capacity of the individual to perform complex tasks under cognitive load. Each of the MET–R scores (rule breaks, number of locations visited, total number of passes, number of tasks completed, and time to complete the test) provides the occupational therapist with information

EXHIBIT 9.5. MET–R: Administrator's Scoring Sheet

Date:_July 29, 2004 Examiner: Tracy Client ID: JDR75	Start Time: 2:00pm Meet Time: 2:15pm End Time: 2:30pm Total Time: 30 minutes	All Tasks Completed_____ Partial Task Completion___X____ No Task Completion_____	Spoke to Examiner (frequency:) I I I I $ Spent____$5.25_____

Areas Visited & Tasks Attempted (refer to Map locations) (e.g., 1: bought a coca-cola)		**Tasks Completed:**	**Pass #**	**MAP**
	Revisit	___ Collect something for examiner _____		View: II
1 - coke		___ Collect - do necessary _____		
2- bonnie where				
- bonnie who		_X__ Buy 4 pieces of candy	3	Mark: III
A1 - none		___ Buy card _____		
3 - closing time uniform, opening time gift		_X_ Buy a Coca-Cola	1	
1- Pringles	R	_X__ Price of Pringles	2	Total Use:___5
3- none	R			
4 - meet examiner		_X__ Telephone Bonnie	1	**Task List/Rules**
3 - candy	R	_X__ Bonnie: where	1	
		_X__ Bonnie: who	1	View: I
		___ Bonnie: time _____		
				Mark: III
		___ Address card WITH stamp _____		
		___ Leave something mailed to _____ Alex		
		_X__ Closing time - uniform	1	Total Use:___4___
		_X__ Opening time - gift shop	1	
		___ Location of chapel _____		**Bag of Task Items**
				View:

Source. Based on "Multiple Errands Test–Revised (MET–R): A Performance-Based Measure of Executive Function in People With Mild Cerebrovascular Accident," by M. T. Morrison et al., 2013, *American Journal of Occupational Therapy, 67*, pp. 460–468. Copyright © 2013 by the American Occupational Therapy Association. Used with permission.

TABLE 9.2. MET–R: Scoring Items and Definitions

SCORING ITEM	DEFINITION
Total time to complete	Total time elapsed from start to when the test taker tells the test administrator they are finished
Total number of locations visited	Total number of locations visited, regardless of whether the locations are related to a task
Total number of tasks completed	Number of tasks assigned that were finished
Total number of passes	Number of times the test taker visited any location relevant to the test tasks
Total number of rule breaks	Number of instructions violated

Source. Adapted from "Multiple Errands Test–Revised (MET–R): A Performance-Based Measure of Executive Function in People With Mild Cerebrovascular Accident," by M. T. Morrison et al., 2013, *American Journal of Occupational Therapy, 67*, p. 464. Copyright © 2013 by the American Occupational Therapy Association. Used with permission.

about the capacity of the individual to safely perform complex instrumental activities without cognitive support. A perfect performance on the MET–R results in a score of 1, whereas imperfect values approach a score of 0.

The performance efficiency score is particularly valuable for the assessment of individuals with subtle but significant deficits in EF ability. Performance efficiency is a quantitative ratio reflecting the number of tasks completed and the number of locations visited. For the study of individuals after mild stroke (Morrison et al., 2013), a perfectly efficient performance reflects the completion of 17 tasks in 5 locations

(17/5 = 3.4). The perfect ratio value of 3.4 may change depending on the specific location and the number of tasks included in the test.

In this example, this value was determined through analysis of all of the test tasks (17) and the least number of locations (5) required to complete the test (see Table 9.2). The perfect value becomes the denominator to determine the participant's performance efficiency score. If the participant executes all 17 tasks in 5 locations, then the value equates to a score of 1, but if the participant executes only some of the 17 tasks in more than 5 locations, then the value approaches a score of 0.

Most often, the test administrator must score for less than perfect performance. For example, for a test taker who visits 6 locations to complete 12 tasks, the performance efficiency score is .59. This value is the result of dividing the number of tasks completed by the number of locations visited (12/6), then by the perfect value of 3.4—in this case, (12/6)/3.4 = .59. The practitioner may consider the performance efficiency value in combination with the frequency of rule breaks (high or low) and the total time to complete the test (long or short) in determining the adequacy of an individual test taker's performance.

Individuals in community-based settings who have inadequate executive abilities are more likely to experience functional-cognitive problems, including falls, motor vehicle accidents, medication errors, and financial mistakes (Morrison et al., 2013). Clinical interviews of individuals who have performed poorly on the MET–R indicate that poor performance was associated with increased frequency of occupational performance problems when compared with the individuals' premorbid functioning (Morrison et al., 2013). Additionally, these individuals report significant changes in their occupational performance patterns, including at-harm behaviors, such as poor time management, reclusive and socially avoidant behaviors, falls in the home, motor vehicle accidents, excessive rushing through tasks, and increased errors in meaningful activities (e.g., IADLs).

Individuals with executive impairment often maintain an awareness about their functional changes and often experience significant decreases in mood and increased anxiety. Occupational therapists are the most appropriate resource for these individuals because of their in-depth knowledge regarding task analysis and occupational performance. People with executive impairments benefit from educational, remedial, and compensatory treatment approaches.

References

Alderman, N., Burgess, P. W., Knight, C., & Henman, C. (2003). Ecological validity of a simplified version of the Multiple Errands Shopping Test. *Journal of the International Neuropsychological Society, 9*(1), 31–44. https://doi.org/10.1017/S1355617703910046

Baum, C. M., Connor, L. T., Morrison, T., Hahn, M., Dromerick, A. W., & Edwards, D. F. (2008). Reliability, validity, and clinical utility of the Executive Function Performance Test: A measure of executive function in a sample of people with stroke. *American Journal of Occupational Therapy, 62,* 446–455. https://doi.org/10.5014/ajot.62.4.446

Berg, E. A. (1948). A simple objective technique for measuring flexibility in thinking. *Journal of General Psychology, 39,* 15–22. https://doi.org/10.1080/00221309.1948.9918159

Burgess, P. W. (2000). Strategy application disorder: The role of the frontal lobes in human multitasking. *Psychological Research, 63,* 279–288. https://doi.org/10.1007/s004269900006

Burns, S. C., & Neville, M. (2016). Cognitive assessment trends in home health care for adults with mild stroke. *American Journal of Occupational Therapy, 70,* 7002290020. https://doi.org/10.5014/ajot.2016.016543

Burns, S. P., Pickens, N. D., Dawson, D. R., Perea, J. D., Vas, A. K., Marquez de la Plata, C., & Neville, M. (2018). In-home contextual reality: A qualitative analysis using the Multiple Errands Test Home Version (MET–Home). *Neuropsychological Rehabilitation.* https://doi.org/10.1080/09602011.2018.1431134

Cipresso, P., Albani, G., Serino, S., Pedroli, E., Pallavicini, F., Mauro, A., & Riva, G. (2014). Virtual Multiple Errands Test (VMET): A virtual reality–based tool to detect early executive functions deficit in Parkinson's disease. *Frontiers in Behavioral Neuroscience, 8,* 405. https://doi.org/10.3389/fnbeh.2014.00405

Clark, A., Anderson, N. D., Arshad, S., & Dawson, D. R. (2012). Improving the discriminability of the Baycrest Multiple Errands Test. *Stroke, 43,* E120.

Clark, A. J., Anderson, N. D., Nalder, E., Arshad, S., & Dawson, D. R. (2017). Reliability and construct validity of a revised Baycrest Multiple Errands Test. *Neuropsychological Rehabilitation, 27,* 667–684. https://doi.org/10.1080/09602011.2015.1117981

Dawson, D. R., Anderson, N. D., Burgess, P., Cooper, E., Krpan, K. M., & Stuss, D. T. (2009). Further development of the Multiple Errands Test: Standardized scoring, reliability, and ecological validity for the Baycrest version. *Archives of Physical Medicine and Rehabilitation, 90*(Suppl.), S41–S51. https://doi.org/10.1016/j.apmr.2009.07.012

Diamond, A. (2013). Executive functions. *Annual Review of Psychology, 64,* 135–168. https://doi.org/10.1146/annurev-psych-113011-143750

Folstein, M. F., Folstein, S. E., & McHugh, P. R. (1975). "Mini-Mental State": A practical method for grading the cognitive state of patients for the clinician. *Journal of Psychiatric Research, 12,* 189–198. https://doi.org/10.1016/0022-3956(75)90026-6

Gioia, G. A., Isquith, P. K., Guy, S. C., & Kenworthy, L. (2000a). *Behavior Rating Inventory of Executive Function.* Lutz, FL: PAR.

Gioia, G. A., Isquith, P. K., Guy, S. C., & Kenworthy, L. (2000b). Behavior Rating Inventory of Executive Function. *Child Neuropsychology, 6,* 235–238. https://doi.org/10.1076/chin.6.3.235.3152

Granger, C. V., Hamilton, B. B., Linacre, J. M., Heinemann, A. W., & Wright, B. D. (1993). Performance profiles of the Functional Independence Measure. *American Journal of Physical Medicine and Rehabilitation, 72,* 84–89. https://doi.org/10.1097/00002060-199304000-00005

Knight, C., Alderman, N., & Burgess, P. W. (2002). Development of a simplified version of the Multiple Errands Test for use in hospital settings. *Neuropsychological Rehabilitation, 12,* 231–255. https://doi.org/10.1080/09602010244000039

Manchester, D., Priestley, N., & Jackson, H. (2004). The assessment of executive functions: Coming out of the office. *Brain Injury, 18,* 1067–1081. https://doi.org/10.1080/02699050410001672387

Morrison, M. T., Giles, G. M., Ryan, J. D., Baum, C. M., Dromerick, A. W., Polatajko, H. J., & Edwards, D. F. (2013). Multiple Errands Test–Revised (MET–R): A performance-based measure of executive function in people with mild cerebrovascular accident. *American Journal of Occupational Therapy, 67,* 460–468. https://doi.org/10.5014/ajot.2013.007880

Nasreddine, Z. S., Phillips, N. A., Bédirian, V., Charbonneau, S., Whitehead, V., Collin, I., . . . Chertkow, H. (2005). The Montreal Cognitive Assessment, MoCA: A brief screening tool for mild cognitive impairment. *Journal of the American Geriatrics Society, 53,* 695–699. https://doi.org/10.1111/j.1532-5415.2005.53221.x

O'Keefe, J., & Nadel, L. (1979). Précis of O'Keefe & Nadel's The hippocampus as a cognitive map. *Behavioral and Brain Sciences, 2,* 487–494. https://doi.org/10.1017/S0140525X00063949

Roth, L. I. P., Gioia, G. A., Besnard, R. J., & Le Gall, D. (2013). E–BRIEF. *Human Development, 89,* 865–874.

Saliba, D., Buchanan, J., Edelen, M. O., Streim, J., Ouslander, J., Berlowitz, D., & Chodosh, J. (2012). MDS 3.0: Brief Interview for Mental Status. *Journal of the American Medical Directors Association, 13,* 611–617. https://doi.org/10.1016/j.jamda.2012.06.004

Shallice, T., & Burgess, P. W. (1991). Deficits in strategy application following frontal lobe damage in man. *Brain, 114,* 727–741. https://doi.org/10.1093/brain/114.2.727

Steverson, T., Adlam, A. R., & Langdon, P. E. (2017). Development and validation of a modified Multiple Errands Test for adults with intellectual disabilities. *Journal of Applied Research in Intellectual Disabilities, 30,* 255–268. https://doi.org/10.1111/jar.12236

Stroop, J. R. (1935). Studies of interference in serial verbal reactions. *Journal of Experimental Psychology, 18,* 643–662. https://doi.org/10.1037/h0054651

Tariq, S. H., Tumosa, N., Chibnall, J. T., Perry, M. H., III, & Morley, J. E. (2006). Comparison of the Saint Louis University Mental Status examination and the Mini-Mental State Examination for detecting dementia and mild neurocognitive disorder—A pilot study. *American Journal of Geriatric Psychiatry, 14,* 900–910. https://doi.org/10.1097/01.JGP.0000221510.33817.86

Valls-Serrano, C., Verdejo-García, A., Noël, X., & Caracuel, A. (2018). Development of a contextualized version of the Multiple Errands Test for people with substance dependence. *Journal of the International Neuropsychological Society, 24,* 347–359. https://doi.org/10.1017/S1355617717001023

10

Complex Task Performance Assessment

ANNA E. BOONE, MSOT, PhD, OTR/L,
AND TIMOTHY J. WOLF, OTD, PhD, OTR/L, FAOTA

LEARNING OBJECTIVES

After completing this chapter, readers should be able to

- Understand the background and theoretical basis for the Complex Task Performance Assessment (CTPA),
- Describe the standardized procedure for administering the CTPA,
- Identify clients in practice for whom the CTPA is an appropriate assessment, and
- Interpret CTPA results and implications for treatment planning.

KEY TERMS AND CONCEPTS

- Complex Task Performance Assessment • Functional–cognitive assessment • Mild cognitive impairment
- Prospective memory

Introduction

The Complex Task Performance Assessment (CTPA; Wolf et al., 2008, 2017) was developed in response to 3 needs:

1. Limitations of traditional neuropsychological assessments

2. A lack of a performance-based functional–cognitive test based on work tasks

3. Limitations of the Multiple Errands Test (MET; Shallice & Burgess, 1991; Wolf et al., 2017).

The **Complex Task Performance Assessment** is a performance-based test (PBT) of functional cognition in work tasks. A **functional–cognitive assessment** evaluates collective cognitive processes in real-world activities and contexts. In contrast, traditional **neuropsychological assessments** evaluate isolated components of cognition and are poor predictors of daily life functioning (see Chapter 4, "The Cognitive–Functional Evaluation Framework," for further detail; Lezak, 1982). Until the development of the CTPA, no other performance-based assessment evaluated executive function (EF) in the context of work-related tasks.

Rigorous evaluation of EF in work tasks is essential for people of working age, especially for those who have sustained a mild neurological injury or disorder. In some cases, cognitive deficits may not be apparent on global screening measures or PBTs of routine ADL tasks. An example population is clients with mild stroke.

The age of first-time stroke seems to be decreasing, with nearly half reported as younger than 65 years and nearly one-third younger than 55 years. Younger individuals with stroke coupled with rising retirement age yields a growing number of individuals returning to the work environment after stroke (Mermin et al., 2007; Wolf et al., 2009).

Clients with profound neurological impairment typically have cognitive impairments that are easily detectable with gross screening measures. However, clients with milder neurological impairment often score within the cognitively intact range on screening measures and require use of PBTs for detection (Lezak, 1982). Mild cognitive impairment (MCI) often accompanies mild neurological impairment. MCI is a subtle decrement in cognitive function that is not typically identified by traditional global screening measures but can have a profound impact on occupational performance. PBTs are required for determining not only potential for return to work but also return to the home and community.

The CTPA was also developed to address limitations of the MET. The MET was originally developed by Shallice and Burgess (1991) to address gaps in assessment of high-level cognitive function. Shallice and Burgess acknowledged that there was a gap between the clinical presentation of some individuals with neurological injury and their performance on standardized neuropsychological measures of EF. The neuropsychological measures indicated little to no cognitive impairment; however, the individuals were experiencing profound deficits in everyday life.

The basis for the MET was rooted in ecological psychology and the concept of *ecological validity* originally described by Egon Brunswik (1955). Brunswik argued that to understand behavior, practitioners need to evaluate using an ecological approach in everyday life, to observe free behavior in an unrestricted environment. Since 1991, the MET has been rigorously evaluated, and multiple versions are now in practice and development (see Chapter 9, "The Multiple Errands Test–Revised," for more detail). However, some practical limitations of the MET restrict its wide adoption in clinical practice. These include

- The time and space required;

- A lack of alternative forms, which precludes repeated testing because of learning effects; and

- The environmental component, which requires that the MET be redeveloped at each site where it is used (Wolf et al., 2017).

The CTPA was established on the basis of the same theory, scoring, and multitasking criteria as the MET (see Table 10.1). However, it was developed to be administered in a clinical setting in a practical amount of time (Burgess, 2000).

CTPA Structure

The CTPA consists of 2 main tasks that are performed simultaneously: (1) Bookkeeping–Current Inventory Control, and (2) Telephone Messaging (Wolf et al., 2008). To complete the Bookkeeping–Current Inventory Control task, the client calculates current fines and replacement costs of overdue books and videos as if they were performing clerical duties in a library. The client must then decide whether the book or video borrower is more likely to pay a fine or a replacement fee.

To complete the Telephone Messaging task while completing the Bookkeeping–Current Inventory Control task, the participant listens and responds appropriately to voice messages with 3 levels of challenge:

1. Level 1 voice messages require the recording of a note.

2. Level 2 messages require an additional sequential step: The client must listen to the message and record a change of address or name.

3. Level 3 messages are from a caller questioning the legitimacy of the fine. The client has to compare the mailing list and the database to make a judgment about the accuracy of the message, then decide whether to include the fine in calculations of the bookkeeping task.

The CTPA includes 2 task components that require the use of **prospective memory,** or the ability to recall an intended action at a point in the future (Smith et al., 2017):

1. The first is an event-based prospective memory component, for which the client is instructed to immediately deliver a message to the examiner when "Katie Huiell" calls.

2. The 2nd prospective memory component is time based; the client must verbalize when 10 minutes have passed and when they have completed the assessment.

According to the structure of the MET, there are rules the client must adhere to. The CTPA implements 5 rules. The client

1. May not talk to the examiner;

2. May not use a cell phone to talk to anyone during the assessment;

3. May replay a message only once by asking the examiner, and may not touch the audio player;

4. May review the instruction sheet as many times as needed but may not mark on the instruction sheet; and

5. May not mark on any index cards, the mailing list, or the database (sticky notes are supplied for making notes).

The CTPA was first piloted with a small group of individuals with mild stroke and healthy control participants (Wolf et al., 2008). The CTPA was able to discriminate between individuals with mild stroke and control participants on

- Inventory control accuracy ($p = .03$),

- Number of executive decisions ($p = .02$),

- Number of tasks completed ($p = .01$), and

- Performance efficiency ($p = .01$).

After the pilot, the CTPA was revised to improve clinical feasibility. Revisions included decreasing the total possible testing time from 1 hour to 40 minutes, decreasing the number of phone messages, and decreasing the number of titles the client is required to evaluate. After revisions, the assessment was psychometrically evaluated with a larger sample of individuals with mild stroke and community control participants with equivalent education levels (Wolf et al., 2017).

In Wolf et al.'s (2017) study, the CTPA was found to have high interrater reliability for the total score (intraclass correlation [ICC] = .991) and for subscores (ICCs = .889–.977). Furthermore, it demonstrated acceptable concurrent validity with

TABLE 10.1. Burgess (2000) Multitasking Constructs and Their Link to the CTPA

MULTITASKING CONSTRUCT	OPERATIONAL DEFINITION	CTPA COMPONENT
Many tasks	A number of discrete and different tasks have to be completed.	Use the inventory control sheet, answer all phone messages, respond to appropriate phone messages, and perform time and event prospective memory tasks.
Interleaving required	Performance on these tasks needs to be dovetailed to be time-effective.	Phone messages are dovetailed with inventory-control activity.
1 task at a time	Because of either cognitive or physical constraints, only 1 task can be performed at a time.	The test taker cannot physically write the phone message while recording on inventory control.
Interruptions and unexpected outcomes	Unforeseen interruptions, sometimes of high priority, will occasionally occur, and things will not always go as planned.	Phone messages are spaced intermittently throughout the CD.
Delayed intentions	The time for a return to a task that is already running is not signaled directly by the situation.	Time and event prospective memory tasks (e.g., tell the examiner when 10 minutes has passed).
Differing task characteristics	Tasks usually differ in terms of priority, difficulty, and the length of time they take to complete.	All tasks require a different amount of time. The inventory control is the main focus of the activity.
Self-determined targets	People decide for themselves what constitutes adequate performance.	The participant informs the examiner when they are finished.
No immediate feedback	There is no minute-by-minute performance feedback of the sort that participants in many laboratory experiments receive. Typically, failures are not signaled at the time they occur.	The participant receives no feedback from the examiner on correct or incorrect performance during the assessment. The participant makes their own determination.

Note. CTPA = Complex Task Performance Assessment.
Source. From "Initial Development of a Work-Related Assessment of Dysexecutive Syndrome: The Complex Task Performance Assessment," by T. J. Wolf, T. Morrison, & L. Matheson, 2008, *Work, 31,* p. 224. Copyright © 2008 by IOS Press. Adapted with permission of IOS Press. The article is available at IOS Press through https://content.iospress.com/articles/work/wor00726.

neuropsychological tests of EF, including the Delis–Kaplan Color–Word subtest Condition 4 ($r = -.43$; Delis et al., 2001) and the Wechsler Test of Adult Reading ($r = -.49$; Wechsler, 2001). The CTPA was also able to discriminate between individuals with mild stroke and healthy control participants on the

- Total score ($p = .007$),
- Total number of task failures ($p = .02$),
- Total number of inefficiencies ($p = .045$), and
- Total number of rule breaks ($p = .042$),

thereby establishing known-groups validity.

To help minimize learning effects of the CTPA and to allow for use as an outcome measure, the researchers then developed an alternate form of the CTPA (CTPA–Alt). A repeated-measures study was conducted, with community control participants completing each of the CTPA forms 1 week apart (Saa et al., 2017). The CTPA–Alt is similar in structure and scoring to the CTPA but differs in the base tasks, which are

- Completing a calendar for scheduling appointments, and
- Telephone messaging.

Clients must schedule 16 appointments and tasks of varying flexibility for a bank manager in the schedule. They complete the scheduling while responding to 4 telephone messages.

The CTPA and the CTPA–Alt were found to be moderately correlated ($r_s = .44$), which indicates that performance on the 2 measures was related. However, they seem to be sufficiently different, according to different scoring patterns in task failures (Saa et al., 2017). Few functional–cognitive assessments have alternate forms available; however, practitioners continue to use them for longitudinal assessment despite probable learning effects.

Target Population

An occupational profile helps practitioners determine whether they should use the CTPA with a client. The CTPA is particularly relevant for clients expecting to return to a work environment. It may also be appropriate for clients who have responsibilities for managing a budget or other high-level multitasking activities, such as managing a calendar in the work environment or home environment. The CTPA may also be useful to evaluate clients' capacity to perform other complex tasks after they have demonstrated difficulty in performing certain IADLs.

The CTPA is suitable for clients with mild to moderate neurological deficits. For example, on a cognitive screener such as the Montreal Cognitive Assessment (Nasreddine et al., 2005), the CPTA is indicated for individuals classified as cognitively intact or as having limited impairment, with scores of 22 to 30. In essence, the CTPA is most typically appropriate for individuals who

- Are higher functioning,

- Are highly educated, and

- Have milder neurological impairments, so that they are experiencing challenges with complex IADL tasks in everyday life but showing few to no deficits on standardized neuropsychological testing.

Often, occupational therapists' clinical judgment detects deficits in functional cognition during treatment tasks, such as cooking; they may use the CTPA as a way to objectively verify these clinical judgments and to quantify them. Because of the time required to administer the CTPA, it is most relevant for use in the inpatient rehabilitation setting, outpatient settings, or community-based settings.

Administration

The CTPA requires approximately 45 minutes to complete. The ecologically valid nature of functional–cognitive assessments means they generally take more time to complete. Space and material constraints for the CTPA are minimal, which thus increases its clinical utility. The measure requires only a moderate amount of table space and the printed materials (which are freely available), along with a few other readily available materials (e.g., calculator, clock; see Exhibit 10.1).

The CTPA is available for free at https://www.ot.wustl.edu/mm/files/CTPA.zip. This includes the manual, step-by-step testing kit instructions, inventory labels, mailing list, master database, and recorded voice messages. See Exhibit 10.2 for step-by-step instructions for administering the assessment.

The CTPA was developed with the intention that it would be administered and interpreted by licensed occupational therapy professionals. Beyond this, no additional formal training is needed to administer the CTPA in practice or research. However, the developers of the CTPA are willing to provide any support necessary to use and interpret the CTPA. All information needed may be found in the manual. Please see Video 10.1 for an example of the setup and administration instructions for the CTPA.

After preparing the materials, the examiner asks the client the pretest questions. The examiner then reads the instructions aloud (scripted words are in *italics*). The client must comprehend the instructions before beginning, and the examiner may answer questions as needed. To ensure understanding, the client should repeat these instructions back to the examiner. The use of this teach-back method is imperative to limit deficiencies in interpretation of instructions. After the assessment, the client rates perceived performance on a scale of 1–10.

For valid testing results, the testing environment should have limited auditory and visual distractions. Additional major distractions will lead to increased cognitive load for the participant. Furthermore, for standardized administration, the test taker must adhere to all instructions in full. To assist in this, examiners should ensure that all testing materials are present before initiation of testing. Similarly, the examiner

EXHIBIT 10.1. Setup for Administering the CTPA

STEP	MATERIALS AND TASKS	
1. Gather materials.	• 64 index cards (4 in. × 6 in.) • 64 white shipping labels (2 in. × 4 in.) • 2 3-ring binders (0.5 in.) with clear cover pocket • 1 metal book ring • 2 pieces of colored paper (8.5 in. × 11 in.) • Printer paper	• MP3 player • Clock • Sticky notes • Pen or pencil • Calculator • CTPA testing packet
2. Prepare index cards.	• Print inventory control labels document. • Place labels 1 at a time on index cards. • Place index cards on metal book ring.	
3. Prepare mailing list and master database binders.	• Print title page document on each of the 2 pieces of colored paper. • Place each sheet in the cover pocket of the binders. • Print mailing list and master database documents and place in appropriate binder.	
4. Prepare phone messages.	• Download files from phone messages folder onto an MP3-compatible device.	

Note. CTPA = Complex Task Performance Assessment.

EXHIBIT 10.2. Instructions for Administering the CTPA

1. Place materials in front of the participant. The index cards should be off of the metal book ring and presented in a random order.
2. Ask pretest questions.
3. Read the task instructions, with scripted words *italicized*. This step familiarizes the client with the materials and procedures to follow during the assessment. Make sure the participant understands the instructions before beginning the assessment. Ask the client to repeat the instructions back to you in their own words.
4. Start the assessment, and tell the client to begin. Note the time.
5. As soon as the assessment has begun, begin playing the MP3 messages.
6. Record any observations during the testing on the scoring sheet.
7. After assessment completion or after 40 minutes, ask the final question: "On a scale of 1 to 10, how well do you believe you did on the assessment?"
8. Transfer data from the pretest questions and the final question to the scoring sheet.

Note. CTPA = Complex Task Performance Assessment.

should use the precise language included in the scripted text during standardized administration. If multiple individuals in a facility are using the CTPA, it is important to first calibrate between raters to ensure reliability in administration and scoring.

Scoring Criteria

The CTPA total score is based on inefficiencies, rule breaks, interpretation failures, task failures, and the accuracy of inventory control (see Table 10.2). Each of these subscores, with the exception of inventory control accuracy, is based on criteria developed by Shallice and Burgess (1991) as part of the MET scoring. The total score is the sum of all of the subscores. Higher scores indicate more severe impairment.

If a task is not completed because of misinterpretation of the task, it is an interpretation failure; however, if a task is not completed for any other reason (e.g., the test taker did not attempt it, believed the test to be completed, or reached the time limit), it is a task failure. At the end of administration, scoring data are compiled, with answers to questions asked of the client, on the CTPA scoring sheet. Normative data are not yet available for the CTPA, and cutoff scores have not been

established. Scores can be interpreted with control participant data reported by Wolf and colleagues (2017).

Documentation

The CTPA is intended to be used as a standardized assessment. Assessment results (see the "Scoring Criteria" section) should be placed in the objective portion of documentation. Objective results include inefficiencies, rule breaks, interpretation failures, task failures, inventory control accuracy, and total score. Time of administration is also monitored and can be reported as well.

Interpretation of these results and implications of the client's functional cognition in the context of client-centered goal performance should also be documented in the assessment section of the documentation. It is critically important to interpret the scoring in the context of the client's occupational profile and premorbid level of occupational performance (see Chapter 5, "Occupational Profile," for further detail). Assessment results may also inform discharge environment, potential for return to work, or needed support.

Although it is not the intended use, the CTPA could serve as the basis for a treatment session. For instance, the occupational therapist could use it as a method to assess awareness by asking a client how successful they will be or what types of errors they think they will make. Comparison of the client's estimates with their actual performance will indicate awareness of deficits.

Occupational therapists could use this method to determine where in the Pyramid Model of Awareness a client falls (see Chapter 17, "Intervention Selection," for further detail; Crosson et al., 1989). Depending on the client's level of awareness, the assessment could inform treatment planning, including but not limited to the following:

- Development of skills related to identification of errors made and potential errors

- Decisions about when to apply a cognitive strategy

- Development of a cognitive strategy

- Implementation of a cognitive strategy.

TABLE 10.2. CTPA Scoring

SCORING CATEGORY	DESCRIPTION
Inefficiencies	When a more effective or efficient method could have been applied
Rule breaks	When a rule from the list of rules provided to the client is broken
Interpretation failures	When requirements of a task are misinterpreted
Task failures	When a task is not completed
Inventory control accuracy	Reflects number of inaccurate or incomplete items (15 possible)

Note. CTPA = Complex Task Performance Assessment.

Interpretation and Intervention Considerations

Results of any assessment, including functional–cognitive assessments and the CTPA, are to be interpreted in the context of occupational performance goals developed collaboratively with a client and the client's support system. Functional–cognitive changes related to complex IADLs are most apparent in unstructured activities that are not routinized. Difficulties encountered with the CTPA likely are reflective and predictive of other complex IADL tasks the client may have trouble with when returning home, reengaging in the community, or returning to work.

Results of the CTPA can help inform decisions about whether an individual is able to return to a previously held work position, what modifications may be required, or whether a job with more structured duties is necessary. In addition to information about how a client can be safe and independent in the home and work settings, other considerations include how effective, efficient, and satisfactory the occupational performance is to the client.

The occupational therapist should communicate the results and interpretations of the CTPA to other team members and family members, for a cohesive team approach to addressing impairments. For example, clients with higher levels of awareness, for whom cognitive strategy use is indicated, would benefit from team reinforcement of the application of developed strategies and continued development of new cognitive strategies through a global problem-solving approach.

The role of occupational therapy in functional–cognitive assessment and treatment is important and distinct. Therefore, a client's functional cognition is not addressed if therapists do not fulfill this role. Because the client's functional cognition is a primary concern of occupational therapy, not the underlying impairments, further testing after the CTPA may prove unnecessary.

If further assessment is indicated, then the occupational therapist should refer to other cognitive measurement domains outlined in the Cognitive–Functional Evaluation Framework (see Chapter 4, "The Cognitive–Functional Evaluation Framework," for more detail). In brief, these include

- More in-depth testing of the specific cognitive impairments,

- Assessment of the specific impairment in the context of occupational performance, and

- Environmental assessment.

If results of the CTPA indicate profound loss of functional cognition, then behavioral management strategies may be appropriate. In contrast, clients with milder deficits and more intact awareness would benefit from strategy-based interventions (see Chapter 17 for more information).

References

Brunswik, E. (1955). Representative design and probabilistic theory in a functional psychology. *Psychological Review, 62,* 193–217. https://doi.org/10.1037/h0047470

Burgess, P. W. (2000). Strategy application disorder: The role of the frontal lobes in human multitasking. *Psychological Research, 63,* 279–288. https://doi.org/10.1007/s004269900006

Crosson, B., Barco, P. P., Velozo, C. A., Bolesta, M. M., Cooper, P. V., Werts, D., & Brobeck, T. C. (1989). Awareness and compensation in postacute head injury rehabilitation. *Journal of Head Trauma Rehabilitation, 4,* 46–54. https://doi.org/10.1097/00001199-198909000-00008

Delis, D. C., Kaplan, E., & Kramer, J. H. (2001). *Delis–Kaplan Executive Function System.* San Antonio: Psychological Corporation.

Lezak, M. D. (1982). The problem of assessing executive functions. *International Journal of Psychology, 17,* 281–297. https://doi.org/10.1080/00207598208247445

Mermin, G. B., Johnson, R. W., & Murphy, D. P. (2007). Why do boomers plan to work longer? *Journals of Gerontology, Series B: Psychological Sciences, 62,* S286–S294. https://doi.org/10.1093/geronb/62.5.S286

Nasreddine, Z. S., Phillips, N. A., Bédirian, V., Charbonneau, S., Whitehead, V., Collin, I., . . . Chertkow, H. (2005). The Montreal Cognitive Assessment, MoCA: A brief screening tool for mild cognitive impairment. *Journal of the American Geriatrics Society, 53,* 695–699. https://doi.org/10.1111/j.1532-5415.2005.53221.x

Saa, J. P., Doherty, M., Young, A., Spiers, M., Leary, E., & Wolf, T. J. (2017). Development and alternate form reliability of the Complex Task Performance Assessment (CTPA) for people with mild stroke. *American Journal of Occupational Therapy, 71,* 7103190030. https://doi.org/10.5014/ajot.2017.024356

Shallice, T., & Burgess, P. W. (1991). Deficits in strategy application following frontal lobe damage in man. *Brain, 114,* 727–741. https://doi.org/10.1093/brain/114.2.727

Smith, R. E., Hunt, R. R., & Murray, A. E. (2017). Prospective memory in context: Moving through a familiar space. *Journal of Experimental Psychology: Learning, Memory, and Cognition, 43,* 189–204. https://doi.org/10.1037/xlm0000303

Wechsler, D. (2001). *Wechsler Test of Adult Reading: WTAR.* San Antonio: Psychological Corporation.

Wolf, T. J., Baum, C., & Conner, L. T. (2009). Changing face of stroke: Implications for occupational therapy practice. *American Journal of Occupational Therapy, 63,* 621–625. https://doi.org/10.5014/ajot.63.5.621

Wolf, T. J., Dahl, A., Auen, C., & Doherty, M. (2017). The reliability and validity of the Complex Task Performance Assessment: A performance-based assessment of executive function. *Neuropsychological Rehabilitation, 27,* 707–721. https://doi.org/10.1080/09602011.2015.1037771

Wolf, T. J., Morrison, T., & Matheson, L. (2008). Initial development of a work-related assessment of dysexecutive syndrome: The Complex Task Performance Assessment. *Work, 31,* 221–228.

11

The Actual Reality™ Assessment

YAEL GOVEROVER, PhD, OTR/L,
AND JOHN DeLUCA, PhD

LEARNING OBJECTIVES

After completing this chapter, readers should be able to

- Describe the scope and nature of Actual Reality™ (AR), a new performance-based assessment of functional cognition;
- Identify key findings from high-quality studies of the development of AR; and
- Discuss how AR can be integrated into practice and research.

KEY TERMS AND CONCEPTS

- Actual Reality™ • Functional cognition

Introduction

Improving how the clinical manifestations of multiple sclerosis (MS) are assessed has long been a priority for researchers and health care practitioners. It is vitally important to document the progress of the illness and its related disorders and establish the benefits of potential treatments (Goverover et al., 2015; Rudick et al., 1997). MS is a chronic inflammatory disease of the central nervous system that leads to demyelination and neurodegeneration (Pugliatti et al., 2006). It is characterized by damage to both white and gray matter in the brain, which results in

- Impaired muscle coordination and speech,

- Fatigue,

- Numbness, and

- Blurred vision (Sacco et al., 2015).

About two-thirds of those diagnosed with MS have cognitive decline in addition to motor impairments (Chiaravalloti & DeLuca, 2008; Goverover, Sandroff, & DeLuca, 2018). Similarly, up to two-thirds of those with MS have been found to

have limited ADLs and IADLs (Basak et al., 2015; Einarsson et al., 2006). Such impairments have been found to result in decreased quality of life and well-being (Goverover, Genova, et al., 2016; Goverover et al., 2015). By accurately identifying the link between cognitive impairments and limitations in ADLs and IADLs, professionals may be better able to address those limitations and find ways to weaken or strengthen these links (e.g., providing strategies, changing the environment or task).

Assessment of *functional cognition*—how a person uses and integrates their thinking and processing skills to accomplish everyday activities—has many apparent merits in chronic illness outcome measurement. It can be used to measure incremental improvement in a wide range of IADLs directly associated with the patient and across various medical disciplines. However, to date, assessment of functional cognition among persons diagnosed with MS is limited.

This scarcity led us to develop an assessment of actual everyday life performance, which we viewed as necessary for an accurate assessment of potential functional difficulties. We saw a need for an assessment that was not a self-report or proxy report (e.g., the Functional Assessment of Multiple Sclerosis; Cella et al., 1996). *Actual Reality™* (AR; Goverover & DeLuca, 2018; Goverover et al., 2010, 2015) is a new and innovative method for measuring actual, everyday life activities. AR is a performance-based assessment approach that allows clients to use the Internet to perform actual, everyday life activities. This chapter describes the AR assessment process and its uses.

We first detail the background and process of AR's development. We then describe AR and follow with a discussion of research that supports its use, primarily among persons diagnosed with MS or traumatic brain injury (TBI). We conclude with suggestions for how AR can be further integrated into practice and research.

Background and Development

IADLs and functional cognition can be assessed either by observation of task performance or by self- and proxy report (Chiaravalloti & Goverover, 2016). Direct observation of performance seems to provide the most accurate assessment; however, it cannot always be conducted, because of limiting factors such as time or space restrictions, the client's physical or medical condition, or the client's level of familiarity with a task. Therefore, professionals often rely on indirect reports of IADL performance, as reported either by the individual (i.e., self-report) or by a family member or someone else who knows the individual well (i.e., informant report).

Research suggests that these informant reports and self-reports may be biased because depression, anxiety, or other factors (e.g., those linked to self-efficacy) might affect responses (Goverover, Chiaravalloti, & DeLuca, 2005; Goverover et al., 2009; Steene-Johannessen et al., 2016). For example, Goverover, Kalmar, et al. (2005) did not find significant correlations between self-reports of functional status and IADL performance. However, after they controlled for depressive symptoms, IADL performance was significantly associated with self-report of functional status. Thus, self-report is often associated with depressive symptoms and levels of self-awareness (Goverover et al., 2009). Individuals, especially those who have experienced cognitive decline, have difficulty accurately evaluating their everyday competency (Goverover, Kalmar, et al., 2005).

MS presents with a challenging disease course. A few studies have assessed IADLs and functional cognition among participants with MS using performance-based tools, such as the Executive Function Performance Test (EFPT; Kalmar et al., 2008), the Assessment of Motor and Process Skills (AMPS; Doble et al., 1994), and the Timed Instrumental Activities of Daily Living (TIADL; Goverover et al., 2007; Owsley et al., 2001). Although these assessments capture sample behaviors related to IADLs, they do not adequately represent the MS functional profile, because they focus on components of cognitive skills, not the whole complexity required for IADLs.

For example, Doble et al. (1994) examined the relationship between AMPS scores and

- Standard clinical ratings on the Expanded Disability Status Scale (EDSS; Kurtzke, 2015) and

- The subjective ratings of general health status on the Sickness Impact Profile (SIP; Bergner et al., 1976).

Results indicated that MS participants, who would not have been expected to have IADL difficulties on the basis of the ratings of neurological impairments (as in the EDSS or the SIP), actually were found to be impaired on the AMPS. Correlations were significant between the subjective self-reports from the SIP and the motor—but not the process—skills component of the AMPS tool. It should be noted, however, that only occupational therapists who have completed a specific training program can administer the AMPS; thus, its use in practice and research is limited for other professionals.

Goverover et al. (2007) found that participants with MS required significantly more time to complete the TIADL than did those who did not have MS. However, the scoring of the TIADL is based on how much time it takes to complete a simple IADL task, such as locating food items on a small shelf, reading ingredients on a can of food, or counting change. Similar to the EFPT, which focuses on executive function (EF) components while test takers are performing IADLs, the TIADL assesses 1 aspect of cognitive functioning—processing speed in performance of IADLs.

In sum, researchers study performance-based assessment of everyday functioning far less frequently than questionnaire-based methods, and only a few studies have focused on assessing IADLs among persons with MS (e.g., Doble et al., 1994; Goverover, Kalmar, et al., 2005; Goverover et al., 2010; Kalmar et al., 2008). Those studies have provided useful information on how someone performs a task through a focused lens (i.e., EFs or processing speed) and, basically, the functional performance of persons with MS.

However, these performance-based assessment tools have some limitations, such as safety concerns (e.g., when to ask someone to operate a stove or to walk if stability is an issue) and time and space restrictions (e.g., many tasks require a kitchen). Additionally, administration of some tools (e.g., the AMPS) requires special training for both administering and scoring. Last, many of these assessments are not detailed or sensitive enough to capture the complexity of daily functioning among persons diagnosed with MS. Thus, we developed a new assessment tool—the AR—that takes into account more aspects of cognition and that can be administered by various professionals.

Description

The AR assessment tool was designed specifically for use with the Internet to assess the actual IADL performance of persons with disabilities, starting specifically with MS (Goverover et al., 2010). The AR assessment covers a wide range of cognitive processes required to perform everyday life tasks, such as using an actual website to purchase airline tickets, cookies for a child's birthday party, or pizza for a party.

Basically, we want to examine naturalistic Internet navigation skills. To enhance the ecological validity of this innovative approach, we decided to use the actual website for a web-based task in an online shopping environment (without having participants actually make the purchase). This allows us to accurately and reliably quantify participants' navigation skills and efficiency. Participants must navigate the website to identify the correct items, place them in a shopping cart, and successfully check out using a mock credit card.

Administration

Before starting the test, all clients must complete a short tutorial on how to navigate the computer and the Internet, regardless of their computer expertise. Then participants are instructed to use any of the materials provided (e.g., pen, paper, calendar, address book) and to complete the task as independently as possible. The test administrator then reads participants the instructions before they perform each task (see Exhibit 11.1).

Participants begin at the desktop page and are asked to start the task after being read the task instructions. Participants independently and freely navigate the websites. At any time during the task, participants can check out using a mock credit card.

One of the biggest advantages of the AR is that anyone can perform an AR assessment as presently conceptualized, with little to no potential physical risk. Additionally, performance of the task is not restricted by a space or location, because every person who has a computer and an Internet connection can be assessed. The only restriction is that some previous computer and Internet experience is needed.

Scoring

Each of the 3 AR tasks we have used to date requires participants to complete a set of 32 steps involving critical actions required to finish the task, such as selecting and clicking on certain Internet

EXHIBIT 11.1. Task Instructions for the AR Assessment

PURCHASING AIRLINE TICKETS

Please pay careful attention to the following directions. You can either listen to the information or take notes on the instructions if you like. You will need to locate the credit card in the wallet. Let's assume that 1 of your family members wants to go on a trip to Florida, and it's your job to buy plane tickets for them. Do you have anyone in mind? [NOTE: If the participant cannot come up with anyone specific, they are asked to make up someone.] For this task, you will need to use the Internet to go to the website for United Airlines to purchase a nonstop, round-trip airline ticket for a vacation in Orlando, Florida. _____ [THE PERSON THAT WAS IDENTIFIED] will be leaving from Newark Airport in New Jersey. You need to buy a round-trip ticket for the lowest possible price. This vacation should take place in the summer months and will be for 1 week's duration. The departure flight should leave in the morning, and the return flight should leave in the evening. ____ [PERSON] wants to use economy class, and you will choose their seat. You must pay with a credit card, which will be provided to you. Keep in mind that any information you do not know, you can make up. Please try to complete this task as independently as possible. It is important to remember that we want you to complete all steps of the order up until the actual placement of the order. DO NOT ACTUALLY PLACE THE ORDER.

BUYING COOKIES

Please pay careful attention to the following directions before beginning this task. You can either listen to the information or take notes on the instructions if you like. You will need to locate the credit card in the wallet in the drawer beside you and the address book on the desktop. Please use the Internet to go to the website for Cookies by Design to purchase a birthday bouquet of cookies for a 13-year-old boy. Your price range is between $30 and $60, including $15 to $25 for shipping and handling. The boy's birthday is on ____ [PARTICIPANT PROVIDES A DATE], and this gift should arrive on his birthday. You should also remember to include a birthday message. The boy's name is Alan Lowe. His address is 40 West 4th Street, Apt. 11A, New York, NY, 10012, and his telephone number is 718-555-9807. You must pay with a credit card, which will be provided to you. Keep in mind that any information you do not know, you can make up. Please try to complete this task as independently as possible. It is important to remember that we want you to complete all steps of the order up until the actual placement of the order. DO NOT ACTUALLY PLACE THE ORDER.

ORDERING PIZZA

Please use the Internet to order pizza from Pizza Hut for a party today at your friend Steven Smith's house. The guests include yourself, 4 children, and 2 other adults. You should order 2 large pizzas: 1 for the children, who like only plain pizza with thin crust, and 1 for the adults, with hand-tossed crust. You should choose 3 toppings for the adult pizza, 1 being onions. Drinks should include a 2-liter bottle of Diet Pepsi for the party. You should pay no more than $60 for the total order, and do not use coupons. You must pay with the credit card, which is provided to you in the wallet. Keep in mind that any information you do not know, you should make up. You should have the pizza delivered to Steven's address at 95 Bloomfield Way, Apt. 5F, West Orange, NJ 07052. The contact phone number for the pizza is 212-555-4023; the contact email is abc123@hotmail.com. Please try to complete this task as independently as possible. It is important to remember that we want you to complete all steps of the order up until the actual placement of the order. DO NOT ACTUALLY PLACE THE ORDER.

Note. AR = Actual Reality™.

icons when necessary (e.g., selecting time, date, and payment; filling in name, address, and payment method). Scoring of the AR is based on a rater's observation, which is focused on errors the participant made while performing the AR task, cues given or not given to remedy the errors, and actions to complete the task (e.g., choosing the correct pizza, not exceeding the price). As an example, see Video 11.1, which presents administration of the pizza task. The AR yields 4 outcome variables:

1. Total number of errors

2. Sum of errors

3. Cognitive capacities score

4. Latency score.

Total Number of Errors

Each error receives 1 point; thus, the score can range from 0 *(no errors)* to 32 *(error on each step of the task)*. Errors are determined on the basis of observation of each step performance. Errors may be related to the instructions for each part of the task or to the participant's actual performance using the website. For example, forgetting to enter information or entering incorrect information are errors related to the instructions of the task. Forgetting to check a box next to "Agree to terms and conditions of the purchase" is an error related to website performance.

Sum of Errors

Each error is further scored on the basis of whether a participant performed the step correctly and independently or needed a cue to finish a step or steps. The score on this scale is based on the participant's reaction to the cue or to the error:

- If the participant made an error but self-corrected or questioned it, it would receive a score of 1.

- If the participant made an error, did not receive a cue, and did not self-correct, it would receive a score of 2.

- If a participant made an error and corrected it after a cue, it would receive a score of 3.

- If the participant made an error and did not correct it after a cue, it would receive a score of 4.

Lower scores indicate greater independence in the performance of the task (i.e., the participant needed fewer cues to perform the steps accurately). Table 11.1 provides examples of this scoring system.

Cognitive Capacities Score

This variable refers to the observable cognitive capacities required to complete the AR task (e.g., initiation, organization, notice, response). The cognitive capacities are evaluated by a trained rater across all individual steps of the task. The response choices for each cognitive capacity are scored as follows:

- Competent (0)

- Inefficient (1)

- Severe deficit (2).

TABLE 11.1. AR: Sum of Errors Scoring System Examples

SCORE	DEFINITION	EXAMPLE(S)
0	The step was performed correctly and independently.	• Participant entered the correct date of departure, correct time of departure.
1	The step was performed correctly after self-correction or self-questioning.	• Participant entered pizza type and, while in checkout, realized independently that it was not the correct pizza dough and corrected it.
2	The step was performed incorrectly without a cue.	• Participant added to the cart the incorrect pizza type and did not correct it. • Participant made a typo in entering the credit card number.
3	The step was performed correctly after a cue.	• Participant forget to check a box next to "Agree to terms and conditions" and click enter; however, the computer brought the participant back to the same screen with a red mark next to the box. The participant noticed it and corrected their error. • Participant asked the assessor whether they needed to buy a large or medium pie and reacted correctly to the assessor's response.
4	The step was performed incorrectly after a cue.	• Participant forgot to check a box next to "Agree to terms and conditions" and click enter; the computer brought the participant back to the same screen with a red mark next to the box. However, they did not understand and correct the error. • Participant asked the assessor a question, such as what was the budget for buying the cookies. The assessor answered, but the participant did not correct their purchase to stay within the budget.

Note. AR = Actual Reality™.

Latency Score

The latency score is the completion time—the length of time it took the participant to complete the task.

Scoring Training

AR scoring does require some training. We are currently preparing a training manual, along with 10 AR video clips to be posted online. Potential assessors will be required to watch the videos and read the manual to rate their observation. In the interim, material is available from the authors.

Uses

Findings from the various studies suggest that persons with cognitive impairments, such as those typical of MS and TBI, struggle to perform fundamental Internet-based tasks, which may have detrimental downstream effects on their day-to-day household management. To date, we have found that the AR has at least 2 major uses:

1. Evaluation of online household shopping skills (using everyday technology to assess IADL performance, including evaluation of money management)

2. Evaluation of long-term changes (e.g., pretreatment to posttreatment, changes over time).

Evaluation of Online Household Shopping Skills

Advances in Internet technology may provide an especially germane, naturalistic, user-friendly, and contemporary platform on which to develop the next generation of performance-based everyday-functioning assessments for persons with MS and TBI. As we have discussed, AR is a recently developed technique that uses the Internet to measure actual everyday activity. Initial studies have shown that difficulties with AR tasks, such as booking an airline ticket using the Internet, are significantly associated with cognitive impairment among participants

with TBI (Goverover & DeLuca, 2015) and MS (Goverover & DeLuca, 2018; Goverover et al., 2010, 2015).

For example, Goverover and DeLuca (2018) found that participants with MS committed more errors and required significantly more cues to perform the 3 AR tasks successfully compared with the healthy control (HC) group, which supports the discriminant validity of the AR. That study confirmed previously published results for both MS and TBI (Goverover & DeLuca, 2015). Furthermore, our prior studies that examined mildly to moderately disabled persons with relapsing–remitting MS (e.g., Goverover et al., 2010) found that worse and slower performance of the AR task of booking an airline ticket was associated with worse cognitive performance on the neuropsychological tests, with medium to large effect size.

These results were confirmed in a 2nd study (Goverover et al., 2015) examining purchasing both a flight ticket and a decorative arrangement of cookies, and also in our most recent study (Goverover & DeLuca, 2018), in which we found moderate to large associations between AR performance and neuropsychological test scores (see Figure 11.1). Results showed that the MS group had significantly more difficulty than the HC group in accurately and independently completing the AR task, primarily because of cognitive impairment, such as in processing speed, learning and memory, and EFs. Note that self-report of quality of life and functional status were not correlated with AR performance in the MS group (see Figure 11.2). However, the self-report measures were significantly associated with depressive symptoms. These studies represent an important step in determining whether Internet technology can be used to more accurately and effectively determine the real-world impact of cognitive and functional impairments related to MS.

Evaluation of Money Management in Shopping for Cookies Online

Capacity to manage finances is considered an IADL (Graf, 2008). Among IADLs, financial capacity is perhaps most fundamental to maintaining independence during adulthood.

FIGURE 11.1. Relationship between AR scores and cognitive skills (*z* score).

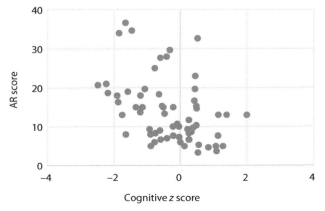

Note. Multiple sclerosis participants = 65; *r* = .42, *p* < .001. AR = Actual Reality™.

FIGURE 11.2. Relationship between depressive symptomatology (*t* score) and AR scores.

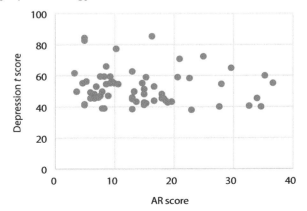

Note. Multiple sclerosis participants = 65; *r* = .15, *p* = .19. AR = Actual Reality™.

Despite its importance, however, few theoretical models of financial functioning exist (Tracy et al., 2017).

All 3 AR tasks require some basic level of managing finances. For example, all 3 tasks require the participant to purchase items online by using a credit card. However, the task of purchasing cookies includes 1 element not in the other 2 AR tasks: It is harder to stay on the particular budget. Participants are required to purchase a bouquet of cookies while keeping in mind that delivery may cost $15 to $25, and they cannot exceed $60 in total.

Therefore, in a recent study (Goverover, Haas, & DeLuca, 2016), we specifically looked at the finance management aspect of this AR task. The study found that individuals with MS reported and demonstrated more problems managing money than did the HC group. Impaired cognitive functioning was significantly correlated with difficulties in money management. Thus, money management is an important IADL that presents problems for individuals with MS. This activity can be assessed by AR and not just by self-report, as it is usually assessed.

Evaluation of Everyday Technology Use

Computer technology—including smartphones and smart homes—is ubiquitous today. In 2013, 83.8% of U.S. households reported owning computers, with 78.5% having a desktop or laptop computer and 63.6% having a hand-held computer (U.S. Census Bureau, 2014). A growing body of research demonstrates how these technological tools can be leveraged for use by people with wide-ranging disabling conditions (Wong et al., 2017).

Whereas computers of all types have proven their usefulness at home, at school, and in the workplace, they can be life changing for people with disabilities. They offer access to the world at large and in many cases substitute for human support by affording increased mobility, safety, and functional independence. Everyday technology can improve activity and participation for persons with neurological disability by removing environmental barriers and supporting physical and mental–cognitive capacities in self-care, work, and play (Larsson Lund et al., 2011). Everyday technology offers some advantages over disability-specific assistive technology, including but not limited to

- Wide availability,

- Affordability, and

- Reduced stigma (Johnson et al., 2009).

As with other assistive technologies, however, research has shown that assessment, adaptation, and training by an occupational therapist can support optimal access to and use of these tools among people with disability (Goverover et al., 2015). Therefore, addressing issues of digital inequality is essential to maximize activity and participation for those with a disability. In addition, understanding how everyday technology can be used to advance the assessment and treatment of persons with neurological disability, in particular those with cognitive

impairments, is crucial to increase their rehabilitation outcomes and quality of life. Using AR can help occupational therapists to explore and understand technology use among persons with neurological disabilities.

In a recent study, we compared the extent to which participants with MS (n = 60) reported problems in everyday technology compared with HC participants (n = 40) and investigated whether cognitive skills or affect symptoms were associated with everyday technology use (Goverover, 2018). Participants diagnosed with MS reported less-frequent computer and Internet use and fewer computer skills than did the HC group. These reports about technology use were associated with self-report of functional status (as measured by the Functional Behavior Profile [FBP]; Baum et al., 1993), with symptoms of depression and anxiety, and with the cognitive domain of processing speed (but no other cognitive domains). Also as anticipated, AR performance was worse for MS participants and was associated mainly with cognitive skills and not with self-report or affect symptoms. It is important to continue to focus on using the AR in studying why persons with disabilities use everyday technologies less frequently than HC participants.

Evaluation of Long-Term Changes

Recently, attention to the assessment and treatment of functional disability has increased. It is widely understood that impairments in ADLs, including independent living skills, social functions, vocational functioning, and self-care, are present among people with cognitive impairments. It is also clear that assessment of these skills can pose substantial challenges in research and clinical practice, including bias and reduced validity of the data. Self-reports and informant reports of IADLs have certain advantages, but they often provide totally different information than direct assessment of skills with performance-based measures, with questionable validity. However, studies using performance-based measures to assess IADLs also have various limitations, as previously discussed.

Even though the field of functional cognition and assessment of IADLs has some performance-based alternatives to assess IADLs, most studies to date have used self-report measures or nothing at all (in particular studies of persons diagnosed with MS). For example, a recent systematic review (Goverover, Chiaravalloti, O'Brien, & DeLuca, 2018) regarding the efficacy of cognitive rehabilitation in MS found few studies, if any, that examined the efficacy of an intervention on IADL performance using a functional cognition assessment.

Recently, Goverover, Chiaravalloti, Genova, and DeLuca (2018) used AR as an outcome measure to document changes in activity limitations after treatment to improve memory among people with MS. This study used a randomized clinical trial design to test the efficacy of using a memory strategy. Outcome was assessed with cognitive measures, activity limitations (measured with the AR), and participation (assessed with the FBP). Although the results indicated improvement on all 3 measures, improvement on the AR was not statistically significant. It is possible that for participants to have a carryover of memory improvement to objective measures of everyday functioning, other cognitive skills may need to be intact, such as EF (Goverover et al., 2013). Alternatively, the relatively low number of treatment sessions in the current protocol might have been a limitation.

A recent study (Goverover & DeLuca, 2018) reported that the AR had moderate to large interrater reliability and that the 3 AR tasks did not differ in the number of errors or the number and quality of cues participants required to complete the AR tasks. A practice effect was observed, however, for cognitive processes and the time it took participants to perform the task. These findings support the AR as an outcome measure that could be used at baseline and follow-up; however, researchers should take the finding of practice effect into consideration.

Final Comments

The American Occupational Therapy Association (n.d.) and the American Occupational Therapy Foundation (n.d.) have stressed the importance of functional cognition across the life course and for individuals with various health conditions. They also have stated that the need for developing measures and effective interventions for functional cognition is high. Additionally, the World Health Organization's (2001) *International Classification of Functioning, Disability and Health* distinguishes body structure and function (i.e., impairment) from activity and participation (i.e., function and successful fulfillment of life roles, respectively).

Thus, it is important to expand on traditional cognitive assessment by identifying relevant domains for an ecologically valid measure of functional cognition. The AR takes this notion into account and defines *functional cognition* as the ability to accomplish everyday activities (in the area of everyday technology) that rely heavily on cognitive abilities. The AR is a functional–cognitive test that includes activities related to computer and Internet use.

References

American Occupational Therapy Association. (n.d.). *Role of occupational therapy in assessing functional cognition*. Retrieved from https://www.aota.org/Advocacy-Policy/Federal-Reg-Affairs/Medicare/Guidance/role-OT-assessing-functional-cognition.aspx

American Occupational Therapy Foundation. (n.d.). *Functional cognition*. Retrieved from https://www.aotf.org/About-AOTF/News/Events/Event-Detail/functional-cognition

Basak, T., Unver, V., & Demirkaya, S. (2015). Activities of daily living and self-care agency in patients with multiple sclerosis for the first 10 years. *Rehabilitation Nursing, 40,* 60–65. https://doi.org/10.1002/rnj.153

Baum, C., Edwards, D. F., & Morrow-Howell, N. (1993). Identification and measurement of productive behaviors in senile dementia of the Alzheimer type. *Gerontologist, 33,* 403–408. https://doi.org/10.1093/geront/33.3.403

Bergner, M., Bobbitt, R. A., Pollard, W. E., Martin, D. P., & Gilson, B. S. (1976). The Sickness Impact Profile: Validation of a health status measure. *Medical Care, 14,* 57–67. https://doi.org/10.1097/00005650-197601000-00006

Cella, D. F., Dineen, K., Arnason, B., Reder, A., Webster, K. A., Karabatsos, G., . . . Stefoski, D. (1996). Validation of the Functional Assessment of Multiple Sclerosis quality of life instrument. *Neurology, 47,* 129–139. https://doi.org/10.1212/WNL.47.1.129

Chiaravalloti, N. D., & DeLuca, J. (2008). Cognitive impairment in multiple sclerosis. *Lancet Neurology, 7,* 1139–1151. https://doi.org/10.1016/S1474-4422(08)70259-X

Chiaravalloti, N. D., & Goverover, Y. (Eds.). (2016). *Changes in the brain: Impact on daily life.* New York: Springer. https://doi.org/10.1007/978-0-387-98188-8

Doble, S. E., Fisk, J. D., Fisher, A. G., Ritvo, P. G., & Murray, T. J. (1994). Functional competence of community-dwelling persons with multiple sclerosis using the Assessment of Motor and Process Skills. *Archives of Physical Medicine and Rehabilitation, 75,* 843–851. https://doi.org/10.1016/0003-9993(94)90107-4

Einarsson, U., Gottberg, K., Fredrikson, S., Von Koch, L., & Holmqvist, L. W. (2006). Activities of daily living and social activities in people with multiple sclerosis in Stockholm County. *Clinical Rehabilitation, 20,* 543–551. https://doi.org/10.1191/0269215506cr953oa

Goverover, Y. (2018, April). *Assessment and the relationship between cognition and everyday technology use.* Paper presented at the AOTA Annual Conference & Expo, Salt Lake City.

Goverover, Y., Chiaravalloti, N., & DeLuca, J. (2005). The relationship between self-awareness of neurobehavioral symptoms, cognitive functioning, and emotional symptoms in multiple sclerosis. *Multiple Sclerosis, 11,* 203–212. https://doi.org/10.1191/1352458505ms1153oa

Goverover, Y., Chiaravalloti, N., & DeLuca, J. (2013). The influence of executive functions and memory on self-generation benefit in persons with multiple sclerosis. *Journal of Clinical and Experimental Neuropsychology, 35,* 775–783. https://doi.org/10.1080/13803395.2013.824553

Goverover, Y., Chiaravalloti, N., Gaudino-Goering, E., Moore, N., & DeLuca, J. (2009). The relationship among performance of instrumental activities of daily living, self-report of quality of life, and self-awareness of functional status in individuals with multiple sclerosis. *Rehabilitation Psychology, 54,* 60–68. https://doi.org/10.1037/a0014556

Goverover, Y., Chiaravalloti, N., Genova, H., & DeLuca, J. (2018). A randomized controlled trial to treat impaired learning and memory in multiple sclerosis: The self-GEN trial. *Multiple Sclerosis Journal, 24,* 1096–1104. https://doi.org/10.1177/1352458517709955

Goverover, Y., Chiaravalloti, N. D., O'Brien, A. R., & DeLuca, J. (2018). Evidenced-based cognitive rehabilitation for persons with multiple sclerosis: An updated review of the literature from 2007 to 2016. *Archives of Physical Medicine and Rehabilitation, 99,* 390–407. https://doi.org/10.1016/j.apmr.2017.07.021

Goverover, Y., & DeLuca, J. (2015). Actual Reality: Using the Internet to assess everyday functioning after traumatic brain injury. *Brain Injury, 29,* 715–721. https://doi.org/10.3109/02699052.2015.1004744

Goverover, Y., & DeLuca, J. (2018). Assessing everyday life functional activity using Actual Reality in persons with MS. *Rehabilitation Psychology, 63,* 276–285. https://doi.org/10.1037/rep0000212

Goverover, Y., Genova, H. M., DeLuca, J., & Chiaravalloti, N. D. (2016). Impact of multiple sclerosis on daily life. In N. D. Chiaravalloti & Y. Goverover (Eds.), *Changes in the brain: Impact on daily life* (pp. 145–165). New York: Springer. https://doi.org/10.1007/978-0-387-98188-8_7

Goverover, Y., Genova, H. M., Hillary, F. G., & DeLuca, J. (2007). The relationship between neuropsychological measures and the Timed Instrumental Activities of Daily Living task in multiple sclerosis. *Multiple Sclerosis Journal, 13,* 636–644. https://doi.org/10.1177/1352458506072984

Goverover, Y., Haas, S., & DeLuca, J. (2016). Money management activities in persons with multiple sclerosis. *Archives of Physical Medicine and Rehabilitation, 97,* 1901–1907. https://doi.org/10.1016/j.apmr.2016.05.003

Goverover, Y., Kalmar, J., Gaudino-Goering, E., Shawaryn, M., Moore, N. B., Halper, J., & DeLuca, J. (2005). The relation between subjective and objective measures of everyday life activities in persons with multiple sclerosis. *Archives of Physical Medicine and Rehabilitation, 86,* 2303–2308. https://doi.org/10.1016/j.apmr.2005.05.016

Goverover, Y., O'Brien, A. R., Moore, N. B., & DeLuca, J. (2010). Actual Reality: A new approach to functional assessment in persons with multiple sclerosis. *Archives of Physical Medicine and Rehabilitation, 91,* 252–260. https://doi.org/10.1016/j.apmr.2009.09.022

Goverover, Y., Sandroff, B. M., & DeLuca, J. (2018). Dual task of fine motor skill and problem solving in individuals with multiple sclerosis: A pilot study. *Archives of Physical Medicine and Rehabilitation, 99,* 635–640. https://doi.org/10.1016/j.apmr.2017.10.012

Goverover, Y., Strober, L., Chiaravalloti, N., & DeLuca, J. (2015). Factors that moderate activity limitation and participation restriction in people with multiple sclerosis. *American Journal of Occupational Therapy, 69,* 6902260020. https://doi.org/10.5014/ajot.2015.014332

Graf, C. (2008). The Lawton Instrumental Activities of Daily Living Scale. *American Journal of Nursing, 108*(4), 52–53. https://doi.org/10.1097/01.NAJ.0000314810.46029.74

Johnson, K. L., Bamer, A. M., Yorkston, K. M., & Amtmann, D. (2009). Use of cognitive aids and other assistive technology by individuals with multiple sclerosis. *Disability and Rehabilitation: Assistive Technology, 4,* 1–8. https://doi.org/10.1080/17483100802239648

Kalmar, J. H., Gaudino, E. A., Moore, N. B., Halper, J., & Deluca, J. (2008). The relationship between cognitive deficits and everyday functional activities in multiple sclerosis. *Neuropsychology, 22,* 442–449. https://doi.org/10.1037/0894-4105.22.4.442

Kurtzke, J. F. (2015). On the origin of EDSS. *Multiple Sclerosis and Related Disorders, 4,* 95–103. https://doi.org/10.1016/j.msard.2015.02.003

Larsson Lund, M., Lövgren-Engström, A. L., & Lexell, J. (2011). Using everyday technology to compensate for difficulties in task performance in daily life: Experiences in persons with acquired brain injury and their significant others. *Disability and Rehabilitation:*

Assistive Technology, 6, 402–411. https://doi.org/10.3109/17483107.2011.574309

Owsley, C., McGwin, G., Jr., Sloane, M. E., Stalvey, B. T., & Wells, J. (2001). Timed Instrumental Activities of Daily Living tasks: Relationship to visual function in older adults. *Optometry and Vision Science, 78,* 350–359. https://doi.org/10.1097/00006324-200105000-00019

Pugliatti, M., Rosati, G., Carton, H., Riise, T., Drulovic, J., Vécsei, L., & Milanov, I. (2006). The epidemiology of multiple sclerosis in Europe. *European Journal of Neurology, 13,* 700–722. https://doi.org/10.1111/j.1468-1331.2006.01342.x

Rudick, R., Antel, J., Confavreux, C., Cutter, G., Ellison, G., Fischer, J., . . . Willoughby, E. (1997). Recommendations from the National Multiple Sclerosis Society Clinical Outcomes Assessment Task Force. *Annals of Neurology, 42,* 379–382. https://doi.org/10.1002/ana.410420318

Sacco, R., Bisecco, A., Corbo, D., Della Corte, M., d'Ambrosio, A., Docimo, R., . . . Bonavita, S. (2015). Cognitive impairment and memory disorders in relapsing–remitting multiple sclerosis: The role of white matter, gray matter and hippocampus. *Journal of Neurology, 262,* 1691–1697. https://doi.org/10.1007/s00415-015-7763-y

Steene-Johannessen, J., Anderssen, S. A., Van der Ploeg, H. P., Hendriksen, I. J. M., Donnelly, A. E., Brage, S., & Ekelund, U. (2016). Are self-report measures able to define individuals as physically active or inactive? *Medicine and Science in Sports and Exercise, 48,* 235–244.

Tracy, V. L., Basso, M. R., Marson, D. C., Combs, D. R., & Whiteside, D. M. (2017). Capacity for financial decision making in multiple sclerosis. *Journal of Clinical and Experimental Neuropsychology, 39,* 46–57. https://doi.org/10.1080/13803395.2016.1201050

U.S. Census Bureau. (2014). *Computer and Internet use in the United States: 2013* (Report Number ACS-28). Retrieved from https://www.census.gov/library/publications/2014/acs/acs-28.html

Wong, D., Sinclair, K., Seabrook, E., McKay, A., & Ponsford, J. (2017). Smartphones as assistive technology following traumatic brain injury: A preliminary study of what helps and what hinders. *Disability and Rehabilitation, 39,* 2387–2394. https://doi.org/10.1080/09638288.2016.1226434

World Health Organization. (2001). *International classification of functioning, disability and health.* Geneva: Author.

12

Performance Assessment of Self-Care Skills

JOAN C. ROGERS, PhD, OTR, FAOTA; MARGO B. HOLM, PhD, OTR/L, FAOTA, ABDA; AND DENISE CHISHOLM, PhD, OTR/L, FAOTA

LEARNING OBJECTIVES

After completing this chapter, readers should be able to

- Discuss the conceptual foundations of the Performance Assessment of Self-Care Skills (PASS),
- Describe the content and structure of the PASS,
- Explain how the PASS is rated and scored, and
- Give examples of how PASS data lead to an intervention plan.

KEY TERMS AND CONCEPTS

- Dynamic–interactive assessment • Observable task behaviors

People may doubt what you say, but they will always believe what you do.

—Anonymous

Introduction

The Performance Assessment of Self-Care Skills (PASS; Rogers et al., 2016a, 2016b) was developed in response to a clinical need: to provide occupational therapy practitioners with a performance-based instrument to observe and document systematically the skills clients need to live independently in the community. At the time of its inception in 1984, multiple instruments were available to evaluate personal care activities (e.g., FIM®; Keith et al., 1987; Barthel Index; Mahoney & Barthel, 1965), such as feeding, dressing, hygiene, bathing, and functional mobility. However, no performance instrument was available to systematically evaluate community-living skills, commonly referred to as *IADLs*. The lack of performance instruments forced a reliance on self-report or proxy report methodologies, with their associated problems in reliability and validity.

The PASS was developed to fill this gap. In addition to emphasizing IADLs, the PASS fulfills 2 other needs. First, it goes beyond providing information on a client's performance status (i.e., performance is rated as independent, safe, and adequate). The PASS provides information that practitioners can use to guide intervention to improve or stabilize the client's occupational performance.

Second, the PASS supports the occupational therapy process by incorporating the test–intervention–retest paradigm typically used by occupational therapy practitioners. When a performance problem occurs during testing, the practitioner interrupts the testing and intervenes—that is, provides assistance for the part of the task that is problematic—so that the client can proceed with the remainder of the task. The practitioner then documents what was problematic for the client and the type of assistance given.

For example, for the PASS Medication Management item, if the client distributes the wrong number of pills for morning and evening on the medication sheet, the occupational therapy practitioner interrupts the client and gives a verbal cue, such as, "Want to check that again?" If multiple verbal cues are given and the client is still unable to self-correct, the practitioner might use a gesture and point to the directions on the medication label. If this solves the problem, the client can proceed with sorting the 2nd medication. In PASS testing, the point of task breakdown (incorrect sorting of medications) is documented, as are the practitioner's interventions (verbal cues, gestures). Helping clients to do better in the context of testing is usually not allowed, which is 1 reason why practitioners tend to shy away from standardized tests.

Psychometrics

The content validity of the PASS—that is, the inclusion of items in both the Clinic and the Home versions of the PASS—was based primarily on the content of 4 validated tools:

1. IADL Scale (Lawton & Brody, 1969)

2. Comprehensive Assessment and Referral Evaluation (Gurland et al., 1978)

3. Older Americans Resources and Services Multidimensional Functional Assessment Questionnaire (Fillenbaum & Smyer, 1981)

4. Functional Activities Questionnaire (Pfeffer, 1987).

These self-report and proxy-report tools delineate critical activity categories for independent living, such as preparing food, managing medications, taking care of the house, handling finances, shopping, using the telephone, doing laundry, using transportation, assembling tax records, and playing a game of skill. With feedback from the clinical community, we chose 26 core items for the PASS representing the activity categories and operationalized them into observable task behaviors. **Observable task behaviors** consist of the sequence of observable steps in a task and are referred to as *subtasks*.

The content of the Home and the Clinic versions of the PASS is the same; however, in the Home version, clients use their own materials. In both versions of the PASS, items are categorized on the basis of their primary emphasis. The majority of items are IADLs with a cognitive emphasis (IADLs–C; 14 items), followed by items focused on

- Functional mobility (FM; 5 items),

- IADLs with a physical emphasis (IADLs–P; 4 items), and

- Basic ADLs (BADLs; 3 items).

The construct validity of the PASS measures (i.e., independence, safety, adequacy) was established with factor analysis and Cattell's scree test (Cattell, 1966; Chisholm, 2005), and the construct validity of the 26 core items was confirmed with Rasch analysis (Chisholm, 2005). Construct validity was also confirmed with known-groups differences (Chisholm, 2005; Goldstein et al., 1992; Holm & Rogers, 1990a, 1990b; McCue et al., 1990; Rogers & Holm, 1990; Rogers et al., 1994). Test–retest reliability with a 3-day interval was adequate to

excellent (PASS Clinic version: independence, $r = .92$, safety = 89%; adequacy, $r = .82$; PASS Home version: independence, $r = .96$, safety = 97%; adequacy, $r = .97$). Interobserver reliability in the Clinic and the Home versions ranged from 92% to 96% for independence, 93% to 97% for safety, and 88% to 90% for adequacy.

Functional Cognition and the PASS

Several research studies have focused on the effectiveness of the PASS IADL–C items for assessing *functional cognition*— that is, the cognitive processes necessary to perform the 14 IADL–C daily tasks. These studies focused on clients with varying degrees of cognitive deficits. Depressive disorders are often associated with problems in attention, memory, and decision making (Rubin & Zorumski, 2016). Therefore, Chisholm (2005), using Rasch analysis, compared patients being treated for depression who performed slower and faster on the Trail Making Test (Reitan, 1958) and found that those who performed slower had significantly lower scores on the PASS IADL–C items. In a related study, again using Rasch analysis, Chisholm (2005) found that the performance of inpatients of a psychiatric hospital was significantly lower on the PASS IADL–C items than the performance of hospital outpatients being treated at the same time.

More recently, Bingham et al. (2018), in a systematic review of 21 functional assessment instruments, recommended 2 instruments, including the PASS, for use with patients with late-life depression. Their recommendation was based on the instruments' "ability to distinguish between late-life depression patients with differing levels of depression severity and neuropsychological impairment" (p. 65).

In 2016, after the *Williams v. Quinn* (2010) consent decree class-action lawsuit, which enabled individuals with serious mental illness to be discharged from state-funded institutions into communities with professional support, the PASS was chosen to assess residents who had been institutionalized for up to 31 years. Of the first 40 residents evaluated on 9 IADL–C items, residents scored highest on safety, followed by independence, and then adequacy. Although the residents were careful about safety and tried to be as independent as possible, they had difficulty meeting community standards of quality and accuracy, possibly because they had been sheltered for so long (Holm, 2017).

Clients with major neurocognitive disorder (NCD), mild cognitive impairment (MCI), and Parkinson's disease are known to have varying levels and forms of cognitive impairment. In 2014, Rodakowski et al. tested whether 8 PASS IADL–C items could distinguish control participants from those with MCI. All 8 items separated the groups with 81% accuracy, but 2 items alone (shopping, checkbook balancing) separated the groups with 80% accuracy.

In 2015, Ciro et al. compared clients with amnesic MCI with age- and gender-matched control participants on the

14 PASS IADL–C items. Participants with MCI scored significantly lower than the control participants overall and significantly lower for 9 of the 14 IADL–C adequacy measures (i.e., measures associated with accuracy and quality).

In 1999, Dr. Rogers and Dr. Holm were informed by the chief of the Office of Science Policy and Public Liaison, National Institute of Nursing Research (NINR), that a study they had conducted (Rogers et al., 1999) would be part of the Congressional Justification documents (D. J. O'Neal III, personal communication, 1999). The study used adapted PASS items and a modified scoring system. It was presented as "one of a few 'science advances' selected by NINR to feature as examples of research that taxpayer money has generated, research which has 'made a difference' in peoples' lives." This same study was later cited by the Health Care Financing Administration (HCFA), now the Centers for Medicare and Medicaid Services, as 1 of 2 studies that changed HCFA policy to allow patients with major NCD to receive and be reimbursed for rehabilitation services.

In addition to items that focus on emotional and physical health, population studies also include items on cognitive health. In a population-based study associated with health policy—the Aging in Manitoba Study—Brown and Finlayson (2013) compared self-report data and PASS data from 6 IADL–C items and 1 FM item. They found that the "odds of receiving health care within the 30-month follow-up period were 30% higher for each increase in the number of dependent PASS tasks" (p. 284). This explained why respondents' overestimation (self-report) of their function in previous years also might have been 1 of the contributors to health care budget deficits.

Content and Structure

The PASS 4.1 (Rogers et al., 2016a, 2016b) consists of 26 core items, which are grouped into 4 functional domains: IADL–C, FM, IADL–P, and BADL. The criterion for each subtask of a task is the behavior that can be expected of persons who are able to live independently in the community. If living independently in the community is not consistent with a client's discharge status, then the PASS can be used to identify the level of support the client needs to participate in each task item.

The IADL–C domain comprises 14 items, 4 of which involve money management—shopping, paying bills, balancing a checkbook, and mailing a payment. Three IADL–C items involve meal preparation—preparing food using the oven, preparing food using the stovetop, and using sharp utensils. The remaining 7 IADL–C items assess using the telephone, managing medications, obtaining information from visual media, obtaining information from auditory media, repairing a flashlight, being aware of safety factors in the home environment, and playing bingo (representative of leisure).

Five items are in the FM domain: (1) moving in bed, (2) using the stairs, (3) managing toileting, (4) managing tub and shower

mobility, and (5) walking indoors. The 3rd functional domain, IADL–P, consists of 4 items representing light and heavy housework: (1) cleaning up after meal preparation, (2) changing bed linens, (3) sweeping the floor, and (4) removing garbage. Three items are in the BADL domain: (1) performing oral hygiene, (2) trimming toenails, and (3) dressing.

The 26 core items of the PASS represent the array of daily living tasks required to live independently in the community (see Exhibit 12.1). When administered in order, the initial items (FM and BADL) are easy for most clients and nonthreatening to perform. The occupational therapy practitioner then administers the more complex IADL–C and IADL–P items, alternating these more difficult tasks with FM and BADL items. The final 4 task items require the client to plan, organize, and follow through with the making of a light meal consisting of soup, muffins, and fruit and to clean up after the meal.

However, each item of the PASS is valid and reliable and can stand alone (Holm & Rogers, 2008; Rogers et al., 2001). Thus, it is not necessary to administer all 26 items of the PASS. Instead, one can administer 1, 3, 5, 10, or any number of items, depending on the referral and the needs of the client.

For the purposes of guiding the practitioner's observation and rating of the client's performance, each of the 26 task items is dissected into its critical subtasks. These subtasks are observed and rated by the practitioner. In this way, the PASS takes advantage of occupational therapists' expertise in task analysis. The yield from focusing on a task's subtasks is that the practitioner knows the exact point of the task where the client's performance is dependent, unsafe, or inadequate, and they can identify a target for intervention.

The PASS assessment process is known as ***dynamic–interactive assessment*** and is based on the work of the Soviet psychologist Lev Vygotsky (Vygotsky, 1978). Dynamic–interactive assessment includes the identification of critical subtasks in daily activities using task analysis. When a client cannot perform a subtask, the practitioner intervenes with ever-more powerful assists until the client can perform the task. The difference between the desired performance (critical subtasks) and the client's performance (assists required) is recorded. Vygotsky named this difference the "zone of proximal development" (p. 84).

Similarly, when a client cannot perform a subtask, the PASS encourages practitioners to intervene directly but systematically. The practitioner provides assistance moving from the least assistive intervention (encouragement) to the most assistive (doing the subtask for the client). When the client has completed the task item, the practitioner can identify potential intervention strategies to improve or stabilize task performance, on the basis of the points of task breakdown as well as the level of intervention that enabled the client to complete the subtask and move on to the next subtask.

This type of assessment process—which mixes intervention with assessment—mirrors that naturally used by occupational therapy practitioners. However, most formal testing procedures prohibit the assessor from assisting clients during

EXHIBIT 12.1. PASS, Version 4.1, Table of Contents (Home Version)

Page	Items Administered	Task	ADL/IADL	
4	_____	# H1	FM:	Bed Mobility
6	_____	# H2	FM:	Stair Use
8	_____	# H3	FM:	Toilet Mobility and Management
10	_____	# H4	BADL:	Oral Hygiene
12	_____	# H5	FM:	Bathtub and Shower Mobility
14	_____	# H6	BADL:	Trimming Toenails
16	_____	# H7	BADL:	Dressing
18	_____	# H8	IADL-C:	Shopping (Money Management)
20	_____	# H9	IADL-C:	Bill Paying by Check (Money Management)
22	_____	# H10	IADL-C:	Checkbook Balancing (Money Management)
24	_____	# H11	IADL-C:	Mailing Bills (Money Management)
26	_____	# H12	IADL-P:	Taking Out Garbage; Key Use (Heavy Housework)
28	_____	# H13	IADL-C:	Telephone Use
30	_____	# H14	IADL-C:	Medication Management
32	_____	# H15	IADL-P:	Changing Bed Linens (Heavy Housework)
34	_____	# H16	IADL-C:	Obtaining Critical Information from the Media (Auditory)
36	_____	# H17	IADL-C:	Obtaining Critical Information from the Media (Visual)
38	_____	# H18	IADL-C:	Flashlight Repair (Home Maintenance)
40	_____	# H19	IADL-P:	Sweeping (Home Maintenance)
42	_____	# H20	FM:	Indoor Walking
44	_____	# H21	IADL-C:	Home Safety
46	_____	# H22	IADL-C:	Playing Bingo
48	_____	# H23	IADL-C:	Oven Use (Meal Preparation)
50	_____	# H24	IADL-C:	Stovetop Use (Meal Preparation)
52	_____	# H25	IADL-C:	Use of Sharp Utensils (Meal Preparation)
54	_____	# H26	IADL-P:	Cleanup after Meal Preparation (Light Housework)

Note. BADL = basic ADL; FM = functional mobility; IADL–C = IADL with a cognitive emphasis; IADL–P = IADL with a physical emphasis; PASS = Performance Assessment of Self-Care Skills.
Source. From *Performance Assessment of Self-Care Skills–Version 4.1*, by J. C. Rogers, M. B. Holm, and D. Chisholm, 2016, Pittsburgh: University of Pittsburgh. Copyright © 2016 by J. C. Rogers, M. B. Holm, and D. Chisholm. All rights reserved. Reprinted with permission.

testing. The PASS encourages systematic intervention, with the practitioner giving cues or prompts in a defined order from least to most assistive as well as recording which assists they gave for which subtasks.

Target Population

The PASS is intended for clients who need an assessment of their ability to perform the daily living tasks they need to live independently in the community. It yields the level of their independence, safety, and task adequacy as they perform tasks that they need to do, are expected to do, or want to do. Within these broad parameters, the PASS is gender neutral, age neutral, and diagnosis neutral. Stated otherwise, the measure is appropriate for both women and men from late adolescence through later adulthood, regardless of medical or psychiatric diagnosis or developmental condition, when the assessment focus is the individual's ability to live independently.

The PASS was devised specifically for Western culture but has been culturally adapted and translated into Arabic, Farsi, Finnish, French, Hebrew, Japanese, Korean, Portuguese, Spanish, Turkish, and Australian and Irish English. It is appropriate for adolescents who are preparing to live independently or who might meet criteria for being accepted into a group home or community-living arrangement. It is appropriate for clients who were living independently in the community before a medical event and wish to return to independent living after the event. It is also appropriate for clients who have been residing in sheltered housing and wish to return or move to the community.

The occupational therapy evaluation should take into account the tasks that clients need to, are expected to, or want to perform in the proposed living situation, as well as caregivers who are willing and able to help. Each of the 26 core PASS items stands alone and has established validity and reliability. Therefore, the practitioner can choose which items are appropriate to administer. If a client has never cooked, for example, it may be appropriate to omit the meal preparation items. Similarly, for some assisted living settings, residents are expected to manage their own medications, so the medication management item would be appropriate, whereas in other settings, this is a provided service and the medication item could be omitted.

As mentioned, there are 2 versions of the PASS: Clinic and Home. The tasks and subtasks are the same, but for the Clinic version materials are provided for the client, and for the Home version clients use their own objects and materials. In the hospital, acute care, or rehabilitation settings the Clinic version is most appropriate, and for home health and community settings the Home version is most appropriate. Because the 2 versions have identical subtasks to rate but different problems to solve, they can also be used for retesting of clients to avoid learning effects.

Administration

The PASS is free and available to occupational therapy practitioners (contact PASS@shrs.pitt.edu). After completing a short survey, the practitioner is given the URL for the PASS Box. The box includes the PASS–Clinic, the PASS–Home, the materials needed to administer the tools, the scoring guidelines (i.e., manual; Rogers et al., 2016b), and access to administration and scoring videos.

The administration videos show a practitioner administering each of the 26 core PASS items and can be used for training. The scoring videos show a practitioner administering each of the 26 core items to a client who demonstrates problems in performance. Attached to the videos are copies of the authors' rating and scoring sheets for the video clients. These videos can also be used for training. The manual also includes information about how practitioners can calculate their interrater reliabilities against the authors' for each PASS item.

Additionally, the PASS Box includes items developed by practitioners and references for practitioners translating the PASS into other languages and adapting or developing items for other cultures. PASS workshops are usually offered once a year, and companies, state associations, and other organizations can arrange for workshops by contacting PASS@shrs.pitt.edu. The same address can be used for questions about scoring or interpretation of results.

The format and structure of PASS items are shown in Exhibits 12.2 and 12.3 (Medication Management item). As shown in Exhibit 12.2, all PASS items include a "Conditions" section in which the standardized items and their placement, as well as the positioning of the client, are described. This is important for reliability, because if pre-assessment–post-assessment data are recorded and the conditions are not the same, then it is unclear whether the client's progress or lack thereof is due to the intervention or the change in testing conditions. Exhibit 12.2 also includes the instructions for what the practitioner needs to say and do when administering the task to the client. Additionally, Exhibit 12.2 includes the PASS scoring template for the 3 PASS scores: Independence, Safety, and Adequacy.

EXHIBIT 12.2. PASS Conditions, Instructions, and Scoring Template (Medication Management Item–Home Version)

Task # H14: IADL-C Medication Management

HOME CONDITIONS: Table and
1. Seven-day medication sheet with 4 subdivisions for each day – Morning, Noon, Evening, Bedtime
2. 2 of Client's prescription medications:
   - If Client is taking only 1 medication, substitute PASS-Home child-proof lid (C-P) medication containing red vitamin pills and a typed label that reads "Take 2 with breakfast and 1 with lunch and dinner";
   - If Client is not taking any prescription medications, add the PASS-Home non-child-proof lid (N-C-P) medication containing yellow vitamin pills and a typed label that reads "Take 1 tablet with lunch and 1 at bedtime."
3. Items 1-2 on table in front of Client
4. Client seated at the table

Client has......	Present 1st	Present 2nd
2 meds	Either med	Either med
1 med	PASS-Home C-P lid med	Client's med
0 meds	PASS-Home C-P lid med	PASS-Home N-C-P lid med

HOME INSTRUCTIONS:

"The next task involves managing medications. Please show me where you keep your medications. [Select 2 medications to use for the assessment, preferably with different time schedules]. I need to borrow these two bottles for the next task. I will put them back as soon as we are done." [Return to the table where the task items are set up]

"Please read the prescription label and find the directions for taking this medication [Hand Client first bottle of own medication or bottle with child-proof lid and wait until Client looks up]. If you were taking this medication today, when would you have to take the next pill?" [Wait for response].

"This medication organizer is like a pillbox. It has the days of the week across the top [Point] and the time of the day [Point] along the side. Using the organizer, distribute the pills to be taken tomorrow and the following day according to the directions on the prescription label. Do you know what you are to do? Do you have everything that you need?" [Wait for response]

"Now, please read the prescription label on this bottle and find the directions for taking this medication [Hand Client second bottle of own medication or bottle with non-child-proof lid and wait until Client looks up]. If you were taking this medication today, when would you have to take the next pill?" [Wait for response]

"Again, using the organizer, distribute the pills to be taken tomorrow and the following day according to the prescription directions on the label. Do you know what you are to do?" [Wait for response]

SCORE	INDEPENDENCE	SAFETY	ADEQUACY	
			PROCESS	QUALITY
3	No assists given for task initiation, continuation, or completion	Safe practices were observed	Subtasks performed with precision & economy of effort & action	Optimal (performance matches the quality standards listed in each subtask)
2	No Level 7-9 assists given, but occasional Level 1-6 assists given	Minor risks were evident but no assistance provided	Subtasks generally performed w/ precision & economy of effort & action; occasional lack of efficiency, redundant or extraneous action; no missing steps	Acceptable (Performance, for the most part, matches or nearly matches the quality standards listed in each subtask)
1	No Level 9 assists given; or occasional Level 7 or 8 assists given; or continuous Level 1-6 assists given	Risks to safety were observed and assistance given to prevent potential harm	Subtasks generally performed w/ lack of precision and/or economy of effort & action; consistent extraneous or redundant actions; steps may be missing	Marginal (Performance, for the most part, does not match the quality standards listed in each subtask)
0	Level 9 assists given; or continuous Level 7 or 8 assists given; or unable to initiate, continue, or complete subtask or task	Risks to safety of such severity were observed that task was stopped or taken over by assessor to prevent harm	Subtasks are consistently performed w/ lack of precision and/or economy of effort & action so that task progress is unattainable	Unacceptable (Performance does not match the quality standards listed in each subtask, perhaps with few exceptions)

Note. IADL–C = IADL with a cognitive emphasis; med(s) = medication(s); PASS = Performance Assessment of Self-Care Skills.
Source. From *Performance Assessment of Self-Care Skills–Version 4.1*, by J. C. Rogers, M. B. Holm, and D. Chisholm, 2016, Pittsburgh: University of Pittsburgh. Copyright © 2016 by J. C. Rogers, M. B. Holm, and D. Chisholm. All rights reserved. Reprinted with permission.

EXHIBIT 12.3. PASS Rating Form for Item Subtasks (Medication Management Item–Home Version) and Summary Scores

Task # H14: IADL-C: Medication Management		INDEPENDENCE DATA											SAFETY DATA	ADEQUACY DATA		SUMMARY SCORES
Assistive Technology Devices (ATDs) used during task: 1. 2. 3. Total # of ATDs used:_____		No Assistance	Verbal Supportive (Encouragement)	Verbal Non-Directive	Verbal Directive	Gestures	Task or Environment Rearrangement	Demonstration	Physical Guidance	Physical Support	Total Assist	INDEPENDENCE subtask scores	Unsafe Observations	PROCESS: Imprecision, lack of economy, missing steps	QUALITY: Standards not met / improvement needed	
Assist level →		0	1	2	3	4	5	6	7	8	9					
Subtasks	Subtask Criteria															
1 Med 1 C-P*	Reports next time first medication is to be taken correctly (based on testing time, matches direction on label)															INDEPENDENCE MEAN SCORE
2 Med 1 C-P	Opens first pill bottle with ease (by second try)															
3 Med 1 C-P	Distributes pills from first pill bottle into correct time slots for the next 2 days (all pills & all slots indicated; days indicated)															
4 Med2 N-C-P*	Reports next time second medication is to be taken correctly (based on testing time, matches direction on label)															SAFETY SCORE
5 Med2 N-C-P	Opens second pill bottle with ease (by second try)															
6 Med2 N-C-P	Distributes pills from second pill bottle into correct time slots for the next 2 days (all pills and all slots indicated; days indicated)															ADEQUACY SCORE

Note. C-P = childproof lid; IADL–C = IADL with a cognitive emphasis; med = medication; N-C-P = nonchildproof lid; PASS = Performance Assessment of Self-Care Skills

Source. From *Performance Assessment of Self-Care Skills–Version 4.1*, by J. C. Rogers, M. B. Holm, and D. Chisholm, 2016, Pittsburgh: University of Pittsburgh. Copyright © 2016 by J. C. Rogers, M. B. Holm, and D. Chisholm. All rights reserved. Reprinted with permission.

Exhibit 12.3 is the data collection form that guides the practitioner's observations. First, if the client requires the use of any assistive technology devices, these are recorded and tallied. Next, the critical subtasks are listed in the usual order of their occurrence, which cues the occupational therapy practitioner to observe them and be ready to assist if the client has a problem performing the task. This is also the form used to rate and score the client's independence, safety, and adequacy of task performance.

Independence Data

Each subtask begins with a double-underlined action phrase—the behavior that is the focus of the independence rating (see Exhibit 12.3). If the occupational therapy practitioner provides no assistance for Subtask 1, they put an X in the "No Assistance" box across from Subtask 1. However, if the client needs assistance with dynamic assessment, it is given in a hierarchical manner, with each level of assistance more powerful and intrusive than the last, until the client is able to perform Subtask 1 and move on to Subtask 2. Levels of assistance are arranged from least to most assistance (1–9), with each level of assistance requiring greater attention by the practitioner and, ultimately, greater cost of care.

Levels 1–3 are categorized as verbal assists. Level 1, verbal supportive, is used to assure and motivate the client to begin, continue, or complete a subtask. Level 2, verbal nondirective, is used to alert the client to a problem and allow the client to self-correct. Level 3, verbal directive, is used if the client cannot self-correct and the practitioner gives verbal directions to the client about how to fix the problem.

Levels 4–6 are categorized as gestural assists. Level 4, gestures, can include verbal statements, but gestures such as pointing are added. Level 5, task or environment rearrangement, means that the practitioner changes the task order or presentation or removes task items from the standardized format to enable the client to proceed. Level 6, demonstration, is used by the practitioner to show the client what is expected; however, not all items are appropriate for demonstration. For example, one cannot put the soup back in the can.

Levels 7–9 are categorized as physical assists. Level 7, physical guidance, is used by the practitioner to guide (hands down) a client's hand onto the next clothing item to put on. Level 8, physical support, is used by the practitioner to lift or support a client's body part or task item (hands up). Last, Level 9, total assist, indicates that the practitioner needed to take over 1 or more of the subtasks for the client to continue (or needed to take over the total task).

As the practitioner provides assists, they enter a check mark across from the subtask that is problematic (e.g., Subtask 2) and under the type of assist provided (e.g., Level 3, verbal directive; see Exhibit 12.3). As a general rule, no more than 3 assists of the same type should be given (e.g., Level 3, verbal directive), because it means that a more powerful assist is needed (e.g., Level 4, gestures). Although the practitioner should provide the lowest assist followed by progressively more powerful assists, at times a more powerful assist is needed immediately (e.g., safety issue). See the PASS manual for more examples.

Safety Data

Subtasks that do not have a shaded box in the "Safety Data" column are rated for safety issues in the "Unsafe Observations" box across from the subtask (see Exhibit 12.3). If the occupational therapy practitioner observes an unsafe action by the client that has the immediate potential for harm to (or that actually harms) the client, the practitioner, or the environment, the practitioner enters a check mark in the "Safety Data" column and makes a note in the margin of the form as to the specific safety issue. If no safety issues are observed, the "Safety Data" box is left blank. See the PASS manual for more examples.

It is important to note that with the PASS, safety is rated for the immediate context. For example, if a client writes a PASS check that will overdraw the bank account, it is not an immediate safety risk, but the lack of understanding about bank balances is a concern and a target for intervention. However, if a client grabs on to a loosened towel rack when exiting the bathtub, this is an immediate safety risk and warrants a check mark in the "Safety Data" column.

Adequacy Data

The adequacy of a client's task performance consists of 2 components: (1) process and (2) quality (see Exhibit 12.3). Task process ratings apply to the double-underlined actions in each subtask. If the client

- Demonstrates imprecision in carrying out the subtask actions (e.g., calculates and recalculates the bank balance several times),

- Lacks economy of effort (e.g., looks in several cupboards for the milk instead of in the refrigerator), or

- Misses steps in the process of a subtask (e.g., leaves out 1 of the muffin ingredients), the practitioner places a check mark across from a subtask in the "Process" column and makes a note in the margin.

Task quality ratings apply to the single-underlined terms in Exhibit 12.3, which are followed by clarifications in parentheses. For example, on Medication Management Subtask 1, task quality would be rated on "correctly (based on testing time, matches direction on label)." Again, if the client has performance problems with the quality of a subtask, the occupational therapy practitioner places a check mark across from the subtask in the Quality column, with a note in the margin. See the PASS manual for more examples.

Medication Management Video: Sandy

The PASS Medication Management item (see Video 12.1 and Exhibit 12.4) addresses critical behaviors that clients need to demonstrate if they are expected to manage their medications at home. **Sandy** is a stroke survivor (right cerebral vascular accident). He lives alone and is responsible for his BADLs and IADLs, including managing his many medications. To fully make use of Video 12.1, you may find it helpful to print Exhibits 12.2 and 12.3 so that you can follow as **Dr. Holm** administers the Medication Management item with Sandy. After you review the video, move on to the section on scoring to see how the PASS is scored and the results of Sandy's performance.

Scoring

Scoring Independence
Scoring of a PASS item begins with the independence data. First, because Sandy did not need any assists for Subtasks, 1, 2, 3, and 5, Dr. Holm entered an *X* in the "No Assistance" column for those subtasks (see Exhibit 12.4). She also entered a score of 3 opposite each of those subtasks in the "Independence Subtask Scores" column. A score of 3 (see the scoring template in Exhibit 12.2) means that no assistance was provided for Subtasks 1, 2, 3, and 5. However, Dr. Holm did provide assistance for Subtasks 4 and 6.

For Subtask 4, "Reports next time second medication is to be taken correctly (based on testing time, matches direction on label)," Dr. Holm gestured toward the medication label because Sandy was reading the wrong information. Thus, there is a check mark for Subtask 4 in the "Gestures" column. In the "Independence Subtask Scores" column, Dr. Holm entered a score of 2 for Subtask 4. According to the scoring template (see Exhibit 12.2), in the "Independence Subtask Scores" column, a score of 2 is given when "No Level 7–9 assists given, but occasional Level 1–6 assists given."

When rating Sandy on Subtask 6, Dr. Holm entered 3 check marks in the "Verbal Directive" column. Although she could have used a verbal nondirective, such as, "Are you sure that is correct?" Dr. Holm chose to use the more powerful verbal directive (i.e., "Let's check the label") because Sandy had already had difficulty with the label directions on Subtask 4. Next, she provided another verbal directive (i.e., "OK. Do you want to check the label again please?"). On Sandy's 3rd attempt, Dr. Holm gave another verbal directive (i.e., "Let's try it again").

EXHIBIT 12.4. Dr. Holm's Rating and Scoring Form for Sandy's Performance on the PASS (Medication Management Item–Home Version)

Task # H14: IADL-C: Medication Management		INDEPENDENCE DATA										INDEPENDENCE subtask scores	SAFETY DATA — Unsafe Observations	ADEQUACY DATA — PROCESS: Imprecision, lack of economy, missing steps	QUALITY: Standards not met / improvement needed	SUMMARY SCORES
Assistive Technology Devices (ATDs) used during task: 1. 2. 3. Total # of ATDs used:_____		No Assistance	Verbal Supportive (Encouragement)	Verbal Non-Directive	Verbal Directive	Gestures	Task or Environment Rearrangement	Demonstration	Physical Guidance	Physical Support	Total Assist					
	Assist level →	0	1	2	3	4	5	6	7	8	9					
Subtasks	**Subtask Criteria**															
1 Med 1 C-P*	Reports next time first medication is to be taken correctly (based on testing time, matches direction on label)	X										3				**2.5** INDEPENDENCE MEAN SCORE ↑
2 Med 1 C-P	Opens first pill bottle with ease (by second try)	X										3				
3 Med 1 C-P	Distributes pills from first pill bottle into correct time slots for the next 2 days (all pills & all slots indicated; days indicated)	X										3				
4 Med2 N-C-P*	Reports next time second medication is to be taken correctly (based on testing time, matches direction on label)				√							2				**3** SAFETY SCORE ↑
5 Med2 N-C-P	Opens second pill bottle with ease (by second try)	X										3				
6 Med2 N-C-P	Distributes pills from second pill bottle into correct time slots for the next 2 days (all pills and all slots indicated; days indicated)				√√ √							1		√	√	**2** ADEQUACY SCORE ↑

#4 Gesture – Dr. Holm pointed to the correct portion of the label that Sandy needed to read to answer the question
NOTE: No check marks were entered into PROCESS or QUALITY because the gesture was not related to the Standard (Reports next time correctly)
#6 Verbal Directive: Dr. Holm says "Let's check the label" and looks at it with Sandy
#6 Verbal Directive: Dr. Holm says "OK. Do you want to check the label again please."
#6 Verbal Directive: Dr. Holm says "mmmm. Let's try it again."

Independence = 2.5 No level 7-9 assist given, but occasional Level 1-6 assists given (15/6=2.5)
Safety = 3 because he had no issues opening/closing the medication containers
Adequacy = 2 (Acceptable (of the 6 subtasks Sandy only had difficulty with one of the subtasks (#4 cue does not count because it does not relate to a Standard)

Note. C-P = childproof lid; IADL–C = IADL with a cognitive emphasis; med = medication; N-C-P = nonchildproof lid; PASS = Performance Assessment of Self-Care Skills.
Source. From *Performance Assessment of Self-Care Skills–Version 4.1*, by J. C. Rogers, M. B. Holm, and D. Chisholm, 2016, Pittsburgh: University of Pittsburgh. Copyright © 2016 by J. C. Rogers, M. B. Holm, and D. Chisholm. All rights reserved. Reprinted with permission.

Thus, for Subtask 6, there are 3 check marks in the "Verbal Directive" column. The score in the "Independence Subtask Scores" column is a 1 (see Exhibit 12.2 in the "Independence" section: "No Level 9 assists given; or occasional Level 7 or 8 assists given; or continuous Level 1–6 assists given").

The final step in scoring independence is calculating the independence summary score. For independence, the summary score is the mean of the independence subtask scores. For Sandy, on the Medication Management item, his independence subtask scores were 3, 3, 3, 2, 3, and 1, for a total of 15. To obtain the mean, the practitioner divides the total by the number of subtasks (i.e., 6 subtasks; 15/6 = 2.5). Note that the independence mean score is rounded down to the nearest decimal. This is because it is better not to overestimate clients' performance and place them at risk. Although Sandy was independent in 4 of the 6 medication management subtasks, the 2 subtasks that were problematic are now targets for intervention.

With an independence summary score range of 0–3, a mean of 2.5 is near the middle of the 2 score, which indicates that Sandy needed assistance for 1 or more subtasks. If Sandy had needed assistance for each of the 6 subtasks, his independence summary score might have been 2 + 2 + 2 + 2 + 2 + 2 for a total of 12 and a mean of 2.0 (12/6). Although his independence summary score would still have been 2, it would mean that he required more powerful assistance across subtasks.

Scoring Safety

Unlike independence data, which require the occupational therapy practitioner to rate each subtask and derive a mean summary score, the summary score for safety data is for the total task. Only 2 of the 6 Medication Management subtasks pose safety risks:

- Subtask 2: "Opens first pill bottle with ease"

- Subtask 5: "Opens second pill bottle with ease."

Because some medication bottles have little "teeth" to hold the cap on, clients can get cut on them—thus the safety risk. Additionally, some clients try to pry off the lid with their teeth or a knife; both of these approaches present a safety risk. None of the other items has an immediate risk to safety for the client. Because Sandy opened the medication bottles safely, neither box in the "Unsafe Observations" column has a check mark, which means that safe practices were observed. According to the scoring template in Exhibit 12.2, the summary safety score is a 3.

What if Dr. Holm had observed risks to safety when Sandy opened 1 of the bottles? She would have placed a check mark in the "Unsafe Observations" column for the subtask on which she observed the safety issue (i.e., Subtask 2 or 5). The scoring template (Exhibit 12.2) is helpful for rating safety because to rate a client's safety as a 3 or a 2, the practitioner provides no assistance, although a score of 2 indicates a minor risk was observed. To rate a client's safety as a 1 or a 0, the practitioner must provide assistance that addresses 1 or more safety concerns during task performance, and the degree of risk determines whether the safety score will be a 1 or a 0.

Scoring Adequacy

Similar to safety, the summary score for adequacy data is for the total task. However, there are 2 components to be rated for the adequacy score: process and quality. Dr. Holm did not enter any check marks in the "Process" or "Quality" columns for the first 5 Medication Management subtasks. However, for Medication Management Subtask 6, she entered a check mark for process and a check mark for quality. When a practitioner calculates the adequacy summary score, if the process and quality scores differ, the practitioner uses whichever is the lowest as the final adequacy summary score. This is because it is better not to overestimate clients' performance and place them at risk.

Task process ratings apply to the double-underlined actions in each subtask; for Subtask 6, this was, "Distributes pills from second pill bottle . . . for the next 2 days." Because Sandy sorted and re-sorted the pills (imprecision in carrying out the task actions) and sorted pills into the wrong times (extraneous actions), Dr. Holm put a check mark in the "Process" column for Subtask 6. A critical criterion for process, as indicated in the scoring template (Exhibit 12.2), is the difference between a score of 2 and a score of 1. For a score of 2, there can be no missing steps. If there are missing steps, the score must be a 1 or a 0. For Sandy, because of Subtask 6, his performance matches a process score of 2.

Task quality ratings apply to the single-underlined terms and the explanations in parentheses, which for Subtask 6 were "correct . . . (all pills and all slots indicated; days indicated)." Again, Dr. Holm put a check mark in the "Quality" column, because Sandy was not correct in the placement of the pills and days even when provided with verbal assistance. Using the scoring template in Exhibit 12.2, Dr. Holm scored Sandy's performance as a 2.

The criteria for a score of 2 in the "Quality" column are as follows: "Acceptable (Performance, for the most part, matches or nearly matches the quality standards listed in each subtask)." Because Sandy had a check mark in the "Quality" column only for Subtask 6 and he met the standards for the other 5 subtasks, a score of 2 for quality is the correct choice. Because Sandy's process and quality scores were a 2, his adequacy summary score is a 2. However, if either the process or the quality score were lower, then the lowest score for process and quality would be used. Again, this is because it is better not to overestimate clients' performance and place them at risk.

Documentation

In the PASS Box are a documentation grid and a report form that practitioners can use to summarize a client's performance on the PASS. The grid includes all 26 core items of the PASS. Practitioners can copy the document and alter it to include only those items they used in a client's evaluation. The practitioner can write recommendations or the intervention plan in the space below the grid and link it to the PASS data.

For example, Sandy's documentation shows that he did not perform the task independently—he needed verbal and gestural assists to successfully complete the task (see Exhibit 12.5). His performance was safe; however, it did not match community standards and therefore was inadequate.

Interpretation and Intervention Considerations

The PASS is easy to interpret, because the PASS rating and scoring form identifies the levels of assistance the client needed when performing each task and the point of task breakdown (i.e., subtasks). This provides a focus for the intervention plan and identifies the starting point for the level of assistance needed. The PASS also identifies whether there were safety issues during task performance and the aspect of the task affected (i.e., subtask). Finally, the PASS identifies the adequacy of the task performance as well as which subtask was not performed adequately and the standard that was not met. Again, the safety and adequacy measures also target a focus for the intervention plan.

The PASS is unique in its separation of independence, safety, and adequacy. Although other assessment tools include safety and sometimes quality (e.g., FIM; Uniform Data System for Medical Rehabilitation, 2012), the safety and quality data are usually subsumed into an overall independence score and are not separated, as with the PASS.

Although Sandy was able to accurately distribute the first, less-complex medication, he needed several assists to finally distribute the 2nd medication accurately. Because Sandy lives alone, there is no one to check on him each time he takes his medications. Therefore, Dr. Holm made 2 recommendations to ensure that Sandy would be able to accurately manage his medications on a daily basis in the future.

First, Dr. Holm recommended the use of blister packs, which are available at many pharmacies for a nominal fee and can be set up each month for each day and each time of day (e.g., breakfast, lunch, dinner, bedtime). This solution would enable Sandy to be independent on a daily basis. The 2nd recommendation was that Sandy's sister could come over once a month and monitor him as he sorts his medications into medication organizers, or sort his medications for him. This approach would make Sandy dependent on his sister and her schedule but would be an acceptable solution. The latter solution would also depend on Sandy's ability to remember the day and time his sister would come. This is a potential problem, because he once forgot Dr. Holm's appointment even though he was called with a reminder the night before.

EXHIBIT 12.5. Sample Grid for Documentation of Sandy's Performance on the PASS (Medication Management Item—Home Version)

DOCUMENTATION

Performance Assessment of Self-care Skills (PASS)	No Assists (Independent)	Verbal Assists (Min. Assist)	Gestures (Mod. Assist)	Physical Assists (Max. Assist)	Total Assist (Dependent)	Performance UNSAFE	Performance INADEQUATE	Not Assessed
	Independence					Safety	Adequacy	
Functional Mobility Domain								
Bed mobility								X
Stair mobility								X
Tub/shower mobility								X
Toilet mobility								X
Indoor walking								X
BADL Domain								
Oral hygiene								X
Dressing								X
Trimming toenails								X
Cognitive IADL Domain								
Shopping – cash exchange						NA		X
Bill paying by check						NA		X
Checkbook balancing						NA		X
Preparing bills to be mailed						NA		X
Telephone use						NA		X
Medication management		X	X				X	
Obtaining critical information – Radio						NA		X
Obtaining critical information – Newspaper						NA		X
Small repairs (flashlight)								X
Home safety awareness						NA		X
Bingo						NA		X
Oven use								X
Stovetop use								X
Use of sharp utensils								X
IADL Domain - Physical emphasis								
Carrying out the garbage								X
Changing bed linens								X
Sweeping the floor								X
Cleanup after meal preparation								X

Comments/Recommendations: Sandy was unable to accurately distribute his medications according to the directions on the label, without verbal and gestural assists to complete the task. It is recommended that he request blister packs for each day and time of day from the VAMC. If blister packs are not an option, then his sister is willing to monitor Sandy as he sorts his medications into medication organizers, or do it for him if necessary.

PASS summary scores for medication management task: Independence = 2.5/3; safety = 3/3; adequacy = 2/3

(Therapist Signature) MBH   (Date) 2/16/2018

Note. BADL = basic activity of daily living; max. = maximum; min. = minimal; mod. = moderate; NA = not applicable; VAMC = Veterans Administration Medical Center.

Summary

The PASS is a unique, performance-based assessment tool that includes 14 functional items with a cognitive emphasis. It is 1 of the most researched instruments available to occupational therapists. The PASS allows for the assessment of a range of essential ADLs and IADLs and can assist practitioners in determining safe discharge options.

Test administrators can customize the PASS to answer specific questions regarding a client's likely ability to function post-discharge, and a template is available for new item development. Specific items, as well as the total PASS, have been translated into 10 additional languages, and there are 2 English-language adaptations. The PASS has contributed to clinical care, clinical research, federal and provincial policies (Brown & Finlayson, 2013; Rogers et al., 1999), and occupational therapy education.

APPENDIX 12.A. Assignment for the PASS

Review Sandy's rating and scoring directions. Using the blank PASS Medication Management form provided in Exhibit 12.A.1, rate and score the video of **Mrs. Desai** as she engages with the PASS Medication Management task (see Video 12.2). Compare your answers with those of the authors (Exhibit 12.A.2). Then calculate your interrater reliability. With the exclusion of the assistive technology device listing, there are 83 possible decisions (observations, ratings, scores) to be made on the PASS Medication Management form (blank cells). Then count how many of your decisions match those of the authors. For example, if you matched 79 of the 83, then your interrater reliability on this PASS task would be 95.1% (excellent).

EXHIBIT 12.A.1. PASS Medication Management Form (Blank)

Task # H14: IADL-C: Medication Management		INDEPENDENCE DATA											SAFETY DATA	ADEQUACY DATA		
Assistive Technology Devices (ATDs) used during task: 1. 2. 3. Total # of ATDs used:_____		No Assistance	Verbal Supportive (Encouragement)	Verbal Non-Directive	Verbal Directive	Gestures	Task or Environment Rearrangement	Demonstration	Physical Guidance	Physical Support	Total Assist	INDEPENDENCE subtask scores	Unsafe Observations	PROCESS: imprecision, lack of economy, missing steps	QUALITY: Standards not met / improvement needed	SUMMARY SCORES
	Assist level →	0	1	2	3	4	5	6	7	8	9					
Subtasks	**MOBILITY/ADL/IADL SUBTASKS**															
1 Med 1 C-P*	Reports next time first medication is to be taken correctly (based on testing time, matches direction on label)															
2 Med 1 C-P	Opens first pill bottle with ease (by second try)															
3 Med 1 C-P	Distributes pills from first pill bottle into correct time slots for the next 2 days (all pills & all slots indicated; days indicated)															
4 Med2 N-C-P*	Reports next time second medication is to be taken correctly (based on testing time, matches direction on label)															
5 Med2 N-C-P	Opens second pill bottle with ease (by second try)															
6 Med2 N-C-P	Distributes pills from second pill bottle into correct time slots for the next 2 days (all pills and all slots indicated; days indicated)															

Summary Scores: INDEPENDENCE MEAN SCORE ↑ ; SAFETY SCORE ↑ ; ADEQUACY SCORE ↑

Note. C-P = childproof lid; IADL–C = IADL with a cognitive emphasis; med = medication; N-C-P = nonchildproof lid; PASS = Performance Assessment of Self-Care Skills.
Source. From *Performance Assessment of Self-Care Skills–Version 4.1*, by J. C. Rogers, M. B. Holm, and D. Chisholm, 2016, Pittsburgh: University of Pittsburgh. Copyright © 2016 by J. C. Rogers, M. B. Holm, and D. Chisholm. All rights reserved. Reprinted with permission.

(Continued)

APPENDIX 12.A. Assignment for the PASS *(Cont.)*

EXHIBIT 12.A.2. PASS Medication Management Form (Authors)

Task # H14: IADL-C: Medication Management	No Assistance (0)	Verbal Supportive (Encouragement) (1)	Verbal Non-Directive (2)	Verbal Directive (3)	Gestures (4)	Task or Environment Rearrangement (5)	Demonstration (6)	Physical Guidance (7)	Physical Support (8)	Total Assist (9)	INDEPENDENCE subtask scores	Unsafe Observations	PROCESS: Imprecision, lack of economy, missing steps	QUALITY: Standards not met / improvement needed
Assist level →	0	1	2	3	4	5	6	7	8	9				
1 Med 1 C-P* — Reports next time first medication is to be taken correctly (based on testing time, matches direction on label)		√√ √√		√√							**1**		√	√
2 Med 1 C-P — Opens first pill bottle with ease (by second try)	X										**3**			
3 Med 1 C-P — Distributes pills from first pill bottle into correct time slots for the next 2 days (all pills & all slots indicated; days indicated)	X										**3**			
4 Med2 N-C-P* — Reports next time second medication is to be taken correctly (based on testing time, matches direction on label)	X										**3**			
5 Med2 N-C-P — Opens second pill bottle with ease (by second try)	X										**3**			
6 Med2 N-C-P — Distributes pills from second pill bottle into correct time slots for the next 2 days (all pills and all slots indicated; days indicated)	X										**3**			

SUMMARY SCORES
- INDEPENDENCE MEAN SCORE: **2.6**
- SAFETY SCORE: **3**
- ADEQUACY SCORE: **2**

#1Gesture: Dr. Holm reaches out and stops Mrs. Desai from distributing the medications
#1Verbal Non-Directive – Repeats question (therefore indicating there is a problem) "So if you were going to take it….according to the directions….when would you take it today?"
#1Verbal Non-Directive - "At?"
#1Gesture: Dr. Holm reaches and points to the directions on the label
#1Verbal Non-Directive - "At?"
#1Verbal Non-Directive - "At?"

Independence = 2.6 – no Level 7-9 assists given, but occasional Level 1-6 assists given (16/6 = 2.6)
Safety = 3 because she had no issues opening/closing the medication containers
Adequacy = 2 Acceptable (of the 6 subtasks, Mrs. Desai only had difficulty with one of the subtasks)

Note. C-P = childproof lid; IADL–C = IADL with a cognitive emphasis; med = medication; N-C-P = nonchildproof lid; PASS = Performance Assessment of Self-Care Skills.
Source. From *Performance Assessment of Self-Care Skills–Version 4.1*, by J. C. Rogers, M. B. Holm, and D. Chisholm, 2016, Pittsburgh: University of Pittsburgh. Copyright © 2016 by J. C. Rogers, M. B. Holm, and D. Chisholm. All rights reserved. Reprinted with permission.

References

Bingham, K. S., Kumar, S., Dawson, D. R., Mulsant, B. H., & Flint, A. J. (2018). A systematic review of the measurement of function in late-life depression. *American Journal of Geriatric Psychiatry, 26,* 54–72. https://doi.org/10.1016/j.jagp.2017.08.011

Brown, C. L., & Finlayson, M. L. (2013). Performance measures rather than self-report measures of functional status predict home care use in community-dwelling older adults. *Canadian Journal of Occupational Therapy, 80,* 284–294. https://doi.org/10.1177/0008417413501467

Cattell, R. B. (1966). The scree test for the number of factors. *Multivariate Behavioral Research, 1,* 245–276. https://doi.org/10.1207/s15327906mbr0102_10

Chisholm, D. (2005). *Disability in older adults with depression.* Unpublished doctoral dissertation, University of Pittsburgh, Pittsburgh.

Ciro, C. A., Anderson, M. P., Hershey, L. A., Prodan, C. I., & Holm, M. B. (2015). Instrumental activities of daily living performance and role satisfaction in people with and without mild cognitive impairment: A pilot project. *American Journal of Occupational Therapy, 69,* 6903270020. https://doi.org/10.5014/ajot.2014.015198

Fillenbaum, G. G., & Smyer, M. A. (1981). The development, validity, and reliability of the OARS Multidimensional Functional Assessment Questionnaire. *Journal of Gerontology, 36,* 428–434. https://doi.org/10.1093/geronj/36.4.428

Goldstein, G., McCue, M., Rogers, J. C., & Nussbaum, P. D. (1992). Diagnostic differences in memory test based predictions of functional capacity in the elderly. *Neuropsychological Rehabilitation, 2,* 307–317. https://doi.org/10.1080/09602019208401416

Gurland, B., Kuriansky, J., Sharpe, L., Simon, R., Stiller, P., & Birkett, P. (1978). The Comprehensive Assessment and Referral Evaluation (CARE)—Rationale, development and reliability. *International Journal of Aging and Human Development, 8,* 9–42. https://doi.org/10.2190/CL3J-0E20-97XX-MV5L

Holm, M. B. (2017). *PASSport to improving function.* Paper presented at the Scholarship of Practice Symposium, University of Illinois–Chicago.

Holm, M. B., & Rogers, J. C. (1990a). Functional assessment outcomes: Differences between settings. *Archives of Physical Medicine and Rehabilitation, 71,* 761.

Holm, M. B., & Rogers, J. C. (1990b). Functional performance differences between the health care setting and the home [Special issue]. *Gerontologist, 30,* 327A.

Holm, M. B., & Rogers, J. C. (2008). The Performance Assessment of Self-Care Skills (PASS). In B. Hemphill-Pearson (Ed.), *Assessments in occupational therapy mental health* (2nd ed., pp. 101–110). Thorofare, NJ: Slack.

Keith, R. A., Granger, C. V., Hamilton, B. B., & Sherwin, F. S. (1987). The Functional Independence Measure: A new tool for rehabilitation. *Advances in Clinical Rehabilitation, 1,* 6–18.

Lawton, M. P., & Brody, E. M. (1969). Assessment of older people: Self-maintaining and instrumental activities of daily living. *Gerontologist, 9,* 179–186. https://doi.org/10.1093/geront/9.3_Part_1.179

Mahoney, F. I., & Barthel, D. W. (1965). Functional evaluation: The Barthel Index. *Maryland State Medical Journal, 14,* 61–65.

McCue, M., Rogers, J. C., & Goldstein, G. (1990). Relationships between neuropsychological and functional assessment in elderly neuropsychiatric patients. *Rehabilitation Psychology, 35,* 91–99. https://doi.org/10.1037/h0079052

Pfeffer, R. (1987). The Functional Activities Questionnaire. In I. McDowell & C. Newell (Eds.), *Measuring health: A guide to rating scales and questionnaires* (p. 108). New York: Oxford University Press.

Reitan, R. M. (1958). Validity of the Trail Making Test as an indicator of organic brain damage. *Perceptual and Motor Skills, 8,* 271–276. https://doi.org/10.2466/pms.1958.8.3.271

Rodakowski, J., Skidmore, E. R., Reynolds, C. F., 3rd, Dew, M. A., Butters, M. A., Holm, M. B., . . . Rogers, J. C. (2014). Can performance on daily activities discriminate between older adults with normal cognitive function and those with mild cognitive impairment? *Journal of the American Geriatrics Society, 62,* 1347–1352. https://doi.org/10.1111/jgs.12878

Rogers, J. C., & Holm, M. B. (1990). In-home safety for persons with cognitive impairment [Special issue]. *Gerontologist, 30,* 217A.

Rogers, J. C., Holm, M. B., Beach, S., Schulz, R., & Starz, T. W. (2001). Task independence, safety, and adequacy among nondisabled and osteoarthritis-disabled older women. *Arthritis Care and Research, 45,* 410–418. https://doi.org/10.1002/1529-0131(200110)45:5<410::AID-ART359>3.0.CO;2-Y

Rogers, J. C., Holm, M. B., Burgio, L. D., Granieri, E., Hsu, C., Hardin, J. M., & McDowell, B. J. (1999). Improving morning care routines of nursing home residents with dementia. *Journal of the American Geriatrics Society, 47,* 1049–1057. https://doi.org/10.1111/j.1532-5415.1999.tb05226.x

Rogers, J. C., Holm, M. B., & Chisholm, D. (2016a). *Performance Assessment of Self-Care Skills—Version 4.1.* Pittsburgh: University of Pittsburgh.

Rogers, J. C., Holm, M. B., & Chisholm, D. (2016b). *Performance Assessment of Self-Care Skills—Version 4.1—Scoring guidelines.* Pittsburgh: University of Pittsburgh.

Rogers, J. C., Holm, M. B., Goldstein, G., McCue, M., & Nussbaum, P. D. (1994). Stability and change in functional assessment of patients with geropsychiatric disorders. *American Journal of Occupational Therapy, 48,* 914–918. https://doi.org/10.5014/ajot.48.10.914

Rubin, E., & Zorumski, C. (2016, June 8). Cognitive impairment in depression: Do cognitive deficits improve when depressive symptoms improve? *Psychology Today.* Retrieved from https://www.psychologytoday.com/us/blog/demystifying-psychiatry/201606/cognitive-impairment-in-depression

Uniform Data System for Medical Rehabilitation. (2012). *The FIM® instrument: Its background, structure, and usefulness.* Buffalo, NY: Author.

Vygotsky, L. S. (1978). *Mind in society: The development of higher psychological processes.* Cambridge, MA: Harvard University Press.

Williams v. Quinn, 1:05-CV-04673 (N.D. Ill., 2010).

SECTION

Assessment

Functional Cognition in the Home and ADLs:
Performance-Based Assessment Tools

13

ADL-Focused Occupation-Based Neurobehavioral Evaluation: The A–ONE

GLEN GILLEN, EdD, OTR, FAOTA

LEARNING OBJECTIVES

After completing this chapter, readers should be able to

- Understand the background and development of the ADL-Focused Occupation-Based Neurobehavioral Evaluation (A–ONE),
- Explain how the A–ONE differs from traditional cognitive assessments, and
- Describe the scoring of the A–ONE.

KEY TERMS AND CONCEPTS

- Activities of daily living • Neurobehavior • Neurobehavioral deficits

Introduction

The ADL-Focused Occupation-Based Neurobehavioral Evaluation (A–ONE), formerly known as the Árnadóttir OT–ADL Neurobehavioral Evaluation, was developed by Icelandic occupational therapist Guðrún Árnadóttir in the late 1980s (Árnadóttir, 1990). At this time in the occupational therapy profession's development, therapists were almost exclusively using out-of-context pen-and-paper assessments that were developed by colleagues in other disciplines as the means to evaluate cognition and perception.

The A–ONE was developed for several reasons:

- To demonstrate the unique perspective of occupational therapists related to the assessment process in this area of practice

- To reject the dichotomy between cognitive–perceptual evaluation and the evaluation of *activities of daily living* (ADLs; i.e., activities oriented toward taking care of one's own body)

- To determine the impact of *neurobehavioral deficits* (i.e., an individual's functional impairments, manifested

as defective task performance, resulting from a neurological processing dysfunction) on ADLs

- To allow practitioners to hypothesize the area of a client's cortex that is damaged on the basis of skilled observations made while observing the errors (i.e., occupational errors) the client made during performance of ADLs.

The A–ONE was 1 of the first performance-based assessments that was developed for use with clients whose neurological damage affects their *neurobehavior* (i.e., behavior based on neurological function). The A–ONE is a standardized, criterion-based, norm-based instrument used by occupational therapists to assess persons with cortical or subcortical brain damage affecting ADLs. The goal of this instrument is to give therapists the ability to determine the impact of neurobehavioral impairments on ADL performance in natural contexts. It allows practitioners to document clients' lack of independence in ADLs and, more important, the underlying reason for the lack of independence (Árnadóttir, 1990, 2010, 2016, 2017). See Exhibit 13.1 for a list of occupations and client factors addressed by the A–ONE.

EXHIBIT 13.1. Occupations and Neurobehavioral Impairments Considered in the A–ONE

OCCUPATIONS AND ADLS	CLIENT FACTORS (NEUROBEHAVIORAL IMPAIRMENTS)
Dressing	Specific impairments
Manipulate fastenings	Decreased motor function
Put on pants	Decreased organization and sequencing
Put on shirt and upper body garments	Ideational apraxia
Put on shoes	Impaired spatial relations
Put on socks	Motor apraxia
Grooming and hygiene	Perseveration
Bathe or shower	Somatoagnosia
Brush teeth	Topographical disorientation
Comb hair	Unilateral body neglect
Perform toilet hygiene	Unilateral spatial neglect
Shave beard or apply cosmetics	Pervasive impairments
Wash face and upper body	Anosognosia
Transfers and mobility	Apathy
Maneuver around	Associative visual agnosia
Sit up in bed	Astereognosis
Transfer to and from bed	Attention (impaired)
Transfer to toilet	Body part identification (impaired)
Transfer to tub	Circumlocution
Feeding	Concrete thinking
Bring food to mouth by fork or spoon	Confabulation
Drink from glass or cup	Confusion
Use fingers to bring food to mouth	Depression
Use knife to cut and spread	Disorientation
Communication	Distractibility
Comprehension	Dysarthria
Expression	Echolalia
	Field dependency
	Frustration
	Initiation (impaired)
	Insight (decreased)
	Irritability
	Jargon aphasia
	Judgment (impaired)
	Lability
	Long-term memory loss
	Motivation (impaired)
	Motor impersistence
	Mutism
	Paraphasia
	Performance latency
	Perseveration
	Restlessness
	Right–left discrimination (impaired)
	Sensory loss
	Short-term memory loss
	Visual object agnosia
	Wernicke's aphasia

Note. A–ONE = ADL-Focused Occupation-Based Neurobehavioral Evaluation.

Background, Theory, and Development

The A–ONE is grounded in core principles of occupational therapy—in particular, the assessment of occupational performance and how various client factors support or limit engagement in specific occupations (Árnadóttir, 1990, 2010, 2016, 2017).

Neurobehavioral Theory also guided the development of the instrument. Llorens (1986) described *Neurobehavioral Theory* as

> conceptualized from an understanding of nervous system functioning that follows a model described as a) stimulation of the sensory systems to facilitate intersensory integration; b) the processing of stimuli, that is, the recognition, interpretation, storage, and retrieval of information to which meaning is attributed from past and present experience; and c) the generation of behavioral response. (p. 104)

See Figure 13.1 for a graphic representation of Neurobehavioral Theory.

Target Population

The A–ONE is appropriate for use with clients older than 16 years who have sustained damage to their central nervous system (CNS). Specific diagnoses include the following:

- Anoxia
- Brain tumor
- Dementia (Alzheimer's disease and frontotemporal)
- Head injury
- Inflammatory disease
- Multiple sclerosis
- Parkinson's disease
- Stroke
- Toxic and metabolic diseases.

The tool is appropriate for those experiencing difficulties with self-care and functional mobility secondary to neurobehavioral dysfunction. Target areas may include increasing the client's independence and safety regarding these areas of occupation as well as decreasing caregiver burden. Because the items on the A–ONE are in alignment with the items that are traditionally scored by occupational therapy practitioners on the FIM® (Keith et al., 1987), poor performance on the FIM combined with a diagnosis of dysfunction of the CNS may trigger use of the A–ONE. In addition, there is a moderate statistical relationship between the A–ONE and the Barthel Index (Mahoney & Barthel, 1965) as well as the Mini-Mental State Examination (Folstein et al., 1983; see Árnadóttir, 1990, 2010, 2016, 2017).

FIGURE 13.1. Schematic representation of Neurobehavioral Theory.

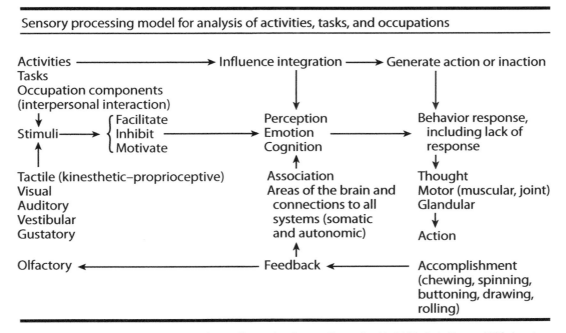

Sensory processing model for analysis of activities, tasks, and occupations

Source. From "Activity Analysis: Agreement Among Factors in a Sensory Processing Model," by L. A. Llorens, 1986, *American Journal of Occupational Therapy, 40,* p. 104. Copyright © 1986 by the American Occupational Therapy Association. Reprinted with permission.

Administration

The A–ONE was published in the textbook *The Brain and Behavior: Assessing Cortical Dysfunction Through Activities of Daily Living* (Árnadóttir, 1990). No specialized equipment is required. Administration requires the client's clothing, grooming implements, a sink, a bed, a chair, feeding equipment, and a table for eating a simple meal. If time or fatigue is of concern, parts of the tool may be administered at different times. For example, 1 session might consist of the observation of transfers and mobility, grooming, and dressing. A 2nd session might then be used to complete the feeding items on the tool (Árnadóttir, 1990).

For reliable administration, a 5-day training course is required (see http://www.a-one.is/about.html for details). Training courses are taught throughout the world and in a variety of languages (Árnadóttir, 2017).

The steps of administration are as follows (Árnadóttir, 1990):

1. The administrator sets up the environment with all necessary items. Items should be placed on both the left and the right sides and within the client's reach.

2. The administrator uses interactive reasoning before the actual assessment to determine language ability, insight, orientation, memory, and so forth. For example, after introductions, the administrator might say, "I was able to review your medical chart and have an understanding of what happened to you. I would like to hear this from you now."

3. The administrator gives the client a set of instructions related to what tasks they will perform.

4. Structured observations begin once the client begins to engage. Most often, the order of the tasks is as follows: bed mobility, transfer, ambulation or wheeled mobility, grooming, dressing, and feeding.

5. The test administrator provides cues as needed, starting with verbal cues followed by physical assistance.

6. The administrator documents the results of the assessment.

Test administrators must consider context for accurate interpretation. Because of the nature of the items in the tool, morning administration in an appropriate environment (e.g., hospital room, home, simulated apartment, ADL room) is preferred (Árnadóttir, 1990).

Scoring

The A–ONE consists of 3 subscales (Árnadóttir, 1990). The first subscale is the Functional Independence subscale, which documents the level of assistance required for each item. The scale ranges from 0 to 4, with higher scores indicating higher levels of independence:

- 4 = *Independent and able to transfer activity to other environmental situations*

- 3 = *Independent with supervision*

- 2 = *Needs verbal assistance*

- 1 = *Needs demonstration or physical assistance*

- 0 = *Unable to perform. Totally dependent on assistance.*

The 2nd subscale is the Neurobehavioral Specific Impairment subscale. This scale indicates which specific impairments are interfering with ADL performance and the severity of each impairment. It is also a 0–4 scale, with higher scores indicating more severe impairment:

- 0 = *No neurobehavioral impairments observed*

- 1 = *Able to perform without additional information, but some neurobehavioral impairment is observed*

- 2 = *Able to perform with additional verbal assistance, but neurobehavioral impairment can be observed during performance*

- 3 = *Able to perform with demonstration or minimal to considerable physical assistance*

- 4 = *Unable to perform due to neurobehavioral impairment. Needs maximum physical assistance.*

The 3rd subscale is the Neurobehavioral Pervasive Impairment subscale. Impairments that may affect performance across ADL domains are scored as present or absent:

- 0 = *Impairment is absent*

- 1 = *Impairment is present.*

The scores on the Functional Independence subscale can be added for each category but should not be added across domains. In other words, the measure yields separate scores for dressing, grooming and hygiene, transfers and mobility, feeding, and communication. These separate scores are not additive.

The scores on the Neurobehavioral Specific Impairment subscale also are not additive. Each impairment is identified separately and scored for severity. Similarly, the Neurobehavioral Pervasive Impairment subscale is not additive. Each impairment is separately scored as present or absent only (Árnadóttir, 1990, 2017). See Exhibit 13.2 for an example of scoring the results of the A–ONE.

Documentation

Documenting the results of the A–ONE is a twofold process. First, the test administrator completes a narrative summary of the specific functional independence scores. As previously noted, the measure does not include a total ADL score. The administrator then completes a summary or checklist of the impairments that are limiting the client's function (see Exhibit 13.3 for an example).

EXHIBIT 13.2. Sample Documentation of the Scoring and Results of the A–ONE

a. Sample from the dressing domain of the Functional Independence scale and the Neurobehavioral Specific Impairment subscale

Functional Independence Scale and
Neurobehavioral Specific Impairment Subscale

Name ___ Mary Wilson _____ Date __ 6/13/2014 ___

Independence score (IP):

4 = Independent and able to transfer activity to
    other environmental situations.
3 = Independent with supervision.
2 = Needs verbal assistance.
1 = Needs demonstration or physical assistance.
0 = Unable to perform. Totally dependent on assistance.

Neurobehavioral score (NB):

0 = No neurobehavioral impairments observed.
1 = Able to perform without additional information, but some
    neurobehavioral impairment is observed.
2 = Able to perform with additional verbal assistance, but
    neurobehavioral impairment can be observed during
    performance.
3 = Able to perform with demonstration or minimal to considerable
    physical assistance.
4 = Unable to perform due to neurobehavioral impairment. Needs
    maximum physical assistance.

List helping aids used:

• Wheelchair
• Nonslip for soap and plate
• Adapted toothbrush
• Velcro fastening on shoes

Primary ADL activity	Scoring	Comments and reasoning
Dressing	**IP score**	
Shirt (or dress)	4 3 2 (1) 0	Include one armhole, fix shoulder
Pants	4 3 2 (1) 0	Find correct leghole
Socks	4 3 2 (1) 0	One-handed technique, unstable
Shoes	4 3 2 (1) 0	Unstable
Fastenings	4 3 2 (1) 0	Match buttonholes, Velcro through loop
Other		

NB Impairment	NB Score	
Motor apraxia	(0) 1 2 3 4	
Ideational apraxia	(0) 1 2 3 4	
Unilateral body neglect	0 1 2 (3) 4	Leaves out left body side
Somatoagnosia	(0) 1 2 3 4	
Spatial relations	0 1 2 (3) 4	Finding correct holes, front/back
Unilateral spatial neglect	0 1 (2) 3 4	Leaves out items in left visual field
Abnormal tone: right	(0) 1 2 3 4	
Abnormal tone: left	0 1 2 (3) 4	Sitting balance/bilateral manipulation
Perseveration	(0) 1 2 3 4	
Organization/sequencing	0 1 (2) 3 4	For activity steps
Other		

Note: All definitions and scoring criteria for each deficit are in the evaluation manual.

© 2014, Guðrún Árnadóttir

(Continued)

EXHIBIT 13.2. Sample Documentation of the Scoring and Results of the A–ONE *(Cont.)*

b. Sample ADL summary sheet

**Activity-Focused Occupation-Based
Neurobehavioral Evaluation
(A-ONE)**

Name __Ms. Mary Wilson__	Date __7-29-2014__
Birthdate __4-15-1954__	Age __60__
Gender __Female__	Ethnicity __Caucasian__
Dominance: __Right__	Profession __Dressmaker__
Therapist: __Jon Jonsson__	A-ONE certification #: __IS89-333__

Medical diagnosis:

Right CVA 6/2/2014

Medications:

Social situation:

Lives alone in an apartment building on third floor.
Has two adult daughters.

Summary of independence:

Needs considerable physical assistance with dressing, grooming and hygiene, transfer and mobility tasks because of left-sided paralysis, perceptual and cognitive impairments (spatial relations, neglect to space and body, organization and sequencing of activity steps, working memory and attention). Is more or less able to feed herself if meals have been prepared. No problems with personal communication, although perceptual impairments will affect reading and writing skills. Also has lack of judgment and insight into own situation which affect task performance. Is not able to live alone at this stage. If personal home support becomes available, will need a home evaluation because of physical limitation and wheelchair use.

Functional independence score

Task	Raw score						Domain score	Aids used for performance
Dressing	1	1	1	1	1		5/20	Velcro fastenings on shoes
Grooming and hygiene	1	2	1	1	1	0	6/4	Adapted toothbrush, nonslip for soap
Transfers and mobility	1	1	1	1			5/20	Wheelchair
Feeding	4	4	4	3			15/16	Nonslip for plate
Communication	4	4					8/8	–
Measure (logit)	0,58							
SE	0,35							

© 2014, Guðrún Árnadóttir

(Continued)

EXHIBIT 13.3. Sample Documentation for the A–ONE: Checklist of Impairments

SPECIFIC IMPAIRMENT	ADL DOMAIN: DRESSING
Decreased motor function	√
Decreased organization and sequencing	√
Ideational apraxia	√
Impaired spatial relations	√
Motor apraxia	
Perseveration	
Somatoagnosia	
Topographical disorientation	
Unilateral body neglect	
Unilateral spatial neglect	

Note. A–ONE = ADL-Focused Occupation-Based Neurobehavioral Evaluation.

Interpretation and Intervention Considerations

Because the A–ONE is a performance-based measure, observation of occupational performance is the foundation of this tool. Although some performance-based measures only indicate the level of assistance the client requires to perform tasks, the A–ONE detects the reason for the lack of independence. This information is critical for intervention planning. The interventions that one would use for a person with decreased occupational performance secondary to apraxia are different from those used for someone living with unilateral neglect. Understanding the patterns of impairments is critical before the development of an intervention plan.

EXHIBIT 13.2. Sample Documentation of the Scoring and Results of the A–ONE *(Cont.)*

c. Sample neurobehavioral summary sheet

List of Neurobehavioral Impairments Observed

Specific impairment	D	G	T	F	C	Pervasive impairment	ADL	Pervasive impairment	ADL
Motor apraxia						Astereognosis	✓	Restlessness	
Ideational apraxia						Visual object agnosia		Concrete thinking	✓
Unilateral body neglect	3	3	3	1		Visual spatial agnosia	✓	Decreased insight	✓
Somatoagnosia						Associative visual agnosia		Impaired judgment	✓
Spatial relations	3	3	3	1		Anosognosia		Confusion	
Unilateral spatial neglect	2	2	3	1		R/L discrimination	✓	Impaired alertness	
Abnormal tone: Right						Short-term memory	✓	Impaired attention	✓
Abnormal tone: Left	3	3	3	1		Long-term memory		Distractibility	✓
Perseveration						Disorientation	✓	Impaired initiative	
Organization	2	2	2	1		Confabulation		Impaired motivation	
Topographic disorientation		3				Lability	✓	Performance latency	
Other						Euphoria		Absentmindedness	
Sensory aphasia						Apathy		Other	
Jargon aphasia						Depression	✓	Field dependency	✓
Anomia						Aggressiveness			
Paraphasia						Irritability			
Expressive aphasia						Frustration			

Use (✓) for presence of specific impairments in different ADL domains (D = dressing, G = grooming, T = transfers, F = feeding, C = communication) and for presence of pervasive impairments detected during the ADL evaluation.

Summary of Neurobehavioral Impairments:
Needs physical assistance for most dressing, grooming, hygiene, transfer, and mobility tasks because of left-sided paralysis, spatial relations impairments (e.g., problems differentiating back from front of clothes and finding armholes and legholes), and unilateral body neglect (i.e., does not wash or dress affected side). Does not attend to objects in the left visual field and needs verbal cues for performance. Also needs verbal cues for organizing activity steps. Does not know her way around the hospital. Does not have insight into how the CVA affects her ADL and is thus unrealistic in day-to-day planning. Has impaired judgment resulting in unsafe transfer attempts. Leaves the water running after hygiene and grooming activities if not reminded to turn it off. Is emotionally labile and appears depressed at times. Is not oriented regarding time and date. Presents with impaired attention, distraction, and defective short-term memory requiring repeated verbal instructions.

Treatment considerations:

Occupational therapist: *Jon Jonsson*

A-ONE certification number: *IS89-333*   © 2014, Guðrún Árnadóttir

Note. A–ONE = ADL-Focused Occupation-Based Neurobehavioral Evaluation; CVA = cerebrovascular accident; R/L = right/left; SE = standard error.
Source. From "Impact of Neurobehavioral Deficits on Activities of Daily Living," by G. Árnadóttir, in *Stroke Rehabilitation: A Function-Based Approach* (4th ed., pp. 605–607), by G. Gillen (Ed.), 2016, St. Louis: Elsevier. Copyright © 2014 by Guðrún Árnadóttir. Reprinted with permission.

The A–ONE is also useful to determine discharge environment and need for caregiver assistance because of its ability to document the severity of ADL and mobility limitations. Research has shown that the A–ONE is able to detect change in status over time. This is particularly useful for determining what setting (e.g., inpatient rehabilitation vs. subacute facility) is appropriate on the basis of the client's response to therapy (Árnadóttir, 1990, 2010, 2017).

Two items on the Neurobehavioral Pervasive Impairment subscale may be of particular help in terms of intervention. The item *insight* in the tool refers to the ability to have insight into one's own condition or disability (Árnadóttir, 2017). A person with impaired insight may make unrealistic comments about their disability, make unrealistic statements about the future, or lack insight into the impact of their impairments.

The item *judgment* refers to the inability to make realistic decisions based on environmental information (Árnadóttir, 2017). Clients with impaired judgment demonstrate unsafe behaviors during the A–ONE, such as not locking wheelchair brakes or mouthing objects inappropriately. Determining insight helps the occupational therapist choose the appropriate intervention.

For example, if a person is developing insight into the impact of their unilateral neglect, they may be a candidate for visual scanning training. If they do not gain insight into their difficulties, an environmental modification approach is a better fit. Finally, if the person presents with impaired

EXHIBIT 13.4. A–ONE Results for Client in Video 13.1

Client: Ed
Diagnosis: Left MCA CVA
Prior Functional Status: Independent at home in the community 1 week prior to this assessment.
Assessment: A–ONE
Domain: Grooming and Hygiene
Tasks: Brush Teeth and Comb Hair

A–ONE Part I
Functional Independence Scale and
Neurobehavioral Specific Impairment Subscale

Name _____ Ed _____   Date _____ 11/14/18 _____

Independence score (IP):

4 = Independent and able to transfer activity to other environmental situations.
3 = Independent with supervision.
2 = Needs verbal assistance.
1 = Needs physical assistance.
0 = Unable to perform. Totally dependent on assistance.

List helping aids used:

Neurobehavioral score (NB):

0 = No neurobehavioral impairments observed.
1 = Patient is able to perform without additional information, but some neurobehavioral impairment can be observed.
2 = Patient is able to perform with additional verbal assistance, but neurobehavioral impairment can be observed during performance.
3 = Patient is able to perform with demonstration or minimal to moderate physical assistance.
4 = Patient is unable to perform due to neurobehavioral impairment. Needs maximum physical assistance.

Grooming and hygiene	Scoring IP score					Comments and reasoning
Wash face and upper body	4	3	2	1	0	N/T
Comb hair	4	3	2	(1)	0	
Brush teeth	4	3	2	(1)	0	
Shave, makeup	4	3	2	1	0	N/T
Continence/toilet	4	3	2	1	0	N/T
Bath	4	3	2	1	0	N/T
Other						

NB impairment (grooming)	Scoring NB score					Comments and reasoning
Motor apraxia	0	1	2	(3)	4	
Ideational; apraxia	0	1	2	(3)	4	
Unilateral body neglect	(0)	1	2	3	4	
Somatoagnosia	(0)	1	2	3	4	
Spatial relations	(0)	1	2	3	4	
Unilateral spatial neglect	(0)	1	2	3	4	
Abnormal tone: Right	0	1	2	(3)	4	
Abnormal tone: Left	(0)	1	2	3	4	
Perseveration	(0)	1	2	3	4	
Organization/sequencing	0	1	2	(3)	4	
Other						

Note. All definitions and scoring criteria for each deficit are in the Evaluation Manual. A–ONE = ADL-Focused Occupation-Based Neurobehavioral Evaluation; CVA = cerebrovascular accident; MCA = middle cerebral artery; N/T = not tested.
Source. Modified from *The Brain and Behavior: Assessing Cortical Dysfunction Through Activities of Daily Living* (pp. 227–228), by G. Árnadóttir, 1990, St. Louis: Mosby. Copyright © 1990 by Guðrún Árnadóttir. Adapted with permission.

judgment, discussions around supervision, level of caregiver assistance, and the use of restraints must become part of the overall management plan.

For an example of administration of the A–ONE, see Video 13.1, as well as Exhibit 13.4, for test results for the client in the video.

References

Árnadóttir, G. (1990). *The brain and behavior: Assessing cortical dysfunction through activities of daily living.* St. Louis: Mosby.

Árnadóttir, G. (2010). *Measuring the impact of body functions on occupational performance: Validation of the ADL-focused Occupation-Based Neurobehavioral Evaluation (A–ONE)* (Umeå University Medical Dissertations, New Series No. 1322). Department of Community Medicine and Rehabilitation/Occupational Therapy, Umeå University, Umeå, Sweden.

Árnadóttir, G. (2016). Impact of neurobehavioral deficits on activities of daily living. In G. Gillen (Ed.), *Stroke rehabilitation: A function-based approach* (4th ed., pp. 573–611). St. Louis: Elsevier. https://doi.org/10.1016/B978-0-323-17281-3.00026-5

Árnadóttir, G. (2017). *A–ONE training course lecture notes.* Umeå, Sweden: Author.

Folstein, M. F., Robins, L. N., & Helzer, J. E. (1983). The Mini-Mental State Examination. *Archives of General Psychiatry, 40,* 812. https://doi.org/10.1001/archpsyc.1983.01790060110016

Keith, R. A., Granger, C. V., Hamilton, B. B., & Sherwin, F. S. (1987). The Functional Independence Measure: A new tool for rehabilitation. *Advances in Clinical Rehabilitation, 1,* 6–18.

Llorens, L. A. (1986). Activity analysis: Agreement among factors in a sensory processing model. *American Journal of Occupational Therapy, 40,* 103–110. https://doi.org/10.5014/ajot.40.2.103

Mahoney, F., & Barthel, D. (1965). Functional evaluation: The Barthel Index. *Maryland State Medical Journal, 14,* 61–65.

14

Cognitive Performance Test

JACQUELINE WESSON, BAppSc (OT), MA, PhD,
AND THERESSA BURNS, OTR

LEARNING OBJECTIVES

After completing this chapter, readers should be able to

- Describe functional cognition as the construct measured by the Cognitive Performance Test (CPT);
- Discuss the Revised CPT as an ecological measure of working memory and executive function;
- Understand differences between the CPT and its practice model, on the one hand, and Allen's Cognitive Disabilities Model, on the other;
- Understand the role of the CPT in contributing to a functional diagnosis in neurocognitive disorders;
- Describe CPT administration and scoring procedures and features of standardization;
- Describe how to interpret CPT results and use them in intervention planning; and
- Describe the measurement properties of the CPT and the populations with whom it has been validated.

KEY TERMS AND CONCEPTS

- Older adults • Performance based

Introduction

The Cognitive Performance Test (CPT; Burns, 2018) is a standardized, occupation-based or "top-down" observational measure of functional cognition for **older adults** (i.e., adults 65 years or older). When administering the measure, occupational therapists directly observe performance in simulated everyday tasks to evaluate working memory and executive functioning (EF) processes that mediate common goal-directed activity. Severity of impairment is rated according to the CPT half-level profile system, which enables therapists to explain and predict functional–cognitive abilities used to perform everyday tasks and occupations. This chapter introduces the Revised CPT and its psychometric properties, including the standardized administration procedures that lead to the CPT evidence-based profiles for intervention.

The CPT is a global measure of information-processing abilities and underlying patterns of performance across a range of everyday activities. In that sense, it differs from other occupational therapy assessments, which highlight specific tasks individuals can or cannot perform. That is, the CPT is not a "traditional" measure of function that quantifies skills in discrete everyday activities, but it provides an overall estimate of functional–cognitive ability.

The CPT consists of 7 subtasks (Medbox, Shop, Toast, Phone, Wash, Dress, and Travel), for which the task cues and working memory requirements are systematically varied. Each CPT subtask repeatedly measures the same construct (as demonstrated by studies of internal consistency; Bar-Yosef et al., 2000; Burns et al., 1994; Douglas et al., 2012). Individuals' working memory and a global construct of EFs are rated during task performance (e.g., task planning, problem solving, divided attention, new learning). At each higher level, subtask cues are increasingly complex, requiring more organized and complex working memory.

Occupational therapists first offer the task details, including distracter props. They then reduce task performance requirements by adjusting task concepts and object cues in response to errors made during the assessment. Subtasks are rated with a performance-level score and then averaged for a CPT total score for use in clinical practice. This score is then interpreted within the CPT profiles, which outline the predicted functional–cognitive ability and support needs at the half-level (see Table 14.1).

The CPT was initially developed as a research instrument (Burns, 1986, 1990) to assess cognition in daily task performance and change over time among people with Alzheimer's disease (AD). Reliability and validity were established as part of a longitudinal study of AD progression conducted by the National Institute on Aging (Burns et al., 1994). The original 6-item battery was based on Allen's (1985; Allen & Allen, 1987) Cognitive Disabilities Theory, which proposes 6 ordinal levels of global cognition, associated motor actions, and corresponding routine task behavior (i.e., planned actions, exploratory actions, goal-directed actions, manual actions, postural actions, automatic actions). However, the CPT is not part of the current Allen's Cognitive Disabilities Model. Although the CPT may seem similar to Allen's scale (Allen et al., 1992) in its scoring hierarchy, they are different in the processes used to arrive at a score and in the theoretical underpinnings.

Discrete interpretations of ability in the CPT are described by its half-level cognitive–functional profiles system. These profiles are founded on early evidence generated by the CPT (Bar-Yosef et al., 2000; Burns et al., 1994, 2004; Ebbitt et al., 1989; Thralow & Rueter, 1993), combined with advances in cognitive neuroscience and the identification of memory systems (i.e., episodic, semantic, procedural, and working memory) associated with neurocognitive disorders (NCDs; Burns, 2013, 2018, 2019; Burns & Levy, 2006; Burns et al., 2018). The CPT has been revised to consider an updated construct and language that is consistent with contemporary cognitive neuroscience and what is known about the progressive stages of impairment in the associated memory systems of mild and major NCDs (American Psychiatric Association, 2013).

The CPT is a cognitive–functional measure that identifies patterns of performance associated with long-term memory stores. The specific tasks that are included are less important than the manner in which clients respond to the task demands of varying complexity. The intent is to measure working memory and EF processing capacities that underlie functional performance. The primary focus of the assessment

TABLE 14.1. CPT Cognitive–Functional Profiles

CPT PROFILE	CHARACTERISTICS OF FUNCTIONAL COGNITION
5.6	Relevant information can be activated and used purposefully to carry out complex activities and IADLs independently. May have other cognitive or behavioral concerns.
5.0	Mild functional decline due to deficits in executive control functions (task planning, problem solving, divided attention, new learning). Difficulties may manifest in the performance of IADLs, including managing finances, job performance, driving, or following a complex medication/co-morbidity regime. Check-in support and assistance with IADLs may be needed. ADLs typically show no change.
4.5	Mild to moderate functional decline due to significant deficit in executive control functions; difficulty with divided attention and solving problems. Complex tasks are performed with inconsistency or error. With IADLs, the person struggles to manage the details. ADLs may show decline in ability to self-initiate. Independent living poses significant risk for mismanaging meals, finances, medications and co-morbidities. Driving poses safety risks, with impaired ability to divide attention between environmental cues. IADL assistance and/or in-home assistance is needed. Assisted living environments provide a good fit.
4.0	Moderate functional decline; from abstract to concrete thought processes. The person relies on familiar routines and environments and uses what they see for cues as to what to do. IADLs need to be done by or with others. ADLs are remembered but typically the quality shows decline. The person benefits from structure and simple routines and may benefit from day activity programs. Hazardous activities require supervision or restriction. The person is not safe to live alone.
3.5	Moderate functional decline; concrete thought processes. ADLs require set-up and often direction during performance. Needs 24-hour care; may benefit from supportive residential placement. May benefit from simple sequencing and repetitive activities to focus attention. May benefit from 1:1 simple socialization, such as singing/listening to music and pets.
3.0	Moderate to severe functional decline; increased cues needed during tasks. One-to-one assistance for all activity. Sensory deprivation; may benefit from sensory programs.
2.5	Severe functional decline; from object-centered to movement/sensory processes. Poor use of familiar objects. Total assist with ADLs. May be resistant with cares. Little speech. Sensory deprivation; may benefit from sensory programs.
1.0	Late-stage dementia. Unresponsive to surroundings. Comfort/hospice approach to care.

Source. From *Cognitive Performance Test (CPT) Revised Manual* (p. 2), by T. Burns, 2018, Pequannock, NJ: Maddak. Copyright © 2018 by Theressa Burns. Reprinted with permission.

is on the degree to which specifically defined deficits in working memory capabilities compromise performance in daily occupations.

Individuals present in clinical situations with impairments in memory that align with the cognitive–functional profiles seen in the CPT. For example, individuals at CPT Profile 5 show episodic memory impairment for verbal and visual information, but they can perform sufficiently using repeated directions, because their semantic memory is relatively intact.

For individuals performing at CPT Profile 4, both episodic and semantic memory are impaired. Their attention is impaired for task details and competing cues, and they have difficulty processing the conceptual and semantic information provided during the test. This level of impairment relates directly to difficulty with IADLs.

Reliance on procedural memory to use the objects provided during the test is characteristic of performance of individuals at CPT Profile 3. Difficulty initiating and sequencing task steps is prominent among individuals at this level. Table 14.2 describes the CPT performance patterns that correspond to subtask scores.

Cross-sectional studies support the concurrent validity of the CPT. The Mini-Mental State Examination (MMSE; Folstein et al., 1975) has a moderate to strong relationship with the CPT (range of correlation coefficients = .47–.88; Bar-Yosef et al., 2000; Burns, 2006; Douglas et al., 2012), as does the Assessment of Motor and Process Skills (AMPS) Process Scale (Fisher, 2010; r = .53; Douglas et al., 2012).

CPT scores have also been associated with basic ADLs for people with moderate to severe cognitive impairment living in residential care (Schaber et al., 2013; Thralow & Rueter, 1993) and for informant-rated ADLs and IADLs among community-dwelling people in mild to moderate stages of major NCD (Bar-Yosef et al., 2000; Burns et al., 1994). The CPT showed good ability to predict the need to retire from driving at a cutoff below 4.7 (sensitivity = 89%), in contrast with a need for driving restrictions (specificity = 75%), when the current 7-item battery was used (Burns et al., 2018).

A recent study (Burns et al., 2018) demonstrated that the CPT was able to accurately discriminate functional–cognitive abilities in the upper range of test scores. The CPT differentiated between individuals with a mild NCD and those with major NCD (early AD or other major NCDs). CPT scores in the low Level 5 range (i.e., 5.1–4.8) aligned with mild NCD (i.e., insignificant impairment in daily life), whereas CPT scores in the Level 4 range (4.8–4.5) were associated with major NCD and significant functional decline. Overlap in CPT scores with mild and (early) major NCD were also observed in this study.

The CPT was used in an inpatient rehabilitation setting as a predischarge measure to predict time to incidence of harm among people with suspected cognitive impairment once they left the hospital to return to community living (Douglas et al., 2013). Clients were followed over 6 months, and findings demonstrated preliminary evidence that the CPT was able to correctly identify people who did not have an incident of harm (i.e., specificity = 0.91), although AMPS Process scores were the best single predictor of time to incident of harm (Douglas et al., 2013). Both the AMPS Process scores and the CPT were better predictors than other clinical measures in the study, including the MMSE.

The earlier longitudinal study (Burns et al., 1994) showed that the CPT was able to predict risk of institutionalization among people with mild to moderate AD, with lower baseline scores indicating greater risk. Longitudinal testing demonstrated a significant decline in mean CPT scores with disease progression, and, in contrast to the MMSE, initial CPT scores predicted the risk of institutionalization over the 4-year follow-up period. All participants with an initial CPT score of 4.2 or less were institutionalized within 3.6 years of the

TABLE 14.2. Performance Patterns by CPT Score

CPT TASK SCORE	CPT TASK PERFORMANCE PATTERNS
6 or 5/5	The client demonstrates efficient and error-free execution of the task.
5 of 6	The client is able to process multiple written, verbal, visual, and contextual cues, but with relatively mild working memory/executive function impairments they may be slow, inefficient, impulsive, or make overt errors they can correct.
4.5 or 4.0	Executive dysfunction manifests in testing: The client cannot act on multiple task details and contextual directions without task reductions and cues. Although the person retains the main goal of each task, they cannot pay simultaneous attention to the details, nor inhibit the distracter props. Semantic memory impairment interferes here.
3.5 or 3.0	Working memory/executive function impairments are severe: The client relies on implicit procedural recognition cues to use the objects employed in the test but has trouble sequencing or loses sight of the intended outcome of the task.
2.5	The client touches or holds the objects but cannot perform the associated actions.

Source. From *Cognitive Performance Test (CPT) Revised Manual* (p. 8), by T. Burns, 2018, Pequannock, NJ: Maddak. Copyright © 2018 by Theressa Burns. Reprinted with permission.

baseline assessment, whereas 40% of the participants whose initial scores were above 4.2 remained in the community (Burns et al., 1994).

Several reliability studies have been completed with the CPT. Internal consistency has been reported to be high (α = .84) for the original 6-item battery (Burns et al., 1994), as well as for the original 6-item battery with 3 subtasks using substituted cultural task props (α = .95; Bar-Yosef et al., 2000). It was also acceptable both for the 7-item version with the medication subtask added (Burns et al., 2008) and when the 7-item version was used but only 6 items were included (the phone subtask was dropped; α = .71; Douglas et al., 2012).

Interrater reliability studies have often used videotaped performances (Bar-Yosef et al., 2000; Schaber et al., 2016), which may neutralize the "dynamic component of the CPT" (Bar-Yosef et al., 2000, p. 75) to some extent, thus inflating reliability coefficients, because scoring with videos is not done in real time. Nevertheless, these studies and the original study using real-time direct observation (Burns et al., 1994) consistently have reported high values for interrater reliability (from .91 to .98). Reliability among raters on the 7-item version (Burns, 2013) remains high irrespective of whether the raters are novice or experienced CPT administrators (Schaber et al., 2016). Test–retest reliability is similar. The original version of the CPT reported a high correlation coefficient (r = .89; Burns et al., 1994).

As the CPT has developed over time and revisions have been made (Burns, 2002, 2006, 2013, 2018), studies assessing the psychometric properties with several populations have consistently reported sound results for validity and reliability (Bar-Yosef et al., 2000; Burns et al., 1994, 2018; Douglas et al., 2012, 2013; Schaber et al., 2013, 2016). Research is continuing into the performance of the CPT with different clinical settings, but the existing psychometric properties of the CPT have strong foundations.

Target Population

Older adults (usually older than 65 years, but this may vary in indigenous populations) with suspected cognitive impairment are the principal target group for the CPT. Such individuals may present to therapists with self- or informant-reported difficulties in either IADLs or ADLs, depending on the clinical context. The CPT has been validated with older adults with NCDs across the continuum of care.

The original version of the CPT was developed for older adults with AD living in the community in the United States (Burns, 1986). Subsequent research has continued in this population, mostly in the United States in similar community-based outpatient settings (Burns et al., 1994, 2008, 2018; Schaber et al., 2016), with 1 cross-cultural replication study conducted in Israel (Bar-Yosef et al., 2000). The CPT has also been validated with older adults in a Canadian inpatient rehabilitation setting (Douglas et al., 2012, 2013) and with people with major NCD

living in residential care (in the United States; Schaber et al., 2013; Thralow & Rueter, 1993).

The CPT is anecdotally reported by experts in the field to be used with people who have mental health conditions, often in context of a suspected comorbid NCD (Burns, 2019; Burns & Haertl, 2018). There are no reports in the literature on the use of the CPT with adults with stroke or traumatic brain injury (Schaber et al., 2016), with children or adolescents, or with non-English-speaking people (other than the Israeli study by Bar-Yosef et al., 2000).

The CPT is able to identify deficits and predict function (Douglas et al., 2012). Examples of different purposes and contexts are provided in the next several sections.

Clients Without a Diagnosis

Individuals often present to occupational therapy with concern for cognitive or functional impairment but without a formal diagnosis. The CPT can be used to identify functional cognition impairment at the time of assessment, with the qualification that the assessment is cross-sectional and the individual may improve, especially if the acute event (e.g., delirium) is resolving. The CPT can help determine the level and type of supports the client requires to live in the community and whether supported residential accommodation is indicated. Follow-up reassessment or a formal diagnostic investigation for dementia may be indicated. The CPT is not a bedside evaluation and must not be administered if individuals are unable to participate in the subtasks according to the standardized instructions.

Outpatient Clinics

In outpatient clinics, the CPT can be used to provide a baseline or serial assessment of functional cognition and may include the family or caregivers, who provide collateral information and actively participate in the session. This is a complex, comprehensive process that requires the occupational therapist to administer the standardized assessment while simultaneously providing education to the individual and their caregiver.

Residential Settings

In residential care settings, people may have severe cognitive disabilities, and the CPT can be used to tailor assistance from staff as ability to perform self-care activities progressively declines. It can also help determine how best to engage clients in meaningful occupation.

Range of Abilities

The CPT is able to differentiate performance across the continuum of ability. There is evidence of its ability to differentiate between individuals with mild or major NCDs (Burns et al., 2018), and discriminative validity to differentiate healthy older adults from adults with moderate to severe stages of NCD has been demonstrated (Bar-Yosef et al., 2000; Burns et al., 1994). Research indicates that scores on the Standardized MMSE (Folstein et al., 1975) correlate moderately with CPT scores (Bar-Yosef et al., 2000; Burns et al., 1994; Douglas et al.,

2012), and participants perform within the expected range for MMSE, depending on diagnostic stage:

- Mean MMSE scores for healthy older adults range from 27.7 to 29.1 of 30.

- Mean MMSE scores for adults with dementia range from 10.9 to 20.3 of 30 (Bar-Yosef et al., 2000; Burns et al., 1994).

The focus of the CPT is on cognitive abilities, and the measure was constructed to minimize the influence of motor skills and sensory functions (Burns, 2018). A study with an inpatient rehabilitation sample (Douglas et al., 2012) supported this assertion, indicating that there was no influence of overall comorbidities on CPT scores. The influence of specific pathologies and of number of pathologies is unknown; however, further research is required. Although impaired motor functioning may influence test performance (Burns, 2018), during testing the therapist can provide physical assistance to the test taker without this having an effect on scoring.

Demographics

Age, gender, education, and comorbidities do not influence performance on the CPT among older adults with major NCD (Bar-Yosef et al., 2000) or those with suspected cognitive impairment (Douglas et al., 2012). Test administrators should, however, consider English literacy, because individuals are required to interpret test stimuli (e.g., reading medication labels, using a telephone book; Schaber et al., 2016). Cultural bias may also skew scores if clients have no familiarity with or concept of the usual routine performance of the activity.

Administration

The Revised CPT manual (Burns, 2018) using the 7-item battery is the current version of the CPT. This Revised CPT manual replaces previous manuals and, in particular, the original 6-item battery (Burns, 1992), all of which should no longer be used. The addition in 2002 of the CPT Medbox subtask changed the quality of the tool by adding another high-level task with multiple objects and semantic-knowledge-based cues. For example, concepts such as "take every other morning" and "take as needed" require intact semantic memory for performance—and evidence indicates that this is impaired at CPT Profile 4 (Burns et al., 2018).

Video 14.1 demonstrates the practice model and CPT administration. It starts with the occupational profile interview, followed by the CPT evaluation and client education. Viewers should note that the occupational profile interview matches the client's performance on the CPT Medbox subtask in terms of its score of 4.0 and in terms of support needs; however, the overall cognitive–functional level score (4.6) indicates capacities beyond what would be expected at lower scores (see Table 14.1).

For example, **George,** the veteran who consented to participate, passed a Veterans Administration driving exam. He was a police officer and drove nighttime duty for more than 30 years. People who function in CPT 4 have a wide range of abilities. The CPT Medbox subtask is not a stand-alone assessment, either as an indication of capacity to manage medications (with reliability) or for staging function on the CPT. The whole CPT battery should be administered to determine CPT profile. This is then used, in conjunction with the complexity of the person's own medication regimen, and their occupational profile to determine likely medication management ability.

CPT administration requires a private room set up with the standardized environmental props. All test protocols and most test items are provided in the kit, with some subtasks requiring therapists to gather additional supplies that are location specific. For example, the kit does not supply the coats used in the Dress subtask; a toaster for the Toast subtask; or a phone, cash, and stationery items for the Shop subtask. Perishable and local items are additional requirements.

Occupational therapists outside the United States need to localize test stimuli—that is, convert cash into equivalent amounts and establish culturally equivalent items. This may restrict the subtasks that are offered. For example, certain items may not be available in warmer climates, such as graded weightings of outdoor coats or the range of rainwear required in the Dress subtask. Therapists should contact the test author (theressa.burns@va.gov) to discuss equivalent stimuli that can be substituted, because the test is standardized and the specific properties are an important part of the standardization process.

For example, the CPT Phone subtask includes using a phone book and has been updated to a simulated call (Burns, 2018). Test administrators use clinical reasoning to score the client's performance in using the complex written cues contained in the phone book, including understanding the book's alphabetical organization, maintaining focus at the top of the book, and using semantic knowledge and memory for whom to call. The CPT props are meant to be basic and universal, such that the test has a relatively low bar or ceiling for typical adult performance.

All 7 subtasks should be administered in cases of mild to moderate cognitive impairment when a full assessment is necessary for accurate results—for example, when administration is to support diagnostic investigation or driving ability (Burns et al., 2018). Acceptable to good internal consistency has been reported (α = .71–.95 for different versions; Bar-Yosef et al., 2000; Burns et al., 1994; Douglas et al., 2012), which indicates that the construct being tested is global ability to perform activities, not discrete, domain-specific functional tasks (Burns et al., 1994). These studies on various versions of the CPT show that therapists need to administer multiple subtasks to maintain this reliability (Bar-Yosef et al., 2000; Burns et al., 1994; Douglas et al., 2012).

Another option is to administer the 5-item CPT subtask battery (Medbox, Shop, Wash, Toast, and Phone). This 5-task version has been compared with the 7-item CPT for concurrent validity with an Altman–Bland comparison method

(Schaber et al., 2016). The bias (20.01; potential for the score between the 2 versions to increase or decrease) and limits of agreement (20.30 to 0.27) indicate that the 5-task CPT version can be used effectively in lieu of the 7-task version. With fewer subtasks to score and average, however, the 5-item CPT typically yields a total score that is a few decimal points lower.

All subtasks are administered during a single assessment session, but the sequence can be varied according to the needs of the occupational therapist for efficient administration, such as ease in moving around the clinic from task to task. It may be helpful to start with the more challenging tasks (e.g., Medbox, Shop) and end with the easier tasks or alternate the two. The therapist first offers the whole task and its details, then reduces the performance requirements or adjusts the task props as they observe difficulty with task concepts and object cues. Once the therapist identifies (i.e., scores) the performance pattern, they tactfully end the subtask and move to the next task.

The CPT imposes stated and implied goals with written, verbal, and multistep contextual task requirements, and the test administrator observes patterns of performance that relate to each CPT level. They use multiple subgoals within each task to detect and objectively measure and quantify executive dysfunction (e.g., CPT Shop subgoals include selection by size, price, and available money in the wallet). Working memory difficulties and other executive dysfunctions may be reflected in performance errors relating to decision making, problem solving, and subgoal initiation and completion. The occupational therapist may observe the client having difficulty retaining all of the relevant information imposed during the test and difficulty staying on track long enough to produce the specific outcome as stated in the test instructions, while simultaneously inhibiting distractions (e.g., distracter props) and overriding their usual "familiar" method to perform the task.

The CPT performance levels range from intact performance (Level 6 or 5) to profound disability (Level 2). The manner in which the individual responds to the task contexts and the cognitive–functional demands of varying complexity is the primary concern. Table 14.2 describes the performance patterns associated with CPT subtask scores.

Scoring

Each CPT subtask performance is rated with a gross performance-level score (e.g., 6.0, 5.0, 4.5, 4.0, 3.5, 3.0, 2.5). Four subtasks (Medbox, Shop, Phone, Travel) scale to Level 6, and 3 (Wash, Toast, Dress) scale to Level 5 because these involve less-complex processing requirements. An advantage of the CPT is that the scoring criteria are organized by types of cues, and this is easy to follow on the score sheets. After initial directions are provided,

- General semantic cues,

- Specific semantic cues,

- Task setup, and

- Demonstrations

are structured into a descending hierarchy, with task reductions representing lower ability. Therapists work their way down the task reductions until the subtask performance score is identified. Subtask scores are summed, then divided by the number of subtasks completed to provide an overall score, ranging from 5.6 (*intact functioning*) to 1.0 (*severe impairment*).

CPT total scores represent an average performance or mean score and should not be confused with the Allen (1992) "modes of performance" interpretive system or scale. The Allen scale describes discrete levels of cognitive functions and associated IADL capacities at each mode. These levels do not align with CPT scores in the upper range (i.e., CPT Profiles 5 and 4), where significant variability in cognitive functions and IADL capacities is observed. Also, Allen scores scale up to Level 6 (*intact functioning*), whereas CPT scores scale to 5.6. Therefore, Allen scores in Levels 5 and high 4 describe impairment that is inconsistent with the CPT. Thus, these are 2 different scales and are not interchangeable.

The cognitive–functional profiles (Burns, 2018; see Table 14.1) are used to interpret test scores. These decrease in ordinal intervals; descriptions of cognitive processes, expected patterns of occupational performance, and details of the type and amount of assistance are provided at each level. For example, CPT Profile 4.5 is described as mild to moderate functional decline, and working memory, divided attention, and other EFs are significantly impaired (Burns, 2018). Individuals may therefore have difficulty with complex IADLs, because ability to manage details is impaired, but basic ADL performance is usually intact, with some reduced ability to initiate routines (Burns et al., 2018; Schaber et al., 2013). Individuals at this level are likely to need assistance with all IADLs, monitoring of ADLs, and help with potential safety hazards.

Occupational therapists can enhance the activation of clients' occupational performance by using concrete cues to tap into familiar and well-learned routines and environmental simplification (Burns et al., 2004; Ebbitt et al., 1989). Therapists can use these cognitive–functional profiles to help "benchmark" decline in occupational performance according to stages of neurocognitive progression (Schaber et al., 2013)— for example, when driving performance and management of finances are likely to become problematic—thereby linking declines in cognitive processes with functional performance.

The CPT cognitive–functional profiles (Burns, 2018) are used in the context of the individual's own activities and environments and their own individual mediating factors. These could include

- The individual's level of insight or awareness of disability;

- Specific activities that the individual does, needs to do, or wants to do;

- Experience and skill or lack of skill in specific tasks;

- Excess disability due to motor or visual impairments or focal brain deficits; and

- The level of caregiver and environmental support.

Diagnosis, prognosis, and specific brain pathology also influence the intervention plan. Thus, CPT interpretations vary on the basis of whether the cognitive–functional level is stable or changing (either improving or declining) and the idiosyncratic characteristics of the client.

Documentation

The purpose, the clinical context of the assessment, and the audience for the report are primary considerations that shape documentation. For example, clinical case notes in medical files may be shorter notes written to inform multidisciplinary teams of scores and cognitive–functional profiles, when the team is familiar with the CPT and its interpretation. Reports to external agencies may contain more detailed information regarding the implications of test results. However, in all cases, the following information should be included:

- Reason for assessment and referral source;

- A brief account of client presentation, including any specific behaviors, such as impulsivity or cooperation with assessment;

- A statement identifying the CPT as a measure of functional cognition that provides information about individuals' "cognitive integration with functioning in an IADL environmental context" (Burns et al., 2018, p. 2) that is standardized and **performance based** (i.e., an objective assessment based on direct observation of the client's ability to complete tasks) and is not an assessment of specific ADL and IADL domains;

- The version of the CPT and subtasks used, with any variations;

- Test score and CPT cognitive–functional profile, with a brief explanation of what this means for the individual's occupational performance (not specific scores for subtasks, which might endorse the perception that these represent a domain-specific ability in ADLs or IADLs);

- Recommendations for future steps for care planning, including any further assessment with focal or domain-specific measures;

- Statement regarding the degree of certainty of results on the basis of contextual factors that may influence performance.

Test administrators should schedule 1 hour for the CPT consultation and should use *Current Procedural Terminology (CPT®)* Code 96125, "Standardized Cognitive Performance Testing"

(American Medical Association, 2019).[1] This 1-hour service code, which can be billed only once per day, can include education and plans for care. Code 96125 also includes face-to-face time, time spent interpreting test results, and time to prepare the report. Occupational therapists should check with their companies to ensure that Code 96125 is covered under payer policy.

Additional information could include the qualitative aspects of task performance, such as error type, details of where task breakdown occurred, and the amount and type of assistance that helped the individual complete the tasks. The occupational therapist can document a comparison of test performance with observations of unstructured everyday activities to provide further confirmation of the functional–cognitive profile and expected patterns of performance.

For example, an individual who performs at 4.0 (moderate cognitive–functional disability; abstract to concrete thought processes) does not follow written directions on the medication labels during the Medbox subtask and does not correct errors in performance but does place some pills in the box. Family members have also observed the individual to ignore written electricity bills, and the individual is unable to understand how this behavior is linked to having their power shut off and why this might be problematic. The individual is unable to interpret or pay attention to written cues, identify or correct errors, or anticipate potential future consequences of actions. Inclusion of examples from individuals' everyday occupational performance helps validate findings of the formal CPT assessment, can help families and caregivers understand performance, and provide information to guide intervention planning.

The aim of the CPT is to evaluate the functional cognition and information-processing skills that are enlisted during occupational performance. It is also important to highlight individuals' strengths and abilities as well as their impairments in formal reports. When this emphasis on what individuals can do is combined with a cognitively oriented task analysis, highly sensitive assistance can be tailored that allows individuals to use their abilities optimally. For example, the therapist might eliminate specific steps in a task if the individual is unable to use higher-level thinking abilities, instead of disallowing them to participate in the task at all.

Interpretation and Intervention Considerations

To accurately interpret results of the CPT, occupational therapists must have a clear understanding that these results are an

---

[1] The code shown refers to *CPT 2019* (American Medical Association, 2019, *CPT 2019 standard*, Chicago: American Medical Association Press) and does not represent all of the possible codes that may be used in occupational therapy evaluation and intervention. After 2019, refer to the current year's *CPT* code book for available codes. *CPT* codes are updated annually and become effective January 1. *CPT* is a trademark of the American Medical Association. *CPT* 5-digit codes, 2-digit codes, modifiers, and descriptions are copyright © 2019 by the American Medical Association. All rights reserved.

estimate of functional cognition, representing global patterns of occupational performance, and not domain-specific functional indicators (Burns, 2006). That is, scores do not represent ability in the specific tasks tested. Rather, emphasis is on the extent of impairment in information processing that may compromise the client's performance of everyday activities, in particular executive control functions and working memory (Burns et al., 2018).

The actual tasks that are used are "less important than the manner in which patients respond to demands of varying complexity" (Burns et al., 1994, p. 46). Instead, the profiles are able to provide "prediction about anticipated level of occupational performance" (Schaber et al., 2013, p. 176). Therapists can then apply these predictions to individual situations, ensuring that the team considers a holistic view of client factors in interpretation. This may include limitations in motor skills, physical impairment, or previous experience with various subtasks.

CPT test scores are interpreted according to the measure's half-level profile system provided in the test manual (see Table 14.1). These descriptions allow therapists to explain and predict individuals' ability to function. Information about working memory and EF processes that clients use while performing tasks is detailed and can be generalized to other areas of occupational performance according to task analysis principles. The cognitive–functional profiles range from 5.6 (intact functioning indicating an absence of cognitive–functional disability) to 1.0 (severe cognitive–functional disability or late-stage dementia; Burns, 2018; see Table 14.1).

The CPT should always be interpreted in the context of the specific situation of the client during the assessment—for example, whether the client is medically stable or their condition is improving or declining. The therapist needs to include in the interpretation other factors that may influence performance, reasserting the statement regarding the degree of certainty of results. Many individual, environmental, and other contextual factors may mediate performance and should be acknowledged. CPT test scores should always be considered in the light of clinical observations and other concurrent measures of cognition and function that may be administered, because classification of impaired functioning can vary among instruments used (Douglas et al., 2012).

A significant advantage of the CPT and the cognitive–functional profiles is the explanation of performance breakdown and identification of support strategies. Insights into why individuals respond in certain ways allow family members, carers, and the health care team to better understand the individual's experience and help provide tailored strategies based on their intimate knowledge of the person. This information frequently comes with a sense of relief, because impaired functional cognition often manifests as limitations in occupational performance.

There is also a tendency to assign negative labels to individuals whose abilities are unclear, and terms such as *difficult* and *oppositional* are often used. This can undermine such individuals' confidence and may result in restrictions being imposed without objective reasons, limiting opportunities for participation. Understanding functional cognition is key to enabling clients, families, caregivers, and staff alike.

Specific recommendations for assisting task performance are key components of the cognitive–functional profiles and form the cornerstone of intervention across the continuum of ability. Individuals are given assistance that is within their information-processing capacity. Strategies may include use of verbal language-based cues at higher levels, visuospatial cues (written, pictorial, or demonstrated), proprioceptive cues, and tactile cues (hand over hand).

Intervention is then directed to specific tasks or everyday activities. Therapists analyze information-processing requirements and either modify the task, adjust the cues, or reconfigure the environment to better support function. This approach to intervention allows the team to capitalize on individuals' strengths and abilities and compensate for impairments, resulting in maximal participation in desired activities.

The CPT and the cognitive–functional profiles have been used to develop care plans and intervention programs for people with major NCD in residential care (Sevier & Gorek, 2000; Thralow & Rueter, 1993). The CPT was used to develop specific care plans focusing on ADL performance for a group of older men with dementia in a residential facility (Thralow & Rueter, 1993). The men functioned at lower levels, and the ability of the CPT to capture and measure behavioral responses was highlighted—an advantage in assessing people living with severe dementia when verbal abilities are impaired. Many assessments are mediated primarily by verbal skills, whereas the CPT accounts for both verbal and motor actions, providing an accurate representation of performance and clear guidance regarding assistance.

A second, anecdotal description of the measure's use in a residential care setting stated that the CPT was effective in guiding care planning for ADLs, IADLs, communication, socialization, and challenging behaviors (Sevier & Gorek, 2000). Occupational therapists assessed individuals, provided direction to individual and group-based activity programs, and trained care staff and families in how to provide assistance to clients. Stated outcomes included a reduction in agitated behaviors, improved engagement in activities, and more-effective use of staff time because the model allowed them to "decrease the amount of time staff spend trying ineffective approaches to care" (Sevier & Gorek, 2000, p. 96). No formal outcome measures were reported, however.

The CPT was used in 2 small studies (*Ns* = 7 and 9) reporting on a community-based, adapted work-style intervention for men with major NCD attending a day center (Burns et al., 2004; Ebbitt et al., 1989). The program was designed to individually assign and adapt tasks on the basis of the men's CPT profile. This program was shown to be feasible and satisfying and reduced depressive symptoms for participants with mild to moderate dementia.

Burns et al. (2004) also suggested that the program might have had a role in delaying decline in AD. When the program ended and the men were transitioned to an alternative "traditional-style" day program, predicted scores on the CPT and MMSE were lower than expected (Han et al., 2000), and significant declines in ADLs were reported by caregivers 4 months later. This finding highlights the role of occupational therapists in using standardized, performance-based measures such as the CPT to evaluate functional cognition among people with major NCD and to help inform detailed and tailored intervention programs to improve occupational performance. This approach in general has been successful for therapists in a number of studies (Gitlin et al., 2008; O'Connor et al., 2017; Wesson et al., 2013).

Summary

The CPT is a standardized, performance-based measure of functional cognition that has been validated in older populations with suspected and diagnosed NCDs. It uses common everyday activities to allow therapists to evaluate the cognitive processes that clients use during functional performance and draw conclusions about their global abilities. Occupational therapists evaluate clients for cognitive–functional impairment and are skilled in observing the effects of such impairment in the context of complex daily tasks. The advantage of the CPT as a standardized evaluation is that the psychometric foundations are strong, and test results can be interpreted with some confidence. That is, scores are reliable and valid and can be generalized for real-world functioning.

The CPT can be purchased in the United States from Maddak.com (https://shop.maddak.com/p/cpt-cognitive-performance-test) and its vendors, including the American Occupational Therapy Association's Online Store. For locations outside the United States, accessing the instrument is more difficult. Suppliers will order the test kit—it is not generally a stocked item, so it can take a minimum of 6 to 8 weeks for it to be shipped after an order is placed.

References

Allen, C. K. (1985). *Occupational therapy for psychiatric diseases: Measurement and management of cognitive disabilities*. Boston: Little, Brown.

Allen, C. K. (1992). Modes of performance within the cognitive levels. In C. K. Allen, C. A. Earhart, & T. Blue (Eds.), *Occupational therapy treatment goals for the physically and cognitively disabled* (pp. 85–102). Bethesda, MD: AOTA Press.

Allen, C. K., & Allen, R. E. (1987). Cognitive disabilities: Measuring the social consequences of mental disorders. *Journal of Clinical Psychiatry, 48*, 185–190.

Allen, C. K., Earhart, C. A. & Blue, T. (1992). *Occupational therapy treatment goals for the physically and cognitively disabled*. Bethesda, MD: AOTA Press.

American Medical Association. (2019). *Current procedural terminology (CPT®) 2019 standard*. Chicago: American Medical Association Press.

American Psychiatric Association. (2013). *Diagnostic and statistical manual of mental disorders* (5th ed.). Washington, DC: Author.

Bar-Yosef, C., Weinblatt, N., & Katz, N. (2000). Reliability and validity of the Cognitive Performance Test (CPT) in an elderly population in Israel. *Physical and Occupational Therapy in Geriatrics, 17*, 65–79. https://doi.org/10.1080/J148v17n01_06

Burns, T. (1986). *Cognitive Performance Test (CPT) manual: A measure of cognitive capacity for the performance of routine tasks*. Minneapolis: Minneapolis Veterans Affairs Medical Center.

Burns, T. (1990, December 27). The Cognitive Performance Test: A new tool for assessing Alzheimer's disease. *OT Weekly, 4*, 51.

Burns, T. (1992). Evaluation instruments: Part III: The Cognitive Performance Test: An approach to cognitive level assessment in Alzheimer's disease. In C. K. Allen, C. A. Earhart, & T. Blue (Eds.), *Occupational therapy treatment goals for the physically and cognitively disabled* (pp. 46–50). Bethesda, MD: AOTA Press.

Burns, T. (2002). *Cognitive Performance Test (CPT) manual*. Pequannock, NJ: Maddak.

Burns, T. (2006). *Cognitive Performance Test (CPT) manual*. Pequannock, NJ: Maddak.

Burns, T. (2013). *Cognitive Performance Test (CPT) manual*. Pequannock, NJ: Maddak.

Burns, T. (2018). *Cognitive Performance Test (CPT) Revised manual 2018*. Pequannock, NJ: Maddak.

Burns, T. (2019). Using the Cognitive Performance Test Neurocognitive Practice Model. In B. J. Hemphill-Pearson & C. K. Urish (Eds.), *Assessments in occupational therapy mental health: An integrative approach* (3rd ed., pp. 179–192). Thorofare, NJ: Slack.

Burns, T., & Haertl, K. (2018). Cognitive Performance Test: Practical applications and evidence-based use. *AOTA SIS Quarterly Practice Connections, 3*(4), 17–20.

Burns, T., Lawler, K., Lawler, D., McCarten, J. R., & Kuskowski, M. (2018). Predictive value of the Cognitive Performance Test (CPT) for staging function and fitness to drive in people with neurocognitive disorders. *American Journal of Occupational Therapy, 72*, 7204205040. https://doi.org/10.5014/ajot.2018.027052

Burns, T., & Levy, L. L. (2006). Neurocognitive practice essentials in dementia: Cognitive disabilities reconsidered model. *OT Practice, 11*(3), CE-1–CE-8.

Burns, T., McCarten, J. R., Adler, G., Bauer, M., & Kuskowski, M. A. (2004). Effects of repetitive work on maintaining function in Alzheimer's disease patients. *American Journal of Alzheimer's Disease and Other Dementias, 19*, 39–44. https://doi.org/10.1177/153331750401900109

Burns, T., McCarten, J. R., & Kuskowski, M. (2008). P3-006: Cognitive performance test: Validity of the new Medbox subtask. *Alzheimer's and Dementia, 4*(Suppl.), T518. https://doi.org/10.1016/j.jalz.2008.05.1569

Burns, T., Mortimer, J. A., & Merchak, P. (1994). Cognitive Performance Test: A new approach to functional assessment in Alzheimer's disease. *Journal of Geriatric Psychiatry and Neurology, 7*, 46–54. https://doi.org/10.1177/089198879400700109

Douglas, A., Letts, L., Eva, K., & Richardson, J. (2012). Use of the Cognitive Performance Test for identifying deficits in hospitalized older adults. *Rehabilitation Research and Practice, 2012*, 638480. https://doi.org/10.1155/2012/638480

Douglas, A. M., Letts, L. J., Richardson, J. A., & Eva, K. W. (2013). Validity of predischarge measures for predicting time to harm in older adults. *Canadian Journal of Occupational Therapy, 80*, 19–27. https://doi.org/10.1177/0008417412473577

Ebbitt, B., Burns, T., & Christensen, R. (1989). Work therapy: Intervention for community-based Alzheimer's patients. *American Journal of Alzheimer's Disease and Other Dementias, 4*(5), 7–15. https://doi.org/10.1177/153331758900400506

Fisher, A. G. (2010). *Assessment of Motor and Process Skills user manual* (7th ed.). Ft. Collins, CO: Three Star Press.

Folstein, M. F., Folstein, S. E., & McHugh, P. R. (1975). "Mini-Mental State": A practical method for grading the cognitive state of patients for the clinician. *Journal of Psychiatric Research, 12*, 189–198. https://doi.org/10.1016/0022-3956(75)90026-6

Gitlin, L. N., Winter, L., Burke, J., Chernett, N., Dennis, M. P., & Hauck, W. W. (2008). Tailored activities to manage neuropsychiatric behaviors in persons with dementia and reduce caregiver burden: A randomized pilot study. *American Journal of Geriatric Psychiatry, 16,* 229–239. https://doi.org/10.1097/01.JGP.0000300629.35408.94

Han, L., Cole, M., Bellavance, F., McCusker, J., & Primeau, F. (2000). Tracking cognitive decline in Alzheimer's disease using the Mini-Mental State Examination: A meta-analysis. *International Psychogeriatrics, 12,* 231–247.

O'Connor, C. M., Clemson, L., Brodaty, H., Low, L. F., Jeon, Y. H., Gitlin, L. N., . . . Mioshi, E. (2017). The Tailored Activity Program (TAP) to address behavioral disturbances in frontotemporal dementia: A feasibility and pilot study. *Disability and Rehabilitation, 41,* 299–310. https://doi.org/10.1080/09638288.2017.1387614

Schaber, P., Klein, T., Hanrahan, E., Vencil, P., Afatika, K., & Burns, T. (2013). Using cognitive–functional assessment to predict self-care performance of memory care tenants. *American Journal of Alzheimer's Disease and Other Dementias, 28,* 171–178. https://doi.org/10.1177/1533317512470206

Schaber, P., Stallings, E., Brogan, C., & Ali, F. (2016). Interrater reliability of the Revised Cognitive Performance Test (CPT): Assessing cognition in people with neurocognitive disorders. *American Journal of Occupational Therapy, 70,* 7005290010. https://doi.org/10.5014/ajot.2016.019166

Sevier, S., & Gorek, B. (2000). Cognitive evaluation in care planning for people with Alzheimer disease and related dementias. *Geriatric Nursing, 21,* 92–97. https://doi.org/10.1067/mgn.2000.107130

Thralow, J. U., & Rueter, M. J. S. (1993). Activities of daily living and cognitive levels of function in dementia. *American Journal of Alzheimer's Disease and Other Dementias, 8*(5), 14–19. https://doi.org/10.1177/153331759300800505

Wesson, J., Clemson, L., Brodaty, H., Lord, S., Taylor, M., Gitlin, L., & Close, J. (2013). A feasibility study and pilot randomised trial of a tailored prevention program to reduce falls in older people with mild dementia. *BMC Geriatrics, 13,* 89. https://doi.org/10.1186/1471-2318-13-89

15

Assessment of Motor and Process Skills

LOU ANN GRISWOLD, PhD, OTR/L, FAOTA

LEARNING OBJECTIVES

After completing this chapter, readers should be able to

- Identify the purpose and unique focus of the Assessment of Motor and Process Skills (AMPS),
- Explain the value of the AMPS in conducting a performance analysis,
- Describe the administration process for the AMPS from interview through documentation, and
- Identify the client characteristics that occupational therapists should consider when determining whether the AMPS is an appropriate assessment tool to choose.

KEY TERMS AND CONCEPTS

- Client centered • Occupation based • Occupation focused • Performance analysis • Performance skills
- Top-down reasoning

Introduction

The Assessment of Motor and Process Skills (AMPS; Fisher & Jones, 2012, 2014) was developed by Anne G. Fisher in the late 1980s, on the basis of preliminary work with Susan Doble (1991). Fisher (1992) saw the need for a valid and reliable assessment based on observations of a person's performance during ADL tasks, particularly IADLs, that were familiar and relevant for the person's daily life. In particular, Fisher developed the AMPS to provide an assessment tool that was *client centered* (i.e., addressing desires and priorities of the client), performance-based, and focused on the quality of a person's ADL task performance. In other words, the AMPS

- Was designed to address tasks that are important to the client,

- Is based on the client's ability to perform desired tasks, and

- Focuses on occupational performance, not factors that might influence the performance.

Fisher (1997) wanted the assessment to provide information that was different from that yielded by other assessment tools and that would allow occupational therapists to evaluate a person's

- Physical effort,

- Efficiency,

- Safety, and

- Need for assistance during ADL performance.

The AMPS enables the occupational therapist to conduct a *performance analysis*—that is, to evaluate the quality of occupational performance skills and the observable actions that make up occupational performance, not underlying body function, such as cognition or physical capacities.

Because the AMPS focuses on occupational performance before considering evaluation of suspected impairment in body function, the measure supports top-down reasoning, as described in the Occupational Therapy Intervention Process Model (OTIPM) developed by Fisher (1998, 2009) and recently expanded by Fisher and Marterella (2019). Furthermore, the AMPS is *occupation focused,* because the proximal focus of the evaluation is on occupation. The AMPS is also *occupation based,* because the evaluation is based on the person engaging in an occupation that is relevant in their life (for further reading on these concepts, see Fisher, 2013).

Fisher (1992) recognized that persons might want to perform a range of ADL tasks, especially IADLs, and that these tasks would pose different levels of challenge. To consider tasks merely on the basis of the number of steps would not allow the occupational therapist to compare the performance of various tasks. As a result, Fisher saw the need to develop a tool based on a conceptualized continuum of ADL ability. The continuum of ADL ability assumes that some tasks are more difficult than other tasks, thus creating a hierarchy of task challenge.

To create an assessment tool that could be used to evaluate the quality of performance of many different tasks and that was very sensitive, Fisher (1997) proposed evaluating the quality of small actions that could be observed in any task performance. She called these "universal actions" *performance skills* because they are universal, observable, goal-directed actions of any ADL task performance. The AMPS includes 36 performance skills (i.e., the AMPS items). The AMPS items also have a hierarchy of difficulty—that is, some skills are easier than others. The hierarchies of task difficulty and AMPS items are 2 of the facets included in the many-faceted Rasch analysis[1] that the Occupational Therapy Assessment Package (OTAP; Center for Innovative OT Solutions, 2016) software uses to generate an ADL motor ability measure and an ADL process ability measure. The results provide a thorough *performance analysis,* indicating the quality of a person's ADL performance.

Although multiple research editions were developed, Fisher published the first edition of the AMPS manual in 1995; this version included 56 IADL tasks. The first edition included computer-scoring software that provided computer-generated reports. Over the years, new tasks have been added, so there are now 142 standardized task options, which include personal ADL (PADL) and IADL tasks. The computer-scoring software, OTAP, has become more sophisticated and easier to use in more recent editions of the AMPS.

More than 200 articles on the AMPS support its reliability, validity, sensitivity, and utility to guide intervention planning and to report change after intervention (Center for Innovative OT Solutions, 2018). AMPS courses have been offered in more than 25 countries, and the *AMPS User Manual* (Fisher & Jones, 2014) has been translated into 8 additional languages. The standardization sample in the current version of OTAP includes more than 250,000 persons with and without identified disabilities, 2 to 103 years of age, from more than 35 countries (Fisher & Merritt, 2012) in the following regions:

- North America
- The United Kingdom and the Republic of Ireland

- Europe
- Nordic countries
- Australasia
- South America
- The Middle East.

The AMPS has been shown to be free of bias associated with gender, ethnicity, and country (Fisher & Merritt, 2012; Gantschnig et al., 2012).

Target Population

The AMPS is designed to be used with anyone who experiences or is at risk of experiencing challenges performing ADL tasks. It may be used with children or adults, including those with

- Mental health diagnoses (Ayres & John, 2015; Rojo-Mota et al., 2014),
- Neurological conditions (Björkdahl et al., 2013),
- Physical impairments (Waehrens et al., 2010), or
- Developmental disorders (Gantschnig et al., 2013; Park, 2015).

For research purposes, the AMPS can also be used with persons who are not experiencing difficulty (i.e., healthy people).

Occupational therapists working with clients who report difficulty with ADLs—either PADLs, such as dressing, showering, or grooming, or IADLs, such as preparing a meal, vacuuming, or washing dishes—may choose to administer the AMPS. ADLs frequently support a person's role as a spouse or partner, parent, or son or daughter.

When providing information for an occupational profile, a client might indicate that they have a desire to complete ADL tasks but are currently having difficulty with 1 or more of these. A client's goals might include being able to perform IADL tasks that range from simple to complex: from pouring a beverage from a pitcher to making a pot of coffee, or from making a simple sandwich to preparing a complex meal with a main dish, salad, and beverage. Other goals might include a range of household tasks, such as sweeping, vacuuming, raking leaves, doing laundry, unloading the dishwasher, or shopping.

The AMPS is a logical assessment to administer before other assessments, because it provides an occupation-focused perspective. That is, the focus of the AMPS is on occupation, not factors that might support or limit a person's occupational performance (e.g., environment, body function, motivation, task demands). Additional assessments can later help the occupational therapist confirm or rule out how other factors might be influencing occupational performance.

The occupational therapist may determine whether to administer the AMPS after administering the Canadian Occupational Performance Measure (Law et al., 2014) or similar

---

[1]Many-faceted Rasch analysis creates a measure of probability using a model based on multiple identified conditions, or facets (Bond & Fox, 2007). The facets used to generate ADL ability measures for the AMPS include the difficulty of the ADL skill items, the challenge of the tasks performed, the ability of the person, and the severity of the rater.

assessment tool to screen for the client's reported perspective on their ADL and IADL ability. Therapists who use the AMPS to assess occupational performance would not use screening tools that focus on body function. Evaluating quality of performance before assessing a suspected cause of problems in performance (e.g., body function, environment) is referred to as a ***top-down reasoning*** to assessment.

Clients may do very well or very poorly on such screening assessments of body function yet perform desired and needed occupations quite differently. For example, a client may not do well answering questions, repeating words, or drawing geometric shapes because these are not familiar tasks and lack relevance. However, context often supports a person's performance of familiar tasks and provides natural motivation for a person to engage in relevant and desired tasks. Therefore, a client might not demonstrate good memory on a screening of cognitive ability (a body function) but might demonstrate the ability to make a sandwich (an IADL task). The natural cues of the environment may support the person's performance when they are making the sandwich. Conversely, a client may perform quite well on a screening tool—able to recall facts or words and identify pictures of animals—but be inefficient when performing an ADL or IADL task (Doble et al., 1997). Assessments of occupational performance, or the ability to perform ADL tasks, evaluate a different construct than the underlying body functions that support occupational performance.

Because the focus of the AMPS is on occupational performance, in particular the performance of ADLs, a client's diagnosis is irrelevant. Children and adults all need to do PADLs and IADLs. Adults need and usually want to return to cooking and household cleaning, because these activities support their roles.

When the clients are children, IADLs are often called *chores.* Activities that children might do include making their bed, packing a lunch, unloading the dishwasher, or raking leaves. As children prepare to transition out of school and into adult life, the expected IADLs increase in complexity. The AMPS has been cited as a valuable tool in planning for transition to adulthood for older youth (Kardos & White, 2006).

Depending on the age, diagnosis, level of acuity, and prognosis, adults engage in a range of ADLs. In acute care, PADLs or basic ADLs may be more important to a client who is medically less stable or deconditioned. During inpatient rehabilitation, clients often want to return home. In this case, the occupational therapist should have the client identify the activities that they will need and want to do at home. To prepare for transition to home, asking the person about simple meal preparation and household tasks helps identify the types of tasks to consider for evaluation and intervention. When a client has returned home and is receiving outpatient occupational therapy, they can clearly identify the desired IADL tasks that are easy and those that are challenging.

Administering the AMPS throughout the continuum of care can allow occupational therapists who provide services to track a client's quality of ADL and IADL performance over time and across settings. The tasks will change as the person transitions through the settings of care and becomes more able. An AMPS evaluation can evaluate change and, more important, can guide intervention throughout the continuum of care.

Administration

The AMPS is available from the Center for Innovative OT Solutions (https://www.innovativeOTsolutions.com). To ensure reliable and valid administration and scoring and become a certified AMPS rater, occupational therapists take either a face-to-face course or an online course. The AMPS manual is a 2-volume set. Volume 1 of the AMPS manual describes administration procedures, interpretation of results, standardization, and development of the AMPS (Fisher & Jones, 2012). Volume 2, the *AMPS User Manual,* includes task descriptions and scoring criteria for each of the AMPS skill items (performance skills; Fisher & Jones, 2014). Also included with course registration is the OTAP software and user license, which are necessary to generate reports, including ADL motor ability and ADL process ability measures.

Occupational therapists submit data for 10 persons after completing the course to establish a calibration rating. The therapist's calibration rating (e.g., their strictness as a rater) becomes 1 of the facets in the many-faceted Rasch analyses needed to generate the ADL ability measures for the person evaluated by a certified AMPS rater.

The AMPS is administered in natural contexts that are appropriate for the ADL tasks chosen by the client. For example, cooking tasks are performed in a kitchen, and grooming tasks are completed in a bathroom, whereas vacuuming a car is done out of doors. In a natural environment, the needed tools and materials are typically readily available for the specific tasks that are selected by the client and occupational therapist. In some situations, the therapist may need to supply a few items, particularly if the assessment is conducted in a clinic environment, where supplies may be more limited.

Setup is minimal because the person performs tasks in the way that they would typically do them, which supports the client-centered perspective of the AMPS. The occupational therapist needs to ensure that all required tools and materials are available before the client begins each task for observation. The therapist also ensures that the client is familiar with the setup of the environment and the location of all needed tools and materials.

Each task is standardized on the basis of specified criteria but flexible enough to allow for the wide variation in the ways people around the world perform ADL tasks. For example, when the client is to make a pot of coffee or tea for 1 or 2 persons, they are "expected to prepare a pot of boiled or brewed coffee or tea and serve the coffee or tea into cups or mugs, and serve the coffee or tea with either a container of milk or cream, or a second pot of hot water" (AMPS Task A-3; Fisher & Jones, 2014, p. 44). These criteria make up the standardization of the task.

To allow the task to be culturally relevant and support client-centered practice, the AMPS tasks have options. For the coffee or tea task, the person decides

- Whether to make boiled or brewed coffee or boiled or brewed tea,

- The type of coffee maker to be used or how the water will be heated,

- How many servings to make,

- Whether to put milk in the cups or mugs, and

- Whether to add or serve sweetener.

The decisions the client makes regarding the task options (e.g., brewing tea, adding milk to the cups, serving with sweetener) are considered when the occupational therapist scores the AMPS observation.

Administration of the AMPS reflects the OTIPM (Fisher, 2009; Fisher & Marterella, 2019). The OTIPM is similar to the *Occupational Therapy Practice Framework: Domain and Process* (3rd ed.; *OTPF–3*; American Occupational Therapy Association [AOTA], 2014) in some respects. However, the OTIPM, a true top-down process, emphasizes observing the person perform a task and completing a performance analysis before considering or evaluating possible underlying causes of diminished occupational performance. The *OTPF–3* includes observation as a possible evaluation method but does not require this valuable step.

Administration of the AMPS begins with an occupational therapy interview with the client to learn about the types of activities the person has done, currently does, and would like to do. The occupational therapist gathers information about the types of tasks that are challenging. Most important, the therapist learns about the client's goals. If the person expresses difficulty with ADLs and a desire or need to perform ADLs, the therapist may choose to administer the AMPS. At that point in the interview, the therapist begins to focus the conversation on tasks that the client reported are relevant and challenging and to match these tasks with those in the *AMPS User Manual*.

If a client who has been referred for an occupational therapy evaluation cannot participate in an interview, someone in the client's constellation—that is, a person familiar with the client—may provide that information. Parents, adult children, spouses, or care providers may be included in the client constellation. Throughout the remainder of this chapter, a case example of a woman named Wanda illustrates the administration of the AMPS.

Wanda said she would like to be able to do the tasks that she used to do. The **occupational therapist** working with Wanda heard Wanda's clearly stated desire to return to tasks she used to do at home, including simple meal preparation, and decided to use the AMPS for evaluation. Wanda said that making breakfast for her family was something that she had done in the past that supported her role as a mother but now was difficult for her. Her therapist asked her questions to learn what Wanda typically prepares for breakfast (e.g., coffee, cereal, eggs, pancakes, French toast; these are tasks in the *AMPS User Manual*).

Depending on what a client reports as relevant, the occupational therapist and client determine together what tasks the therapist will observe the client perform. For an AMPS evaluation, the occupational therapist observes the person perform at least 2 AMPS tasks. The therapist considers the difficulty of the task in relation to the hierarchy of task challenge found in the *AMPS User Manual*. For example, making an instant beverage is much easier than making eggs and toast. Choosing tasks that coincide with the client's overall ability is essential to obtaining valid results with the AMPS. It is important that the therapist be aware of the task-challenge hierarchy and potential task options that reflect the client's general ability level before entering into a discussion of AMPS task options with the client.

The occupational therapist prepares for the interview by developing a list of tasks that coincide with the client's background, ability, and culture as well as where the observations will occur (e.g., the person's home, a clinic). The therapist creates a task list with notes on the tasks to allow the interview to flow smoothly, on the basis of information gathered during the occupational therapy interview. The interview concludes with the client identifying 2 tasks that they will do for the AMPS observation.

Once the client has selected 2 tasks, the occupational therapist and client proceed to the first task. The therapist first sets up the task environment with the client. During this phase, the therapist ensures that the person is familiar with the environment and the location of all needed tools and materials. During the setup of the task, the client identifies specific details of the task to be completed.

Wanda wanted to prepare a bowl of puffed rice cereal, with milk and sugar, and a glass of orange juice. Selecting the type of cereal, putting milk and sugar on the cereal, and pouring the glass of orange juice become part of the specific task expectations.

The fact that the specific task is determined by the client allows the evaluation to be client centered. The client chooses the tasks that they want to do and identifies specific criteria for the task to be performed for the evaluation (e.g., puffed rice cereal). The client then performs the task in their usual manner. All of these factors support a client-centered assessment. As the client performs the task, the occupational therapist observes and takes notes of the client's task performance. The notes are used to score the quality of the client's performance.

Often after performing ADL tasks, clients want to talk about how they did when performing the task. The occupational therapist can choose to ask the client questions to gather their perspective using the *Assessment of Compared Qualities* (ACQ; Fisher et al., 2017). The ACQ, a companion tool to the AMPS, includes 11 questions to learn about the person's perspective on their task performance. The 2 perspectives, that of the client and that of the therapist, can help the therapist and the client later determine client-centered goals based on shared agreement regarding areas of difficulty the client experienced during the task.

The client then proceeds to the 2nd task selected for the AMPS evaluation. That task also begins with the occupational therapist and the client setting up the task environment, followed by the client performing that task as they usually would. The entire administration process—conducting the occupational therapy interview, selecting the 2 tasks the person will perform and observing the 2 ADL tasks, administering the ACQ, and scoring the AMPS and ACQ—generally takes an hour.

Scoring

Knowing whether a person can complete a task, the level of safety observed, and the degree of assistance needed is essential for considering discharge planning and determining supports the client needs to live with greater independence. However, occupational therapists also need to consider the quality of the person's performance during a task. In particular, therapists need to evaluate the amount of physical effort and time and space inefficiencies the person experienced during the ADL task performance, conducting a performance analysis.

After the 2 observations, the occupational therapist uses the scoring criteria in the *AMPS User Manual* to analyze the quality of the person's performance on 36 skill items—16 motor skills and 20 process skills for each task observed. The same motor skills and process skills are in the *OTPF–3*. The AMPS is criterion-referenced, and the criterion is competence. Each of the skill items is scored on a 4-point rating scale, where a score of 4 indicates competent performance of the skill and a score of 1 indicates severely deficient skill performance. Often the severely deficient skill performance results in a marked impact on the overall task.

The rating criteria are summarized below:

- A score of 4 indicates no increase in physical effort or clumsiness; no inefficiency using time, space, or tools and materials; no safety risks during the performance; and no assistance provided.

- A score of 3 indicates questionable quality of performance—that is, the occupational therapist questioned whether the client demonstrated less than competent performance.

- A score of 2 indicates that the client demonstrated ineffective performance that interfered with the task performance—that is, some clumsiness or physical effort, some inefficiency, or a possible safety risk.

- A score of 1 indicates that the client demonstrated severely deficient performance in a skill item because of unacceptable physical effort or clumsiness or unacceptable use of time, space, tools or materials; had an imminent safety risk; or demonstrated the need for assistance.

Scoring each of the 36 skill items on 2 or more tasks leads to a very sensitive measure of ADL task performance.

The occupational therapist then enters the skill item ratings for the observed tasks into the OTAP software. The OTAP software uses many-faceted Rasch analysis to convert the ordinal scores of the skill items into linear measures of ADL motor ability and ADL process ability, which indicate the person's overall physical effort and overall efficiency during ADL task performance. The ADL motor ability measure and ADL process ability measure are reported in logits, or log-odds probability units.

Many-faceted Rasch analysis takes into account

- Rasch-calibrated skill hierarchy,

- Task hierarchy,

- Ability of the client, and

- Occupational therapist's severity as a rater.

As a result, the ability measures are valid and reliable measures of ADL motor and ADL process ability. Only the Rasch-generated ability measures can be used to report on a client's ADL performance; sums of the raw scores are not valid measures.

Video 15.1 provides an example of performance analysis based on observation of a man named James as he makes an open-faced peanut butter sandwich. The video also illustrates an AMPS score form and reports that are generated by the OTAP software.

Documentation

The OTAP software generates several reports that the occupational therapist can use to document the results of the AMPS evaluation. The most relevant report is the AMPS Results Report, which can be shared with the client, family, or team members. The AMPS Results Report includes brief, general information on the AMPS. More important, the AMPS Results Report places the client's ADL motor ability measure and ADL process ability measure, reported in logits, on 2 scales (see Figures 15.1 and 15.2, respectively) and provides interpretation of the measures.

The occupational therapist can add information to the AMPS Results Report to support documentation of the evaluation. Often, therapists add information

- To indicate specific skill items that were strengths and those that were most limiting to the person's ADL task performance, and

- To provide specific contextual information based on the observations.

Such specific information helps the client understand their problems in occupational performance. The therapist can also add goals that the client helped to develop.

FIGURE 15.1. Assessment of motor skills: ADL Motor Scale results for Wanda.

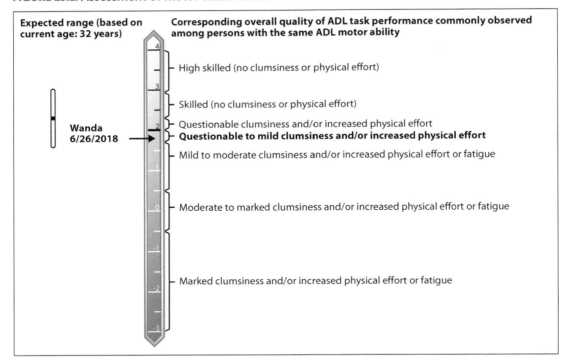

Source. Generated using the *OT Assessment Package* (OTAP software; Three Star Press, 2018).

FIGURE 15.2. Assessment of process skills: ADL Process Scale results for Wanda.

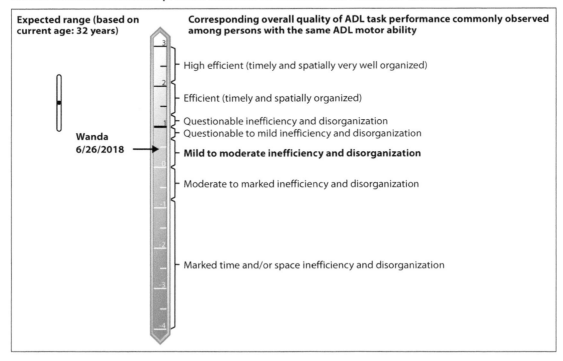

Source. Generated using the *OT Assessment Package* (OTAP software; Three Star Press, 2018).

Wanda's occupational therapist documents the following information in his report for her performance for the cereal task:

> When preparing cereal and a glass of juice, Wanda chose a different type of cereal than she indicated she would, choosing oat cereal rather than puffed rice. She worked slowly and hesitated throughout the task, pausing before each step. Wanda placed objects too close together on the counter and, as a result, bumped into the glass of juice, spilling some juice.

Details of identified problems in ADL task performance also are especially helpful if the occupational therapist also used the ACQ to learn the client's perspective regarding their ADL task performance. When there is agreement between what the client reported during the ACQ interview and what the therapist reported, goal setting and intervention planning become an easy process. When there is not agreement between the client's perspective and the objective perspective of the therapist, based on the performance analysis with the AMPS, the therapist needs to help the client recognize problems that occurred during the task performance and understand the impact of these difficulties before setting goals and planning intervention. Together, the AMPS and the ACQ promote occupation-based, occupation-focused, and client-centered practice.

Interpretation and Intervention Considerations

The ADL motor ability measure is an overall measure of clients' ability to move themselves and task objects throughout the task performance. The ADL process ability measure is an overall measure of clients' ability to efficiently organize and use time, space, tools, and materials during the task as well as to modify their performance in anticipation of and in response to any problems that arise during the task. The results of the AMPS—in particular the ADL motor ability measure and the ADL process ability measure—may be interpreted from a criterion-referenced perspective and a norm-referenced perspective. Both are included in the AMPS Results Report. On the respective ADL Motor Scale and ADL Process Scale, the criterion-referenced interpretation of each ability measure is indicated by darker text to the right of the scale (see Figures 15.1 and 15.2, respectively). The criterion-referenced interpretation corresponds to the level of performance seen for that ability measure.

Wanda's ADL Motor Scale in the AMPS Results Report, shown in Figure 15.1, indicates that her ADL motor ability measure was 1.8 logits, corresponding to questionable to mild clumsiness, increased physical effort, or both. Her ADL Process Scale in the report, shown in Figure 15.2, indicates that her ADL process ability measure was 0.4 logits, corresponding to mild to moderate inefficiency and disorganization during the observed tasks. The ADL Motor Scale and ADL Process Scale of the AMPS provide visual images that

are easily understood by clients and their families as well as team members. Seeing the measures can help motivate the client during therapy.

The occupational therapist can also interpret the ADL motor and ADL process ability measures from a norm-referenced perspective. To the left of each scale, a vertical bar indicates the range of ADL motor ability or ADL process ability measures for persons in the same age group as the client who was evaluated. The dot in the middle of the bar is the mean, and the top and bottom of the bar indicate 2 standard deviations above and below the mean.

The AMPS Results Report also includes a table that reports the person's ADL motor ability measure and ADL process ability measure as standardized z scores, normalized standard scores, and percentile rank. The norm-referenced interpretations are particularly helpful in working with younger clients, when norm-referenced interpretations are used to determine eligibility for occupational therapy services. The norm-referenced interpretations are not to be used in evaluations of progress or change after intervention; only the ADL motor ability measure and the ADL process ability measure provide reliable and valid measures of change.

Multiple measures from different evaluation times are plotted on an AMPS Progress Report to visually indicate a change in occupational performance. Using the AMPS to determine the effectiveness of intervention can be extremely powerful and supports evidence-based practice, focusing on occupation.

The ADL motor ability measure and ADL process ability measure can also indicate the level of assistance a person needs to live in the community (Merritt, 2010, 2011). For example, persons with an ADL motor ability measure below 1.0 logit and ADL process ability measure below 0.7 logit likely need moderate to maximum assistance (Fisher & Jones, 2014, p. 371).

Finally, and of clinical importance, is the use of the AMPS to set observable and measurable goals with the client and to guide intervention. If the occupational therapist used the ACQ, the client's perspective can assist them in setting goals and planning intervention.

During the ACQ interview, Wanda stated that she did not prepare the type of cereal that she had said she would and that she spilled the juice. She did not state that her work space was crowded. She stated that she worked slowly, but she did not report pausing during the task. Thus, there was minimal discrepancy between what Wanda reported and what the occupational therapist observed.

The occupational therapist and Wanda set goals using the baseline performance observed during the desired ADL tasks. Wanda said she wanted to prepare the type of cereal that she had said she would prepare, because cereal type was important to her children when she prepared breakfast for them. She also wanted to prepare cereal and a glass of juice more quickly, without pauses during the task. Had Wanda not indicated the problems observed, the therapist would have needed to point out the difficulties that Wanda had during the tasks before setting goals. Intervention would have changed as well, to address strategies to support Wanda in first identifying the task expectations.

Because the AMPS focuses on occupation, the occupational therapist may decide that using the AMPS provides sufficient information to establish baseline performance of desired tasks, set client-centered goals, and determine intervention. In these situations, the AMPS may be the only assessment needed. In some cases, the therapist may decide it would be helpful to consider factors that limited the person's occupational performance. For example, the therapist may decide that there is a reason to confirm that memory is a problem.

In Wanda's case, the occupational therapist decided confirming memory problems would not change the intervention approach and therefore determined that his performance analysis was sufficient to set goals and plan intervention. Aware of Wanda's desire to return quickly to the tasks that support her role as a mother, the therapist and Wanda chose a compensatory approach for intervention and developed a step-by-step checklist for preparing cereal and juice. They then proceeded to create other step-by-step checklists to support other tasks that Wanda wanted to return to doing in her home. Through discussion of strategies that Wanda said she thought might be helpful, she and the therapist decided to have Wanda listen to music with a strong rhythmic beat when she did routine tasks, to help her keep tasks progressing without hesitations.

In summary, the AMPS provides a standardized way to conduct a performance analysis during ADL tasks as the client performs at least 2 tasks that are relevant for them to support their roles. The number of standardized tasks in the AMPS reflects a variety of tasks people might need or want to do, offering a range of difficulty and cultural relevance and supporting client-centered practice. Administration of AMPS provides a sensitive measure on which to establish baseline performance and measure change after intervention. Because the AMPS focuses on occupation, determining client-centered goals flows easily, as does planning intervention to address the tasks that are important to the client. When the AMPS is used, the role of the occupational therapist is clear to the client, family members, and team members.

References

American Occupational Therapy Association. (2014). Occupational therapy practice framework: Domain and process (3rd ed.). *American Journal of Occupational Therapy, 68*(Suppl. 1), S1–S48. https://doi.org/10.5014/ajot.2014.682006

Ayres, H., & John, A. P. (2015). The Assessment of Motor and Process Skills as a measure of ADL ability in schizophrenia. *Scandinavian Journal of Occupational Therapy, 22,* 470–477. https://doi.org/10.3109/11038128.2015.1061050

Björkdahl, A., Åkerlund, E., Svensson, S., & Esbjörnsson, E. (2013). A randomized study of computerized working memory training and effects on functioning in everyday life for patients with brain injury. *Brain Injury, 27,* 1658–1665. https://doi.org/10.3109/02699052.2013.830196

Bond, T. G., & Fox, C. M. (2007). *Applying the Rasch model: Fundamental measurement in the human sciences* (2nd ed.). Mahwah, NJ: Erlbaum.

Center for Innovative OT Solutions. (2016). *Occupational Therapy Assessment Package (OTAP) reporting software.* Retrieved from https://innovativeotsolutions.com/software

Center for Innovative OT Solutions. (2018). *AMPS reference list.* Retrieved from https://www.innovativeotsolutions.com/wp-content/uploads/2018/06/ampsReferenceList.pdf

Doble, S. E. (1991). Test–retest and inter-rater reliability of a process skills assessment. *OTJR: Occupation, Participation and Health, 11*(1), 8–23. https://doi.org/10.1177/153944929101100102

Doble, S. E., Fisk, J. D., MacPherson, K. M., Fisher, A. G., & Rockwood, K. (1997). Measuring functional competence in older persons with Alzheimer's disease. *International Psychogeriatrics, 9,* 25–38. https://doi.org/10.1017/S1041610297004171

Fisher, A. G. (1992). Functional measures, Part 2: Selecting the right test, minimizing the limitations. *American Journal of Occupational Therapy, 46,* 278–281. https://doi.org/10.5014/ajot.46.3.278

Fisher, A. G. (1995). *Assessment of Motor and Process Skills (AMPS).* Ft. Collins, CO: Center for Innovative OT Solutions.

Fisher, A. G. (1997). Multifaceted measurement of daily life task performance: Conceptualizing a test of instrumental ADL and validating the addition of personal ADL tasks. *Physical Medicine and Rehabilitation, 11,* 289–303.

Fisher, A. G. (1998). Uniting practice and theory in an occupational framework (Eleanor Clarke Slagle Lecture). *American Journal of Occupational Therapy, 52,* 509–521. https://doi.org/10.5014/ajot.52.7.509

Fisher, A. G. (2009). *Occupational Therapy Intervention Process Model: A model for planning and implementing top-down, client-centered, and occupation-based interventions.* Ft. Collins, CO: Three Star Press.

Fisher, A. G. (2013). Occupation-centred, occupation-based, occupation-focused: Same, same or different? *Scandinavian Journal of Occupational Therapy, 20,* 162–173. https://doi.org/10.3109/11038128.2012.754492

Fisher, A. G., Griswold, L. A., & Korttorp, A. (2017). *Assessment of Compared Qualities.* Ft. Collins, CO: Three Star Press.

Fisher, A. G., & Jones, K. B. (2012). *Assessment of Motor and Process Skills: Vol. 1. Development, standardization, and administration manual* (7th ed., rev.). Ft. Collins, CO: Three Star Press.

Fisher, A. G., & Jones, K. B. (2014). *Assessment of Motor and Process Skills: Vol. 2. User manual* (8th ed.). Ft. Collins, CO: Three Star Press.

Fisher, A. G., & Marterella, A. (2019). *Powerful practice: An occupation-centered reasoning model for occupational therapy.* Ft. Collins, CO: Center for Innovative OT Solutions.

Fisher, A. G., & Merritt, B. K. (2012). Conceptualizing and developing the AMPS within a framework of modern objective measurement. In A. G. Fisher & K. B. Jones (Eds.), *Assessment of motor and process skills: Vol. 1. Development, standardization, and administration manual* (7th ed., rev.; pp. 14-1–14-22). Ft. Collins, CO: Three Star Press.

Gantschnig, B. E., Page, J., & Fisher, A. G. (2012). Cross-regional validity of the Assessment of Motor and Process Skills for use in middle Europe. *Journal of Rehabilitation Medicine, 44,* 151–157. https://doi.org/10.2340/16501977-0915

Gantschnig, B. E., Page, J., Nilsson, I., & Fisher, A. G. (2013). Detecting differences in activities of daily living between children with and without mild disabilities. *American Journal of Occupational Therapy, 67,* 319–327. https://doi.org/10.5014/ajot.2013.007013

Kardos, M. R., & White, B. P. (2006). Evaluation options for secondary transition planning. *American Journal of Occupational Therapy, 60,* 333–339. https://doi.org/10.5014/ajot.60.3.333

Law, M., Baptiste, S., Carswell, A., McColl, M. A., Polatajko, H., & Pollock, N. (2014). *The Canadian Occupational Performance Measure* (5th ed.). Ottawa: CAOT Publications.

Merritt, B. K. (2010). Utilizing AMPS ability measures to predict level of community dependence. *Scandinavian Journal of Occupational Therapy, 17,* 70–76. https://doi.org/10.3109/11038120903165107

Merritt, B. K. (2011). Validity of using the Assessment of Motor and Process Skills to determine the need for assistance. *American Journal of Occupational Therapy, 65,* 643–650. https://doi.org/10.5014/ajot.2011.000547

Park, M. O. (2015). Comparison of motor and process skills among children with different developmental disabilities. *Journal of Physical Therapy Science, 27,* 3183–3184. https://doi.org/10.1589/jpts.27.3183

Rojo-Mota, G., Pedrero-Pérez, E. J., Ruiz-Sánchez de León, J. M., & Miangolarra Page, J. C. (2014). Assessment of motor and process skills in daily life activities of treated substance addicts. *Scandinavian Journal of Occupational Therapy, 21,* 458–464. https://doi.org/10.3109/11038128.2014.922610

Three Star Press. (2018). *OT assessment package* (OTAP software; Version 3.11) [Computer software]. Ft. Collins, CO: Author.

Waehrens, E. E., Amris, K., & Fisher, A. G. (2010). Performance-based assessment of activities of daily living (ADL) ability among women with chronic widespread pain. *Pain, 150,* 535–541. https://doi.org/10.1016/j.pain.2010.06.008

16

Cognitive Domain–Specific Testing to Support Interpretation of Performance Assessment

MUHAMMAD O. AL-HEIZAN, MS, OT,
AND DOROTHY FARRAR EDWARDS, PhD

LEARNING OBJECTIVES

After completing this chapter, readers should be able to

- Describe the contribution of neuropsychological tests to the assessment of occupational performance,
- Discuss the importance of ecological validity in selection of assessments to determine the capacity of an individual to perform complex ADLs in context,
- Identify measures of cognitive performance associated with the comprehensive assessment of functional cognition, and
- Select reliable and valid measures of cognitive function that contribute to clinical evaluation of functional cognition.

KEY TERMS AND CONCEPTS

- Attention • Ecological validity • Executive function • Memory • Metacognition • Neuropsychological tests

Overview of the Clinical Neuropsychological Assessment Process

People need many cognitive skills to perform complex daily occupations effectively. These domains include attention, memory, executive functions (EFs), language comprehension, and visual–perceptual skills. Understanding whether any of these cognitive domains are impaired helps clinicians establish clients' baseline abilities and design tailored interventions.

Clinical neuropsychologists focus their evaluations on the practical or functional consequences of cognitive impairment on an individual's ability to engage in basic and instrumental ADLs as well as the capacity to fully participate in leisure, work, and social activities (Evans, 2010). Assessment of cognitive strengths and weaknesses helps clinicians create a preliminary picture of a client's capacity to fully engage in meaningful and necessary occupations.

Assessment of specific cognitive domains is best done with standardized psychometric tests. *Psychometric tests* are tasks designed to evaluate specific cognitive functions and are administered and scored in a highly standardized way. The test creators have systematically administered these tests to sample

groups to provide a means of comparing the performance of an individual assessed in a clinical setting with a representative sample or control group. This information allows the test administrator to determine how a test taker's scores differ from those of the normative group (Michell, 1999). Often, adjusted norms are available to account for the known effects of educational achievement, age, or gender on test performance.

Characteristics of Standardized Neuropsychological Tests

The use of standardized **neuropsychological tests** provides insight into specific types of cognitive impairment. These tests have been shown to be less useful in predicting the capacity of a given individual to successfully perform complex IADLs in their own home or community setting (Law et al., 2012; Manchester et al., 2004). Thus, these measures are said to have low levels of ecological validity (Dawson & Marcotte, 2017). **Ecological validity** refers to the degree to which assessment results relate to, predict, or resemble everyday life behavior or context (Dawson & Marcotte, 2017).

The sole focus on isolated cognitive capacities rather than on the integration of cognitive skills and strategies in the performance of complex everyday life activities may fail to provide realistic estimates of the functional cognitive capacity needed for optimal occupational performance in real-world settings. In addition, occupational therapists should take into account other factors that may affect functional cognitive performance, such as environmental features or task demands, when assessing occupational performance.

Nonetheless, psychometric tests can provide valuable information to occupational therapists, who can use psychometric test performance to better estimate the client's cognitive strengths and weaknesses. Therapists can use the test findings in interpreting the outcomes of performance-based testing of functional cognition as well as in designing and implementing interventions. Psychometric tests vary in their

- Representation of theoretical constructs,

- Complexity of cognitive functions evaluated,

- Length and ease of administration,

- Potential biases based on age and education, and

- Quality of normative standards.

Clinical psychologists typically use either a big battery approach (i.e., always administering the same big battery of tests) or a hypothesis-testing approach, whereby they select measures on the basis of observations of clients' strengths and weaknesses. However, even in the latter case, the psychologist assesses a minimum set of cognitive domains. These typically include

- An estimate of premorbid cognitive function;

- Current intellectual function; and

- Specific areas of cognitive ability, including attention, learning, memory, EF, language and communication skills, and visuospatial perception and constructional skills.

This chapter reviews the primary cognitive domains that support occupational performance and provides an overview of selected assessments for each domain to help inform clinical interpretation of performance-based evaluation of functional cognition.

Estimation of Premorbid Cognitive Capacity and Current Intellectual Functioning

The neuropsychologist uses information elicited during structured clinical interviews of the client and, if necessary, of family members or care providers, together with structured testing to estimate the client's cognitive function before the illness or injury that brought them to the attention of the health care team. This interview is combined with standardized assessments of reading and vocabulary abilities, such as the Wechsler Test of Adult Reading (Wechsler, 2001) and the National Adult Reading Test (Nelson & Willison, 1991).

Other than among clients with aphasia syndromes, both vocabulary and the ability to pronounce words with irregular pronunciations (e.g., *naive, bouquet*) are typically well preserved after neurological insult or illness. As a result, measures that assess vocabulary or word pronunciation can provide an estimate of premorbid abilities, which the practitioner can then compare with clients' postinjury ability on functions that are known to be more susceptible to impairment. This allows the practitioner to estimate the impairment that results from the neurological illness or injury.

General intelligence (i.e., IQ) is evaluated with a battery of tests designed to assess aspects of intellectual ability. The most widely used measure is the Wechsler Adult Intelligence Scale (WAIS; Wechsler, 2008), which is periodically restandardized (the 5th edition of the WAIS is projected for release in 2019). The WAIS has extensive normative data, which the neuropsychologist can use to create a profile of strengths and weaknesses. This process is not diagnostic; rather, the information provides the neuropsychologist with a current estimate of cognitive capacity as part of the diagnostic evaluation.

Neuropsychological Assessment of Attention

Attention is the behavioral and cognitive process of selectively concentrating on a discrete aspect of information, whether deemed subjective or objective, while ignoring other perceivable information. Attention requires the use of mental resources for concentration (Radomski, 2008). Attention has also been described as the allocation of limited cognitive-processing resources (Anderson, 2004). Although there are many ways of categorizing attention, for the purposes of this chapter we focus on tests that evaluate sustained, selective, and divided attention.

Attention is a cognitive domain that encompasses a broad range of abilities, from automatically orienting toward a noise to maintaining focus for a long period of time (i.e., *sustained attention*; Spikman & Van Zomeran, 2010). An example of sustained attention is preparing a meal with several dishes while maintaining focus on the duration of the task (Radomski, 2008; Spikman & Van Zomeran, 2010). *Selective attention* is the ability to attend to relevant information while ignoring irrelevant information or distractions (Sohlberg & Mateer, 2001).

Divided attention is a common skill that people use in everyday contexts when they try to do 2 or more things at once (i.e., multitasking) and is a more complex skill than sustained and selective attention (Spikman & Van Zomeran, 2010). Using a cell phone while walking is an example of a daily task requiring divided attention that can be difficult for all age groups (Farmer et al., 2010). Finally, *alternating attention* is the skill a person uses to flexibly shift attention among different tasks, such as monitoring food cooking on a stove while setting a table and talking on the phone (Radomski, 2008; Sohlberg & Mateer, 2001).

There are many different approaches to assessing attention; the most common include paper-and-pencil tests and computerized batteries. The Trail Making Test (TMT; Reitan, 1992) is a brief paper-and-pencil measure that provides information about attention, visual scanning, and eye–hand coordination. The test has well-developed norms. The TMT assesses both selective and divided attention (Spikman & Van Zomeran, 2010). It is widely used because it has proven useful in documenting brain dysfunction across several diagnostic groups, including traumatic brain injury, attention deficit hyperactivity disorder, and many forms of dementia (Mitrushina et al., 2005).

The Continuous Performance Test (3rd ed.; CPT–III; Conners, 2008) is a widely used computerized test of attention. The CPT–III assesses both selective and sustained attention. The practitioner administers the CPT–III by having the test taker sit in front of a computer monitor, with the instruction to watch a moving display of letters carefully for the occurrence of a specific letter. When the test taker sees the target letter, they are instructed to press a key on the computer keyboard. The test administrator can adjust the speed of the display as well as the frequency of the target letter. The CPT–III requires the test taker to maintain focus over a prolonged period of time, thereby assessing sustained attention (Spikman & Van Zomeran, 2010).

Another commonly used assessment is the Test of Everyday Attention (TEA; Robertson et al., 1996). The TEA evaluates attentional skills while test takers perform tasks that reflect daily activities. The TEA has tasks that assess selective, sustained, and divided attention and is considered to have good ecological validity.

Neuropsychological Assessment of Memory and Learning

Memory is defined as the capacity to encode, store, and retrieve information (Lezak et al., 2012). Psychologists have categorized and described memory skills in many ways and typically assess both visual and verbal aspects of memory, but with a greater emphasis on verbal memory. Although there are many distinct ways to categorize memory systems, the most widely accepted is the distinction among short-term, working, and long-term memory skills.

Short-term and working memory are similar but conceptually distinct systems: Short-term memory has no correlation with intelligence or aptitude, whereas working memory does (Cowan, 2008). *Short-term memory* is the ability to hold but not manipulate a small amount of information in an active, readily available state for a short period of time (Bradley & Kapur, 2010). For example, short-term memory can be used to remember a phone number that has just been recited. The duration of short-term memory is believed to be in the order of seconds. Working memory is also considered to be of

very brief duration. However, *working memory* is defined as the manipulation of stored information, whereas *short-term memory* refers only to the short-term storage of information (Cowan, 2008).

Long-term memory is defined as the ability to hold information in storage indefinitely. It therefore contrasts with short-term and working memory, which persist for only about 18 to 30 seconds. Within long-term memory, psychologists also distinguish between declarative memory (which is further divided into episodic and semantic memory) and procedural (implicit) memory. Declarative (explicit) memory refers to conscious learning, whereas procedural (nondeclarative or implicit) memory refers to unconscious learning (Ball et al., 2010).

Declarative memory, or the memory associated with learned information, is much more susceptible to brain injury and disease as well as the effects of normal aging than is procedural memory. *Episodic memory* consists of knowledge of a previous experience as well as the awareness of or understanding about specific contextual events that the person has experienced (Buckner, 2004; Zoltan, 2007). Episodic memory skills are particularly vulnerable to many forms of brain damage (Budson, 2009; Katz, 2011). Episodic memory skills involve the recall of *temporal* (i.e., when) and *spatial* (i.e., where) information associated with past experiences or events (Ball et al., 2010; Buckner, 2004). They enable a person to remember the day's events, such as consciously recalling the content of a therapy session (Budson, 2009; Gillen, 2009).

Semantic memory is knowledge of facts about the world and of language. The susceptibility of semantic knowledge to insult or injury follows a temporal gradient, with more recently acquired information being more at risk, and material that has been in semantic store for longer periods being more robust. As a result, in primary degenerative dementias, older memories are retained for longer than more recent memories.

Procedural memory involves remembering how to do tasks that are automatic and initiated without conscious awareness. Procedural memory is demonstrated by the use of habit rather than deliberative recall; these types of behaviors include tying a shoe or walking (Ball et al., 2010; Poon, 1985). Both procedural skills and procedural learning remain intact in typical aging as well as in the early stages of neurocognitive disorders, such as Alzheimer's disease (AD; Kuzis et al., 1999). Psychometric tests of memory focus on declarative rather than procedural memory.

Tests of Declarative Memory

Word-list learning and story recall are the most frequently used tests of episodic memory, and there are many standardized tests of verbal memory. A standard approach to testing verbal memory involves the presentation of lists of 12–15 low-frequency (less common) words that are read aloud. The test taker is first asked to repeat the list of words in any order. This part of the test measures immediate verbal recall and the ability to learn the list of unrelated words. After a delay of 20–30 minutes, the participant is asked to again recall the words. This part of the test process assesses delayed recall. Some tests also include presentation of the word list together with distracter words, and the test taker is asked to identify the words on the original list. This part of the test measures recognition memory.

The Hopkins Verbal Learning Test (Benedict et al., 1998) and the California Verbal Learning Test (CVLT; Delis et al., 2017; Lacritz & Cullum, 1998) are among the most common measures used to assess verbal learning and memory. Robust normative data are available for both. Both tests have been found to be sensitive measures of verbal learning, and both have well-established reliability, validity, sensitivity, and specificity in identification of individuals with amnestic mild cognitive impairment (Petersen, 2004). Performance on verbal learning tests may be influenced by age, gender, ethnicity, and education. The test developers have addressed these concerns by providing adjusted norms to correct for the effects of demographic factors.

The most comprehensive multidimensional memory test is the Wechsler Memory Scale (WMS; Wechsler, 2009). The WMS is a more complex test of both verbal and nonverbal memory functions. The most recent version, the WMS–IV, consists of 7 subtests, many of which gauge memory both immediately and after a delay. In addition to word-list learning, the test includes a memory-based test of visual figure reproduction, spatial addition, and symbol memory. A subtest that assesses the ability to remember details of a story read by the examiner (logical memory) measures recall under free recall conditions (Bradley & Kapur, 2010). The Logical Memory Subtest is often administered without the other subtests.

The Rivermead Behavioral Memory Test (RBMT; Wilson et al., 1985, 2008), now in its 3rd edition, is 1 of the most widely used clinical assessments of memory. The measure was designed to predict everyday memory problems among people with acquired, nonprogressive brain injury and to monitor their change over time. Subtests include remembering names, remembering a hidden belonging, remembering an appointment, recognizing a picture, recalling prose (i.e., logical memory), recalling a short route, remembering an errand, demonstrating orientation, and recognizing dates and faces.

This test is thought to have good ecological validity because the subtests reflect everyday memory skills. Furthermore, measures such as the CVLT and the RBMT provide for assessment of both recall and recognition memory skills, because both are important forms of memory needed for daily life activities. Table 16.1 details the common tests of memory and attention.

TABLE 16.1. Assessments of Memory and Attention

INSTRUMENT AND REFERENCE(S)	DESCRIPTION	PSYCHOMETRICS	STRENGTHS AND WEAKNESSES
Test of Everyday Attention (TEA; Robertson et al., 1996)	Assessment of sustained, selective, and divided attention based on 8 common daily tasks, such as map and telephone search (selective attention), elevator counting and lottery (sustained attention), and telephone dual task (divided attention). Test takes 45–60 minutes to complete.	Moderate correlation between the TEA and other measures of attention ($r = .42–.63$), which supports the concurrent validity of the TEA. Statistically significant differences between healthy older adults and people with stroke on all subtests of the TEA ($p < .001$). Strong test–retest reliability across subtests of parallel forms of the TEA ($r = .66–.90$).	*Strengths* • Developed on the basis of research of the functional–neuroanatomical specialization of attention. • Ecologically valid subtests. *Weaknesses* • May be inappropriate for clients with severe visual deficits. • Lengthy assessment for 1 cognitive domain.
Continuous Performance Test (3rd ed.; CPT–III; Conners, 2008)	The CPT–III is a computerized assessment of sustained attention and response inhibition for individuals 8 years and older. Clients are asked to respond when any letter except X appears. The CPT–III has normative data for comparison for ages 8 and older, which have also been adjusted for race, education, and location. Administration time is about 14 minutes.	The CPT–III had strong split-half reliability across samples (median estimate = 0.92), demonstrating internal consistency. It also had good test–retest reliability (median $r = .67$). The CPT–III was able to distinguish between children with attention deficit hyperactivity disorder and healthy children, supporting discriminant validity.	*Strengths* • Easy to use and portable. • Strong psychometric properties. • Normative data for comparison. *Weakness* • May be expensive.

(Continued)

TABLE 16.1. Assessments of Memory and Attention *(Cont.)*

INSTRUMENT AND REFERENCE(S)	DESCRIPTION	PSYCHOMETRICS	STRENGTHS AND WEAKNESSES
Trail Making Test (TMT; Reitan, 1992)	The TMT consists of Parts A and B. In Part A, clients are asked to connect numbered circles scattered across a page. In Part B, they are asked to connect circles with alternating numbers and letters scattered across a page. The TMT can be administered in paper-and-pencil, computerized, or smartphone versions. Part A and Part B are scored separately. The score for each task is the number of seconds required to complete the task. Timing should start as soon as the instruction is given to begin. Administration time is about 5–10 minutes.	O'Donnell et al. (1994) reported the face validity of the TMT in a sample of 117 community-dwelling clients. The results suggest that the TMT is a complex test that involves aspects of attention. The same study examined the convergent validity of the TMT and 4 other neuropsychological tests: Category Test (CAT; Mack & Carlson, 1978), Wisconsin Card Sorting Test (WCST; Meier, 1974), Paced Auditory Serial-Addition Task (PASAT; Gronwall, 1977), and Visual Search and Attention Test (VSAT; Trenerry et al., 1990). The findings suggest adequate correlations between the TMT and the other measures (CAT, $r = .38$; WCST, $r = .31$; PASAT, $r = .44$; VAST, $r = .30$), with Pearson product–moment correlations. Matarazzo et al. (1974) examined the test–retest reliability for Part A and Part B of the TMT ($r = .78$ and .67, respectively), among participants with diffuse cerebrovascular disease. Interrater reliability was found to be high for both Part A ($r = .94$) and Part B ($r = .90$; Fals-Stewart, 1992).	*Strengths* • Relatively easy to administer. • Short in duration. *Weaknesses* • Could be skewed to more-educated individuals. • The instructions could be confusing for some individuals. • Cannot be administered to illiterate clients, non-English speakers, or individuals with hand impairments.
Rivermead Behavioral Memory Test (RBMT; Wilson et al., 1985, 2008)	Assessment of memory skills necessary for everyday activities, including remembering names, faces, routes, and appointments. Takes 30–45 minutes to complete.	Wilson and colleagues (1989) found statistically significant differences between people with brain injury and healthy control participants on all RBMT subtests ($p < .001$). 40 participants with brain injury were scored simultaneously by 2 raters with 100% agreement, which demonstrates interrater reliability.	*Strengths* • Subtests resemble everyday tasks. • Useful for identifying memory deficits in a wide range of diagnostic groups. *Weakness* • Requires intact visual and verbal skills.
Contextual Memory Test (Toglia, 1993)	Dynamic assessment of recall, awareness of memory capacity, and memory strategy use. Clients try to remember 20 objects related to 1 of 2 themes (ADL routine or restaurant). Takes 30–40 minutes to complete.	High correlations with the RBMT ($r = .80–.84$), which demonstrates concurrent validity. Parallel forms had high correlations ($r = .85–.94$). Test–retest reliability for people with brain injury was high ($r = .85–.94$).	*Strength* • Provides information about memory and self-awareness of memory ability. *Weakness* • Pictures used in the assessment have potential for cultural bias.

(Continued)

TABLE 16.1. Assessments of Memory and Attention *(Cont.)*

INSTRUMENT AND REFERENCE(S)	DESCRIPTION	PSYCHOMETRICS	STRENGTHS AND WEAKNESSES
Hopkins Verbal Learning Test (HVLT; Benedict et al., 1998)	The HVLT is a test of verbal learning and memory. The test was developed for clients age 16 or older. The most widely used version is the HVLT–Revised (HVLT–R; Benedict et al., 1998). The HVLT–R has 3 learning trial tasks: a delayed recall trial, a yes–no delayed recognition trial, and a randomized list trial that includes 12 target words and 12 nontarget words. Scoring is based on indexes for total recall, delayed recall, retention (percentage retained), and recognition discrimination. The HVLT–R takes 5–10 minutes to complete.	The HVLT–R has normative data for comparison based on a sample of healthy community residents. Test–retest reliability was reported to be within the acceptable limits. The HVLT–R had high correlations with other widely used tests of learning and memory, supporting construct validity (Shapiro et al., 1999). Also, the HVLT–R was able to discriminate between clients and control participants, demonstrating discriminant validity (Shapiro et al., 1999).	*Strengths* • Easy to score. • May use software for scoring, comparison with normative data, and report generation of the score and performance. • Well tolerated by significantly impaired individuals. • Has multiple forms. • Is appropriate for repeated testing without effects of learning. *Weaknesses* • Requires training of the administrator on standardized procedures. • May not be appropriate for individuals with hearing difficulty.

Neuropsychological Assessment of Language Skills

Language comprehension skills enable people to communicate with others as well as to comprehend verbal or written information. Deficits in these abilities can significantly affect the ability to perform daily activities. The general name given to the disruption of language skills is *aphasia,* which can cause impairments in speaking, reading, listening, writing, or using appropriate gestures (Cherney, 1995).

Aphasia can be classified in various ways but is often classified as *fluent* and *nonfluent* on the basis of the characteristics of a person's ability to produce speech (Goodglass, 1993). In fluent aphasia, a person may be able to produce speech spontaneously, but there are limitations in auditory comprehension and understanding of language (Woodson, 2008). The most common type of fluent aphasia is Wernicke's aphasia, which is also often called a *receptive aphasia* (Woodson, 2008).

People with Wernicke's aphasia generally have fluent speech articulation but have difficulty conveying meaning (i.e., speech is fluent but insubstantial), and they have difficulty understanding spoken or written language. They have limited ability to name objects, repeat names, or follow commands (Sarno, 1994). Individuals with Wernicke's aphasia typically have difficulty reading and writing (Sarno, 1994).

Nonfluent aphasia is characterized by relatively spared comprehension of spoken or written language but difficulty producing syntactically correct speech output (Sarno, 1994). Broca's aphasia, or expressive aphasia, is the most common type of nonfluent aphasia. Individuals with nonfluent aphasia have slow speech or awkward speech production, with limited use of vocabulary or grammar (i.e., agrammatism; Sarno, 1994).

Individuals with Broca's or expressive aphasia can follow commands but have difficulty naming objects, repeating phrases, conveying ideas, or expressing themselves through writing. However, they might be able to sing familiar songs or speak in other automatic ways, such as praying or swearing (Sarno, 1994). The Frenchay Aphasia Screening Test (Enderby et al., 1986) is a common and quick screening for clients with both fluent and nonfluent aphasia.

Anomia is a mild type of aphasia in which individuals have word-retrieval failures and cannot express the words they want to say, particularly associated with the inability to name common objects (Woollams et al., 2008). Individuals with anomia often can describe an object in detail and may be able to use hand gestures to demonstrate how the object is used but cannot find the appropriate word to name the object. Anomia is often indicative of temporal lobe damage, and tests of anomia have been used widely in diagnostic batteries for AD (LaBarge et al., 1992).

The Boston Naming Test (Kaplan & Goodglass, 1983), a test of confrontation naming that involves identification of 60 objects presented as simple line drawings, is the most widely used anomia assessment. There are also short forms of the test that use 30 or 15 items that most clearly distinguish between healthy individuals and individuals with known cognitive and neurologic impairment. Adjusted norms are available for specific age, gender, and racial and ethnic groups. Table 16.2 details the common tests of language comprehension.

TABLE 16.2. Assessments of Language Comprehension

INSTRUMENT AND REFERENCE(S)	DESCRIPTION	PSYCHOMETRICS	STRENGTHS AND WEAKNESSES
Frenchay Aphasia Screening Test (FAST; Enderby et al., 1986)	The FAST is a quick and simple screening for clients with communication difficulties. Assesses 4 major areas: comprehension, verbal expression, reading, and writing. Testing is focused around a single double-sided stimulus card depicting a scene on 1 side and geometric shapes on the other, as well as 5 written sentences. The client is given instructions or item tasks that are graded in length and difficulty. The FAST takes 3–10 minutes to complete.	The FAST had a high inter-rater reliability (Kendall's W = .97). It also demonstrated excellent test–retest reliability (κ = 1.00). The FAST had high correlations (r = .74–.92) with the Screening for Acquired Language Disorders, demonstrating convergent validity (Al-Khawaja et al., 1996). The FAST had a sensitivity of 100% and a specificity of 79% in identifying people with aphasia after stroke (O'Neill et al., 1990).	*Strengths* • Quick and simple to administer. • Does not require specialized training. *Weaknesses* • Lacks adequate validation studies. • Seems to be adversely affected by the presence of visual-field deficits, visual neglect or inattention, illiteracy, deafness, poor concentration, or confusion and therefore should be used with caution with clients with these conditions.
Boston Naming Test (BNT; Kaplan & Goodglass, 1983; Kaplan et al., 1978)	The BNT is a popular test of visual confrontation naming that has been used to assess aphasia among people with dementia and other geriatric populations. It has several variations, including the original 85-item experimental form (Kaplan et al., 1978). The most widely used version is the 60-item version by Kaplan and Goodglass (1983). The BNT stimuli consist of line drawings of objects that present increasing naming difficulty. The stimuli range from simple, high-frequency vocabulary (e.g., *tree*) to rare, low-frequency words (e.g., *abacus*). The BNT requires a spontaneous response from the client within a 20-second period; if the response is not made, 2 prompting cues (1 phonemic, 1 semantic) can be given. Scoring is based on the number of spontaneously produced correct responses, the number of cues given, and the number of responses after phonemic cueing and after semantic cueing.	Test–retest reliability of the BNT was reported to be .94 among adults with intractable epilepsy (Sawrie et al., 1996). The BNT had an .81 reliability coefficient among healthy adults and .97 among clients with Alzheimer's disease (Huff et al., 1986). It had a sensitivity between 56% and 80% and a specificity between 54% and 70% in distinguishing between individuals with and without dementia (Salmon et al., 1995). The BNT had high correlations with the Visual Naming Test of the Multilingual Aphasia Examination, demonstrating concurrent validity (Axelrod et al., 1994).	*Strengths* • Used with a wide range of populations. • Manual provides a method to distinguish between levels of aphasia by comparing with level of typical adults. *Weakness* • May not be suitable for individuals with visual–perceptual deficits.

Neuropsychological Assessment of Visual-Processing Skills

Visual-processing skills involve processing information associated with the reception, organization, and assimilation of visual information (Toglia et al., 2013). Visual-processing skills range from simple tasks, such as matching shapes, to more complex tasks, such as responding to unfamiliar or subtle visual stimuli in visually crowded arrays. Problems in simple visual processing include difficulty in discriminating between objects,

pictures of objects, and basic shapes and difficulty detecting differences in size, direction, and position. Dysfunction of complex visual processing may include difficulty in detecting subtle differences in shapes, objects, size, location, and position. A person might have difficulty recognizing or interpreting facial expressions or making sense of ambiguous or incomplete visual stimuli.

Hemispatial or *visuospatial neglect* is a condition that can occur after damage to either hemisphere of the brain; however, it is more common after unilateral damage to the right hemisphere (resulting in a neglect of left hemispace). It is a deficit in attention to and awareness of 1 side of the field of vision and is defined as the inability to process and perceive stimuli on 1 side of the body or environment (Unsworth, 2007). This inability is not due to a lack of sensation. Visuospatial neglect is most frequently assessed with line-bisection tasks, letter and symbol cancellation tests, and figure- or clock-drawing tests.

The Behavioral Inattention Test (Wilson et al., 1987) includes 6 Conventional subtests and 9 Behavioral subtests. The Conventional tests include

- A series of cancellation tasks designed to quantify the number of omissions on the neglected (usually left) side, and
- Line-bisection tasks to measure the extent of the bias to the nonneglected (usually right) side.

TABLE 16.3. Assessments of Visual Processing and Apraxia

INSTRUMENT AND REFERENCE	DESCRIPTION	PSYCHOMETRICS	STRENGTHS AND WEAKNESSES
Motor-Free Visual Perception Test (MVPT–3; Colarusso & Hammill, 2003)	The MVPT–3 is a motor-free measure of visual perception (i.e., a measure of isolated visual–perceptual ability independent from motor capability). It was developed to measure 5 interrelated processes: spatial relationships, visual discrimination, figure–ground, visual closure, and visual memory. 65 test items are presented to a client horizontally in a spiral-bound test-plates easel. The MVPT–3 takes 20–30 minutes to complete.	The MVPT–3 has been standardized with a national representative sample. Normative data have been established for comparison for test takers 4 years old through 95 and older. The MVPT–3 has a moderate to strong internal consistency for each age group, with Cronbach's coefficient alphas from .69 to .90. The test–retest reliability of the MVPT–3 is high; for a 34-day retest interval, $r = .87$ for ages 4–10 years, and $r = .90$ for ages 11–84 and older. The validity of the MVPT–3 has been well established, with significant differences between individuals with brain injuries or academic difficulties and healthy peers demonstrating construct validity. The MVPT was more predictive of participants who would fail on-road driving tests than other tests of visual perception, which supports predictive validity.	*Strengths* • Examiner- and examinee-friendly. • Administration is brief and easy. • Designed to be a comprehensive measure of overall visual–perceptual ability. *Weaknesses* • Some psychometric examinations were completed on earlier versions of the MVPT. • Has not been adequately validated in some important clinical populations.
Occupational Therapy Adult Perceptual Screening Test (OT–APST; Cooke, McKenna, & Fleming, 2005)	The OT–APST is a standardized screening measure of visual perception and praxis for occupational therapists, particularly with clients after stroke. It has 25 items in 7 subtests: Agnosia, Visuospatial Relations, Unilateral Neglect, Body Scheme, Apraxia, Acalculia, and Functional Skills. The OT–APST takes 20–25 minutes to administer.	The OT–APST has demonstrated high interrater and intrarater reliability (1.00 for both; Cooke, McKenna, Fleming, & Darnell, 2005). The proportion of agreement between raters ranged from 83% to 99% (Cooke, McKenna, Fleming, & Darnell, 2005). The OT–APST was able to discriminate between individuals with stroke and healthy control participants, demonstrating construct validity (Cooke et al., 2006). It correlated highly with the Loewenstein Occupational Therapy Cognitive Assessment, which supports concurrent validity (Cooke et al., 2006). Some subscales had high correlations with the FIM®, which supports both the convergent and the predictive validity of the OT–APST (Cooke et al., 2006).	*Strengths* • Assesses skills relevant to occupational performance. • Easy to score and administer. *Weaknesses* • Not suitable for individuals with severe cognitive deficits. • Not suitable for individuals with language comprehension problems. • Has not been validated in populations other than stroke.

(Continued)

TABLE 16.3. Assessments of Visual Processing and Apraxia *(Cont.)*

INSTRUMENT AND REFERENCE	DESCRIPTION	PSYCHOMETRICS	STRENGTHS AND WEAKNESSES
Behavioral Inattention Test (BIT; Wilson et al., 1987)	The BIT is a battery of tests to assess the presence and extent of visual neglect on a sample of everyday problems faced by clients with visual inattention. The BIT is divided into 2 sections: Conventional and Behavioral tests. The BIT Conventional section consists of 6 subtests, and the Behavioral section consists of 9 subtests. To minimize practice and learning effects on retesting, parallel versions of the test are available. The BIT takes 30–40 minutes to administer.	Wilson et al. (1987) examined the test–retest reliability of the BIT among clients with stroke and healthy individuals and reported high correlation between administrations within 1 week ($r = .83$). The inter-rater reliability was 100% agreement between raters. The BIT was able to predict functional outcomes among people with stroke, demonstrating predictive validity (Jehkonen et al., 2000). Among clients with stroke, it distinguished between individuals with and without visual neglect (Halligan et al., 1991).	*Strengths* • Easy to administer. • Has cutoff scores to distinguish visual neglect. *Weaknesses* • May be too lengthy. • Expensive.
Screening for Apraxia (Almeida et al., 2002)	The screen requires both panto-miming and imitation of transitive (tool-related), intransitive (communication-related), and meaningless gestures. 5 dimensions are scored for each task on a 3-point scale (see Roy et al., 1998 for scoring). Developed to determine a need for more thorough and comprehensive assessment of apraxia.	Interrater reliability had kappa coefficient ranges from .71 to .78. The validity of the screen has not been established.	*Strength* • Quick 5-item screening test. *Weaknesses* • Scoring is unclear and requires previous knowledge and practice by the examiner. • Has not been assessed for validity.
Assessment of Apraxia (Van Heugten et al., 1999)	Assessment focuses on ideational and ideomotor apraxia. Has 2 subtests: demonstration of object use (3 sets of objects presented under 3 different conditions) and imitation of 6 gestures. Each is scored on a scale of 0 (movement not recognizable) to 3 (performance is correct and appropriate). Maximum score is 54 for object use and 36 for imitation of gestures, with a total possible score of 90. Total scores below 86 are considered to identify apraxia.	The Assessment of Apraxia has good internal consistency (Cronbach's $\alpha = .96$). Had interrater reliability of $\kappa > .60$ on all but 3 items (Zwinkels et al., 2004). The cutoff score of 86 has a sensitivity of 91%.	*Strength* • Subtests are assessed with common daily gestures and objects. *Weaknesses* • Has not been assessed for validity. • Measures only ideational and ideomotor apraxia.

The Behavioral measures include scanning pictures (e.g., identifying items on each side of a picture of a sink and identifying foodstuffs on the picture of a plate of food), reading a menu, sorting coins, and telling and setting the time. Table 16.3 presents 2 measures of visual-processing skills: the Motor-Free Visual Perception Test (3rd ed.; Colarusso & Hammill, 2003) and the Occupational Therapy Adult Perceptual Screening Test (Cooke, McKenna, & Fleming, 2005).

Neuropsychological Assessment of Praxis

Praxis is "the ability to organize and skillfully execute purposeful movements" (Giles, 2014, p. 90). *Apraxia* is a deficit in skilled, purposeful movement that cannot be accounted for by weakness, abnormal tone, sensory loss, cognitive deficit, or noncooperation (Buxbaum et al., 2008). There are 3 major forms of apraxia that affect occupational performance:

1. Limb-kinetic apraxia

2. Ideomotor apraxia

3. Ideational apraxia (Pearce, 2009).

Apraxia is now recognized to have an impact on daily functioning (Hanna-Pladdy et al., 2003), although the severity and nature of the impact might be difficult to measure. There is no single test that captures all types of apraxia (Butler, 2002; Buxbaum et al., 2008).

Limb-kinetic apraxia is a disorder in which the ability to perform fine movements is compromised; it is most apparent in tests of finger movements (Heilman & Rothi, 2011). A person with *ideomotor apraxia* may be unable to perform purposeful motor tasks on command, although they have an understanding of the idea or concept of the task (Giles, 2014). For example, a person might be unable to pick up a toothbrush when asked to brush their teeth, despite clearly demonstrating understanding of what is being asked and despite being able to perform the task at another time spontaneously.

Ideational apraxia causes an individual to have difficulty carrying out a series of actions in a sequence required to achieve a goal (Hécaen, 1968). Individuals with ideational apraxia may have difficulty with the logical sequence of single movements, use objects improperly, or skip or repeat movements in a sequence (Poeck & Lehmkuhl, 1980). Two measures of apraxia are included in Table 16.3: the Screening for Apraxia (Almeida et al., 2002) and the Assessment of Apraxia (Van Heugten et al., 1999).

Neuropsychological Assessment of EF

EFs have been defined in various ways across different disciplines and clinical settings (Cramm et al., 2013). **Executive function** has been defined as "a complex, multifaceted construct that comprises those abilities that allow one to plan, organize, and successfully execute purposeful, goal-oriented, and future-oriented actions" (Suchy et al., 2017, p. 551; see also Lezak et al., 2012). Miyake and colleagues (2000) identified 3 subcomponents of executive functioning: (1) task shifting, (2) inhibition, and (3) updating. Lezak et al. (2012) proposed a 4-component model consisting of volition, planning, purposive action, and effective performance. Suchy (2015) included self-awareness and social cognition in her model of EF. Both are important concepts that are also emphasized by occupational therapists regarding cognition in daily life.

EFs support purposeful and goal-directed actions. The abilities to generate plans, solve problems, and organize thoughts that guide future action are distinct EF skills. Working memory is an important EF capacity that enables people to temporarily process, store, and manipulate information consciously to perform daily activities (Rabinovici et al., 2015). An example of working memory in action is calculating a gratuity on a bill. One needs working memory to process the total charge, store the number, and manipulate that information to calculate the percentage of tip and then add the tip amount to the total.

Another EF skill is *inhibition,* which is "the ability to hold back a predominant, automatic, or previously learned response that may be inappropriate or irrelevant in the present context" (Rabinovici et al., 2015, p. 648). Successful performance of some daily activities might require the inhibition of prepotent (i.e., automatic or habitual) responses to meet a current goal. Individuals with inhibition deficits may have difficulty ignoring irrelevant stimuli or may seem easily distracted or impulsive.

Tests of verbal fluency assess both executive control and verbal ability. A common feature of these tests is the need to retrieve words, which requires the test taker to access a mental lexicon, focus on the task, select words that meet certain constraints, and avoid repetition. All of these actions involve executive control processes (Fisk & Sharp, 2004). Two types of verbal fluency tests are typically used:

1. Category fluency, also known as *semantic fluency* (Benton, 1968)

2. Letter fluency, also referred to as *phonemic fluency* (Newcombe, 1969).

In the standard versions of the tasks, participants are given 1 minute to produce as many unique words as possible that fall in a semantic category (category fluency) or start with a given letter (letter fluency). The participant's score in each task is the number of unique correct words.

The Controlled Oral Word Association Test (Lezak et al., 2012), a measure of letter and phonemic fluency, asks the individual to say as quickly as possible words beginning with the letters *F*, *A*, and *S*, with 60 seconds for each letter (e.g., "Tell me as many words as you can think of beginning with the letter *F*"). Animal naming is a commonly used measure of category and semantic fluency (e.g., "Name as many animals as you can in 1 minute"). In general, performance is better on semantic tasks than on phonemic tasks.

Although the letter and category fluency tasks are clearly similar, the demands of the tasks differ in subtle but important ways. Category fluency tasks resemble everyday production tasks, such as making a shopping list, so that participants can exploit existing links between related concepts (e.g., between the category label and the category members and among associated category members) to retrieve responses. In contrast, for letter fluency, task words must be retrieved from a phonemic category, which is rarely done in everyday speech production, so that participants must suppress the activation of semantically or associatively related words and must resort to novel retrieval strategies (Luo et al., 2010).

These tests have been validated in several neurologically healthy and clinical populations across demographic groups and diagnostic categories. One concern raised about the use of these tests is the variability in the specific tasks selected and administration procedures. Although normative data are available for both adults and children, it is important to make sure that the norms selected are associated with the test that is being administered. Table 16.4 describes 3 common EF assessments:

1. Behavioral Assessment of the Dysexecutive Syndrome (Wilson et al., 1996)

2. Delis–Kaplan Executive Function System (Delis et al., 2001)

3. Behavior Rating Inventory of Executive Function– Adult Version (Roth et al., 2005), a self-report measure.

TABLE 16.4. Assessments of EF

INSTRUMENT AND REFERENCE	DESCRIPTION	PSYCHOMETRICS	STRENGTHS AND WEAKNESSES
Behavioral Assessment of the Dysexecutive Syndrome (BADS; Wilson et al., 1996)	The BADS is a standardized test of everyday EF skills. Specific areas of assessment include problem solving, organizing, and planning. Contains 6 subtests of real-life behaviors and 2 20-item Dysexecutive Questionnaires for the client and a proxy to complete for comparison. The 2 questionnaires focus on emotional or personality changes, motivational changes, behavioral changes, and cognitive changes. The BADS takes about 40 minutes to complete.	The BADS demonstrated high inter-rater reliability (r = .88–1.00) across all 6 subtests. It is standardized to 100, with a standard deviation of 15. The manual provides norms for comparison. The BADS had significant correlations with other common standard EF tests, which supports concurrent validity (Norris & Tate, 2000). In addition, it was able to discriminate between individuals with and without brain damage, demonstrating construct validity (Norris & Tate, 2000).	*Strengths* • Developed to be practical and reflective of everyday situations. • Considered to be a comprehensive assessment. • Kit is provided with purchase and is portable. *Weaknesses* • High cost of test kit and additional sheets. • Lack of organization. • Some subtests may be difficult to score. • Some subtests may require subjective judgment by the administrator to score.
Delis–Kaplan Executive Function System (D–KEFS; Delis et al., 2001)	The D–KEFS is a standardized assessment of EF for children, adolescents, and adults 8–89 years old. The D–KEFS is composed of the following 9 stand-alone tests that can be individually or group administered: Trail Making Test, Verbal Fluency Test, Design Fluency Test, Color–Word Interference Test, Sorting Test, Twenty Questions Test, Word Context Test, Tower Test, and Proverb Test. These tests were developed to assess the range of EF skills. The administration format of the D–KEFS is completed without implication of right–wrong feedback to reduce unproductive discouragement and frustration that might be caused by poor performance.	The D–KEFS is a standardized assessment that has normative data based on a national representative sample. Had a reported medium to high reliability, with test–retest correlations ranging from .62 to .80 on all D–KEFS tests. Has reported moderate to high split-half reliabilities across age groups for the Verbal Fluency Test's Letter Fluency condition (.68–.90), the Color–Word Interference Test (.62–.86), the Sorting Test's Sort Recognition section (.62–.81), the Twenty Questions Test's Initial Abstraction section (.72–.87), and the Proverb Test (.68–.80). The D–KEFS has evidence of convergent validity by correlation with the Wisconsin Card Sorting Test. Also had nonsignificant correlation with the California Verbal Learning Test (2nd ed.), demonstrating discriminant validity. The D–KEFS was able to distinguish among many different types of clinical groups, supporting its sensitivity.	*Strengths* • Normative data based on a large and representative national sample. • Strong validation studies that support the use of the D–KEFS. • Has alternative forms to minimize practice effects during reevaluations. *Weaknesses* • Administration may facilitate understanding of task demands of future versions of the D–KEFS. • Test instructions for some D–KEFS tests seem somewhat complex and repetitive. • Although the primary achievement measures of the D–KEFS have adequate to good reliability coefficients, some of the optional process measures have reported low reliability coefficients. • Normative data for the younger age groups has been critiqued as not representative of population performance on these measures.

(Continued)

TABLE 16.4. Assessments of EF *(Cont.)*

INSTRUMENT AND REFERENCE	DESCRIPTION	PSYCHOMETRICS	STRENGTHS AND WEAKNESSES
Behavior Rating Inventory of Executive Function– Adult Version (BRIEF–A; Roth et al., 2005)	The BRIEF–A is a 75-item self-report of EF across a range of situations. It provides information based on 2 indexes—the Behavioral Regulation Index (BRI) and the Metacognition Index (MI)—and 9 subscales. The BRI measures inhibition, shifting, emotional control, and self-monitoring. The MI measures initiation, working memory, planning and organization, organization of materials, and task monitoring. The BRIEF–A takes about 10–15 minutes to complete.	The BRIEF–A has been standardized and validated for ages 18–90. The MI and BRI indexes have a reported high internal consistency (α = .93–.96). The BRIEF–A had moderate to strong correlations with measures of EF (r = .63–.74), demonstrating construct validity. Significant differences were found between healthy individuals and clients with traumatic brain injury on both BRIEF–A indexes, which supports concurrent validity.	*Strengths* • A reasonably brief measure of EF difficulties. • Does not require formal training to administer or score. • Covers various aspects of EF. *Weaknesses* • Validation based on U.S. sample only. • Scoring has to be done by hand unless the computer scoring program is used. • Self-report may not be accurate.
Self-Awareness of Deficits Interview (SADI; Fleming et al., 1996)	The SADI was designed to collect both qualitative and quantitative data on status of self-awareness. The client is asked about self-awareness of deficits, self-awareness of functional limitations because of deficits, and ability to set realistic goals. A therapist familiar with the client's level of functioning assigns a score from 0–3 on each domain (0 represents full awareness). The SADI takes 10 minutes to complete.	The SADI had strong interrater reliability (intraclass correlation [ICC] = .82) and test–retest reliability (ICC = .94). It had moderate correlations with the Dysexecutive Questionnaire (r = .40, p < .05). It significantly predicted performance on a set of EF measures.	*Strength* • Brief semistructured interview with questions that are relevant to intervention planning. *Weakness* • Potential for bias of subjective judgment of the therapist on the extent to which client responses reflect level of self-awareness disorder.
Awareness of Errors in Naturalistic Action (Hart et al., 1998)	After completing a complex daily task, clients rate their performance on a 9-item questionnaire (5-point scale). Higher scores indicate higher ratings of ability. These ratings were compared with actual performance in terms of ability to detect and correct errors occurring in a stream of naturalistic action.	The questionnaire had a high interrater reliability (κ = 95%). Self-ratings on the questionnaire were significantly different in a sample of individuals with traumatic brain injury than in a control sample, which demonstrates content and construct validity. In addition, people with dementia were less accurate in their self-rating of errors than a control sample (Giovannetti et al., 2002).	*Strengths* • Connected to a real task that examiner can compare with. • Has been validated with various diagnostic populations. *Weaknesses* • Ratings specific to the task may not be reflective of real awareness skills. • Does not assess online awareness.

Note. EF = executive function.

Another important skill associated with EF is metacognition (sometimes referred to as *self-awareness*). **Metacognition** in this context refers to a person's ability to "evaluate and become aware of his or her capabilities" (Katz, 2011, p. 279); this could include cognitive and physical abilities. Neuropsychology and rehabilitation literature has also used the term *self-awareness* to describe metacognition (Katz, 2011). People use metacognition to generate strategies that successfully facilitate task performance.

Toglia and Maeir (2018) described *self-awareness* as a multidimensional construct that includes self-knowledge and online awareness. Self-knowledge is a person's understanding of their own cognitive (and noncognitive) strengths and limitations outside the context of or before performance of a task (Toglia, 2011). *Online awareness* consists of metacognitive skills, such as ability to accurately judge task demands, anticipate and monitor errors, and evaluate performance in the context of an activity (Toglia, 2011). Therefore, online awareness changes within an activity, whereas self-knowledge is stable and changes slowly with experiences (Toglia, 2011).

It is important to distinguish between these 2 types of self-awareness. An individual might demonstrate intact self-knowledge (e.g., acknowledges memory difficulties during an interview) yet demonstrate poor online awareness (e.g., fails to look at a planner to check off items; Toglia, 2011). The assessment of these skills is typically carried out through the clinician's subjective rating of a client's awareness or a questionnaire in which clients rate their own level of awareness. Two assessments of self-awareness are described in Table 16.4:

1. Self-Awareness of Deficits Interview (Fleming et al., 1996)

2. Awareness of Errors in Naturalistic Action (Hart et al., 1998).

Conclusion

Neuropsychological tests can provide important information about the cognitive deficits that influence occupational performance. Many performance-based assessments of functional cognition intentionally incorporate activities that rely on these associated cognitive domains. These cognitive measures should not be used to replace functional–cognitive assessments. However, they can be used to support the interpretation of performance-based assessments of functional cognition through the identification of impairments in very specific areas of impaired cognitive function. Understanding the nature and extent of these specific cognitive deficits can inform the development of individualized therapeutic interventions designed to support occupational performance in context.

The process of creating reliable and valid neurocognitive assessments has also focused on the development of normative criteria that account for known differences in performance associated with demographic and environmental factors. Extensive testing of measures across populations and the creation of specific normative criteria are equally important for measures of functional cognition. As these measures are more widely evaluated, normative values will make the clinical application of test results more effective in the development of individualized therapeutic interventions that take into account the interaction of person and environmental factors on occupational performance.

References

Al-Khawaja, I., Wade, D. T., & Collin, C. F. (1996). Bedside screening for aphasia: A comparison of two methods. *Journal of Neurology, 243*, 201–204. https://doi.org/10.1007/BF02444015

Almeida, Q. J., Black, S. E., & Roy, E. A. (2002). Screening for Apraxia: A short assessment for stroke patients. *Brain and Cognition, 48*, 253–258. https://doi.org/10.1006/brcg.2001.1356

Anderson, J. R. (2004). *Cognitive psychology and its implications: John R. Anderson* (6th ed.). New York: Worth.

Axelrod, B. N., Ricker, J. H., & Cherry, S. A. (1994). Concurrent validity of the MAE Visual Naming Test. *Archives of Clinical Neuropsychology, 9*, 317–321. https://doi.org/10.1093/arclin/9.4.317

Ball, K., Ross, L. A., & Viamonte, S. (2010). Normal aging and everyday functioning. In T. D. Marcotte & I. Grant (Eds.), *Neuropsychology of everyday functioning* (pp. 248–263). New York: Guilford Press.

Benedict, R. H. B., Schretlen, D., Groninger, L., & Brandt, J. (1998). Hopkins Verbal Learning Test–Revised: Normative data and analysis of inter-form and test–retest reliability. *Clinical Neuropsychologist, 12*, 43–55. https://doi.org/10.1076/clin.12.1.43.1726

Benton, A. L. (1968). Differential behavioral effects in frontal lobe disease. *Neuropsychologia, 6*, 53–60. https://doi.org/10.1016/0028-3932(68)90038-9

Bradley, V., & Kapur, N. (2010). Neuropsychological assessment of memory disorders. In J. M. Gurd, U. Kischka, & J. C. Marshall (Eds.), *Handbook of clinical neuropsychology* (2nd ed., pp. 159–183). New York: Oxford University Press. https://doi.org/10.1093/acprof:oso/9780199234110.003.009

Buckner, R. L. (2004). Memory and executive function in aging and AD: Multiple factors that cause decline and reserve factors that compensate. *Neuron, 44*, 195–208. https://doi.org/10.1016/j.neuron.2004.09.006

Budson, A. E. (2009). Understanding memory dysfunction. *Neurologist, 15*, 71–79. https://doi.org/10.1097/NRL.0b013e318188040d

Butler, J. A. (2002). How comparable are tests of apraxia? *Clinical Rehabilitation, 16*, 389–398. https://doi.org/10.1191/0269215502cr493oa

Buxbaum, L. J., Haaland, K. Y., Hallett, M., Wheaton, L., Heilman, K. M., Rodriguez, A., & Rothi, L. (2008). Treatment of limb apraxia: Moving forward to improved action. *American Journal of Physical Medicine and Rehabilitation, 87*, 149–161. https://doi.org/10.1097/PHM.0b013e31815e6727

Cherney, L. R. (1995). Management approaches for aphasia. *Topics in Stroke Rehabilitation, 2*, vi–vii. https://doi.org/10.1080/10749357.1995.11754049

Colarusso, R. P., & Hammill, D. D. (2003). *Motor-Free Visual Perception Test* (3rd ed.). Novato, CA: Academic Therapy.

Conners, K. (2008). *Conners' Continuous Performance Test manual* (3rd ed.). Toronto: Multi-Health Systems.

Cooke, D. M., McKenna, K., & Fleming, J. (2005). Development of a standardized occupational therapy screening tool for visual perception in adults. *Scandinavian Journal of Occupational Therapy, 12*, 59–71. https://doi.org/10.1080/11038120410020683-1

Cooke, D. M., McKenna, K., Fleming, J., & Darnell, R. (2005). The reliability of the Occupational Therapy Adult Perceptual Screening Test (OT–APST). *British Journal of Occupational Therapy, 68*, 509–517. https://doi.org/10.1177/030802260506801105

Cooke, D. M., McKenna, K., Fleming, J., & Darnell, R. (2006). Construct and ecological validity of the Occupational Therapy Adult Perceptual Screening Test (OT–APST). *Scandinavian Journal of Occupational Therapy, 13*, 49–61. https://doi.org/10.1080/11038120500363014

Cowan, N. (2008). What are the differences between long-term, short-term, and working memory? *Progress in Brain Research, 169*, 323–338. https://doi.org/10.1016/S0079-6123(07)00020-9

Cramm, H. A., Krupa, T. M., Missiuna, C. A., Lysaght, R. M., & Parker, K. H. (2013). Executive functioning: A scoping review of the occupational therapy literature. *Canadian Journal of Occupational Therapy, 80*, 131–140. https://doi.org/10.1177/0008417413496060

Dawson, D. R., & Marcotte, T. D. (2017). Special issue on ecological validity and cognitive assessment. *Neuropsychological Rehabilitation, 27*, 599–602. https://doi.org/10.1080/09602011.2017.1313379

Delis, D. C., Kaplan, E., & Kramer, J. (2001). *Delis–Kaplan Executive Function System*. San Antonio: Psychological Corporation.

Delis, D. C., Kramer, J. H., Kaplan, E., & Ober, B. A. (2017). *California Verbal Learning Test* (3rd ed.). San Antonio: Pearson.

Enderby, P. M., Wood, V. A., Wade, D. T., & Hewer, R. L. (1986). The Frenchay Aphasia Screening Test: A short, simple test for aphasia appropriate for non-specialists. *International Rehabilitation Medicine, 8*, 166–170. https://doi.org/10.3109/03790798709166209

Evans, J. J. (2010). Basic concepts and principles of neuropsychological assessment. In J. M. Gurd, U. Kischka, & J. C. Marshall (Eds.), *Handbook of clinical neuropsychology* (2nd ed., pp. 15–27). New York: Oxford University Press. https://doi.org/10.1093/acprof:oso/9780199234110.003.02

Fals-Stewart, W. (1992). An interrater reliability study of the Trail Making Test (Parts A and B). *Perceptual and Motor Skills, 74*, 39–42. https://doi.org/10.2466/pms.1992.74.1.39

Farmer, C. M., Braitman, K. A., & Lund, A. K. (2010). Cell phone use while driving and attributable crash risk. *Traffic Injury Prevention, 11*, 466–470. https://doi.org/10.1080/15389588.2010.494191

Fisk, J. E., & Sharp, C. A. (2004). Age-related impairment in executive functioning: Updating, inhibition, shifting, and access. *Journal of Clinical and Experimental Neuropsychology, 26*, 874–890. https://doi.org/10.1080/13803390490510680

Fleming, J. M., Strong, J., & Ashton, R. (1996). Self-awareness of deficits in adults with traumatic brain injury: How best to measure? *Brain Injury, 10*, 1–16. https://doi.org/10.1080/026990596124674

Giles, G. M. (2014). Cognition and cognitive rehabilitation in neurocognitive disorders. In M. A. Corcoran (Ed.), *Neurocognitive disorder (NCD): Interventions to support occupational performance* (pp. 65–103). Bethesda, MD: AOTA Press.

Gillen, G. (2009). *Cognitive and perceptual rehabilitation: Optimizing function*. St. Louis: Mosby/Elsevier.

Giovannetti, T., Libon, D. J., & Hart, T. (2002). Awareness of naturalistic action errors in dementia. *Journal of the International Neuropsychological Society, 8*, 633–644. https://doi.org/10.1017/S135561770280131X

Goodglass, H. (1993). *Understanding aphasia*. San Diego: Academic Press.

Gronwall, D. M. (1977). Paced Auditory Serial-Addition Task: A measure of recovery from concussion. *Perceptual and Motor Skills, 44*, 367–373.

Halligan, P. W., Cockburn, J., & Wilson, B. A. (1991). The behavioural assessment of visual neglect. *Neuropsychological Rehabilitation, 1*, 5–32. https://doi.org/10.1080/09602019108401377

Hanna-Pladdy, B., Heilman, K. M., & Foundas, A. L. (2003). Ecological implications of ideomotor apraxia: Evidence from physical activities of daily living. *Neurology, 60*, 487–490. https://doi.org/10.1212/WNL.60.3.487

Hart, T., Giovannetti, T., Montgomery, M. W., & Schwartz, M. F. (1998). Awareness of errors in naturalistic action after traumatic brain injury. *Journal of Head Trauma Rehabilitation, 13*, 16–28. https://doi.org/10.1097/00001199-199810000-00004

Hécaen, A. (1968). Suggestions for a typology of the apraxias. In M. L. Simmel (Ed.), *The reach of mind: Essays in memory of Kurt Goldstein* (pp. 37–56). New York: Springer. https://doi.org/10.1007/978-3-662-40265-8_5

Heilman, K. M., & Rothi, L. J. G. (2011). Apraxia. In K. M. Heilman & E. Valenstein (Eds.), *Clinical neuropsychology* (3rd ed., pp. 214–237). New York: Oxford University Press.

Huff, F. J., Collins, C., Corkin, S., & Rosen, T. J. (1986). Equivalent forms of the Boston Naming Test. *Journal of Clinical and Experimental Neuropsychology, 8*, 556–562. https://doi.org/10.1080/01688638608405175

Jehkonen, M., Ahonen, J.-P., Dastidar, P., Koivisto, A.-M., Laippala, P., Vilkki, J., & Molnár, G. (2000). Visual neglect as a predictor of functional outcome one year after stroke. *Acta Neurologica Scandinavica, 101*, 195–201. https://doi.org/10.1034/j.1600-0404.2000.101003195.x

Kaplan, E., & Goodglass, H. (1983). *The Boston Naming Test* (2nd ed.). Boston: Lea & Febiger.

Kaplan, E., Goodglass, H., & Weintraub, S. (1978). *The Boston Naming Test*. Boston: E. Kaplan & H. Goodglass.

Katz, N. (Ed.). (2011). *Cognition, occupation, and participation across the life span: Neuroscience, neurorehabilitation, and models of intervention in occupational therapy* (3rd ed.). Bethesda, MD: AOTA Press.

Kuzis, G., Sabe, L., Tiberti, C., Merello, M., Leiguarda, R., & Starkstein, S. E. (1999). Explicit and implicit learning in patients with Alzheimer disease and Parkinson disease with dementia. *Neuropsychiatry, Neuropsychology, and Behavioral Neurology, 12*, 265–269.

LaBarge, E., Balota, D. A., Storandt, M., & Smith, D. S. (1992). An analysis of confrontation naming errors in senile dementia of the Alzheimer type. *Neuropsychology, 6*, 77–95. https://doi.org/10.1037/0894-4105.6.1.77

Lacritz, L. H., & Cullum, C. M. (1998). The Hopkins Verbal Learning Test and CVLT: A preliminary comparison. *Archives of Clinical Neuropsychology, 13*, 623–628.

Law, L. L. F., Barnett, F., Yau, M. K., & Gray, M. A. (2012). Measures of everyday competence in older adults with cognitive impairment: A systematic review. *Age and Ageing, 41*, 9–16. https://doi.org/10.1093/ageing/afr104

Lezak, M. D., Howieson, D., Bigler, E. D., & Tranel, D. (Eds.). (2012). *Neuropsychological assessment* (5th ed.). Oxford, England: Oxford University Press.

Luo, L., Luk, G., & Bialystok, E. (2010). Effect of language proficiency and executive control on verbal fluency performance in bilinguals. *Cognition, 114*, 29–41. https://doi.org/10.1016/j.cognition.2009.08.014

Mack, J. L., & Carlson, N. J. (1978). Conceptual deficits and aging: The Category Test. *Perceptual and Motor Skills, 46*(1), 123–128.

Manchester, D., Priestley, N., & Jackson, H. (2004). The assessment of executive functions: Coming out of the office. *Brain Injury, 18*, 1067–1081. https://doi.org/10.1080/02699050410001672387

Matarazzo, J. D., Wiens, A. N., Matarazzo, R. G., & Goldstein, S. G. (1974). Psychometric and clinical test–retest reliability of the Halstead Impairment Index in a sample of healthy, young, normal men. *Journal of Nervous and Mental Disease, 158*, 37–49. https://doi.org/10.1097/00005053-197401000-00006

Meier, M. J. (1974). Some challenges for clinical neuropsychology. In R. M. Reitan & L. A. Davison (Eds.), *Clinical neuropsychology: Current status and applications*. Washington, DC: V. H. Winston.

Michell, J. (1999). *Measurement in psychology: Critical history of a methodological concept*. Cambridge, England: Cambridge University Press. https://doi.org/10.1017/CBO9780511490040

Mitrushina, M., Boone, K. B., Razani, J., & D'Elia, L. F. (Eds.). (2005). *Handbook of normative data for neuropsychological assessment* (2nd ed.). New York: Oxford University Press.

Miyake, A., Friedman, N. P., Emerson, M. J., Witzki, A. H., Howerter, A., & Wager, T. D. (2000). The unity and diversity of executive functions and their contributions to complex "frontal lobe" tasks: A latent variable analysis. *Cognitive Psychology, 41*, 49–100. https://doi.org/10.1006/cogp.1999.0734

Nelson, H. E., & Willison, J. (1991). *National Adult Reading Test (NART): Test manual* (2nd ed.). Windsor, England: NFER Nelson.

Newcombe, F. (1969). *Missile wounds of the brain: A study of psychological deficits*. London: Oxford University Press.

Norris, G., & Tate, R. L. (2000). The Behavioural Assessment of the Dysexecutive Syndrome (BADS): Ecological, concurrent and construct validity. *Neuropsychological Rehabilitation, 10*, 33–45. https://doi.org/10.1080/096020100389282

O'Donnell, J. P., Macgregor, L. A., Dabrowski, J. J., Oestreicher, J. M., & Romero, J. J. (1994). Construct validity of neuropsychological tests of conceptual and attentional abilities. *Journal of Clinical Psychology, 50*, 596–600. https://doi.org/10.1002/1097-4679(199407)50:4<596::AID-JCLP2270500416>3.0.CO;2-S

O'Neill, P., Cheadle, B., Wyatt, R., McGuffog, J., & Fullerton, K. (1990). The value of the Frenchay Aphasia Screening Test in screening for dysphasia: Better than the clinician? *Clinical Rehabilitation, 4*, 123–128. https://doi.org/10.1177/026921559000400205

Pearce, J. M. S. (2009). Hugo Karl Liepmann and apraxia. *Clinical Medicine, 9*, 466–470. https://doi.org/10.7861/clinmedicine.9-5-466

Petersen, R. C. (2004). Mild cognitive impairment as a diagnostic entity. *Journal of Internal Medicine, 256*, 183–194. https://doi.org/10.1111/j.1365-2796.2004.01388.x

Poeck, K., & Lehmkuhl, G. (1980). Ideatory apraxia in a left-handed patient with right-sided brain lesion. *Cortex, 16*, 273–284. https://doi.org/10.1016/S0010-9452(80)80062-1

Poon, L. W. (1985). Differences in human memory with aging: Nature, causes, and clinical implications. In J. Birren & K. W. Schaie (Eds.),

Handbook of the psychology of aging (2nd ed., pp. 427–462). New York: Van Nostrand Reinhold.

Rabinovici, G. D., Stephens, M. L., & Possin, K. L. (2015). Executive dysfunction. *Behavioral Neurology and Neuropsychiatry, 21,* 646–659.

Radomski, M. V. (2008). Assessing abilities and capacities: Cognition. In M. V. Radomski & C. A. T. Latham (Eds.), *Occupational therapy for physical dysfunction* (6th ed., pp. 261–283). Philadelphia: Lippincott Williams & Wilkins.

Reitan, R. M. (1992). *Trail Making Test: Manual for administration and scoring.* Tucson, AZ: Reitan Neuropsychology Laboratory.

Robertson, I. H., Ward, T., Ridgeway, V., & Nimmo-Smith, I. (1996). The structure of normal human attention: The Test of Everyday Attention. *Journal of the International Neuropsychological Society, 2,* 525–534. https://doi.org/10.1017/S1355617700001697

Roth, R. M., Isquith, P. K., & Gioia, G. A. (2005). *Behavior Rating Inventory of Executive Function: Adult Version: Examiner's manual.* Lutz, FL: Psychological Assessment Resources.

Roy, E. A., Black, S. E., Blair, N., & Dimeck, P. T. (1998). Analyses of deficits in gestural pantomime. *Journal of Clinical and Experimental Neuropsychology, 20,* 628–643.

Salmon, D. P., Jin, H., Zhang, M., Grant, I., & Yu, E. (1995). Neuropsychological assessment of Chinese elderly in the Shanghai Dementia Survey. *Clinical Neuropsychologist, 9,* 159–168. https://doi.org/10.1080/13854049508401598

Sarno, M. T. (1994). Neurogenic disorders of speech and language. In S. B. O'Sullivan & T. J. Schmitz (Eds.), *Physical rehabilitation: Assessment and treatment* (3rd ed., pp. 633–653). Philadelphia: Davis.

Sawrie, S. M., Chelune, G. J., Naugle, R. I., & Lüders, H. O. (1996). Empirical methods for assessing meaningful neuropsychological change following epilepsy surgery. *Journal of the International Neuropsychological Society, 2,* 556–564. https://doi.org/10.1017/S1355617700001739

Shapiro, A. M., Benedict, R. H. B., Schretlen, D., & Brandt, J. (1999). Construct and concurrent validity of the Hopkins Verbal Learning Test—Revised. *Clinical Neuropsychologist, 13,* 348–358. https://doi.org/10.1076/clin.13.3.348.1749

Sohlberg, M. M., & Mateer, C. A. (2001). *Cognitive rehabilitation: An integrative neuropsychological approach.* New York: Guilford Press.

Spikman, J., & Van Zomeran, E. (2010). Assessment of attention. In J. M. Gurd, U. Kischka, & J. C. Marshall (Eds.), *Handbook of clinical neuropsychology* (2nd ed., pp. 81–96). New York: Oxford University Press. https://doi.org/10.1093/acprof:oso/9780199234110.003.05

Suchy, Y. (2015). *Executive functioning: A comprehensive guide for clinical practice.* Oxford, England: Oxford University Press.

Suchy, Y., Ziemnik, R. E., & Niermeyer, M. A. (2017). Assessment of executive functions in clinical settings. In E. Goldberg (Ed.), *Executive functions in health and disease* (pp. 551–569). San Diego: Academic Press. https://doi.org/10.1016/B978-0-12-803676-1.00022-2

Toglia, J. P. (1993). *Contextual Memory Test.* Tucson, AZ: Therapy Skill Builders.

Toglia, J. P. (2011). The Dynamic Interactional Model of Cognition in cognitive rehabilitation. In N. Katz (Ed.), *Cognition, occupation, and participation across the life span: Neuroscience, neurorehabilitation and models of intervention in occupational therapy* (3rd ed., pp. 161–201). Bethesda, MD: AOTA Press.

Toglia, J. P., Golisz, K. M., & Goverover, Y. (2013). Cognition, perception, and occupational performance. In B. A. Schell, G. Gillen, M. Scaffa, & E. S. Cohn (Eds.), *Willard and Spackman's occupational therapy* (12th ed., pp. 779–815). Philadelphia: Lippincott Williams & Wilkins.

Toglia, J. P., & Maeir, A. (2018). Self-awareness and metacognition: Effect on occupational performance and outcome across the lifespan. In N. Katz & J. P. Toglia (Eds.), *Cognition, occupation, and participation across the lifespan: Neuroscience, neurorehabilitation, and models of intervention in occupational therapy* (4th ed., pp. 143–163). Bethesda, MD: AOTA Press.

Trenerry, M. R., Crosson, B., DeBoe, J., & Leber, W. R. (1990). *Visual Search and Attention Test.* Odessa, FL: Psychological Assessment Resources.

Unsworth, C. A. (2007). Cognitive and perceptual dysfunction. In T. J. Schmitz & S. B. O'Sullivan (Eds.), *Physical rehabilitation* (pp. 1149–1185). Philadelphia: Davis.

Van Heugten, C. M., Dekker, J., Deelman, B. G., Stehmann-Saris, F. C., & Kinebanian, A. (1999). A diagnostic test for apraxia in stroke patients: Internal consistency and diagnostic value. *Clinical Neuropsychologist, 13,* 182–192. https://doi.org/10.1076/clin.13.2.182.1966

Wechsler, D. (2001). *Wechsler Test of Adult Reading: WTAR.* San Antonio: Psychological Corporation.

Wechsler, D. (2008). *Manual for the Wechsler Adult Intelligence Scale* (4th ed.). San Antonio: Pearson.

Wechsler, D. (2009). *Wechsler Memory Scale–IV.* San Antonio: Pearson.

Wilson, B. A., Alderman, N., Burgess, P. W., Emslie, H., & Evans, J. J. (1996). *Behavioural Assessment of the Dysexecutive Syndrome.* Bury St. Edmunds, England: Thames Valley Test Company.

Wilson, B. A., Cockburn, J., & Baddeley, A. (1985). *The Rivermead Behavioral Memory Test.* Reading, England: Thames Valley Test.

Wilson, B., Cockburn, J., Baddeley, A., & Hiorns, R. (1989). The development and validation of a test battery for detecting and monitoring everyday memory problems. *Journal of Clinical and Experimental Neuropsychology, 11,* 855–870. https://doi.org/10.1080/01688638908400940

Wilson, B., Cockburn, J., & Halligan, P. (1987). Development of a behavioral test of visuospatial neglect. *Archives of Physical Medicine and Rehabilitation, 68,* 98–102.

Wilson, B. A., Greenfield, E., Clare, L. E., Baddeley, A., Cockburn, J., & Watson, P., . . . Crawford, J. D. (2008). *The Rivermead Behavioural Memory Test* (3rd ed.). London: Pearson Assessment.

Woodson, A. M. (2008). Stroke. In M. V. Radomski & C. A. T. Latham (Eds.), *Occupational therapy for physical dysfunction* (6th ed., pp. 1001–1041). Philadelphia: Lippincott Williams & Wilkins.

Woollams, A. M., Cooper-Pye, E., Hodges, J. R., & Patterson, K. (2008). Anomia: A doubly typical signature of semantic dementia. *Neuropsychologia, 46,* 2503–2514. https://doi.org/10.1016/j.neuropsychologia.2008.04.005

Zoltan, B. (2007). *Vision, perception, and cognition: A manual for the evaluation and treatment of the adult with acquired brain injury* (4th ed.). Thorofare, NJ: Slack.

Zwinkels, A., Geusgens, C., Van de Sande, P., & Van Heugten, C. (2004). Assessment of Apraxia: Inter-rater reliability of a new apraxia test, association between apraxia and other cognitive deficits and prevalence of apraxia in a rehabilitation setting. *Clinical Rehabilitation, 18,* 819–827. https://doi.org/10.1191/0269215504cr816oa

SECTION

Intervention

The point of occupational therapy assessment is to identify areas of impaired occupational performance and to determine the methods most likely to assist clients in improving their occupational performance. In terms of intervention, one size does not fit all, and occupational therapy practitioners need to tailor the interventions provided to the client's specific needs. Section III begins with a chapter that describes the principles of functional–cognitive intervention. Chapter 17 covers fundamental principles related to Learning Theory and models of awareness that are foundational in all intervention frameworks that address functional cognition. This chapter also provides the necessary context for occupational therapists to use the information obtained from the Cognitive–Functional Evaluation process to select the appropriate intervention approach and develop a targeted and individualized treatment plan for each client on the basis of identified functional–cognitive abilities.

The remaining chapters (Chapters 18–21) review specific intervention frameworks. Similar to the chapters of Section II, focused on assessment, these chapters follow a uniform format focused on the pragmatic application of the interventions described. Each chapter includes an introduction that reviews the intervention approach—why it was developed and the theoretical basis for the approach. The remainder of the chapter is focused on the target population for the approach (including typical testing profiles for individuals for whom this intervention would be relevant), the components of the intervention and how it is delivered, information related to training (if necessary), how to document goals and progress using the approach, and finally examples of what treatment activities or sessions would look like when the approach is being used. These chapters have associated video content to demonstrate examples of administration of the interventions to supplement information provided in the text.

17

Intervention Selection: Learning and Concepts of Transfer

PEGGY P. BARCO, OTD, OTR/L, SCDCM, CDRS, FAOTA;

GLEN GILLEN, EdD, OTR, FAOTA;

AND TIMOTHY J. WOLF, OTD, PhD, OTR/L, FAOTA

LEARNING OBJECTIVES

After completing this chapter, readers should be able to

- Describe the importance of Learning Theory as the foundation for cognitive intervention approaches, how learning occurs, and how skills are transferred;
- Understand how person, environment, and occupation factors influence the selection of a cognitive intervention approach to be used with a client;
- Identify the level of awareness at which a client is functioning and how this relates to the type of intervention approach an occupational therapist will use in treatment; and
- Determine when to appropriately use different cognitive intervention approaches (e.g., task/habit training, strategy training, indirect approaches) when treating clients with cognitive and learning challenges.

KEY TERMS AND CONCEPTS

- Anticipatory awareness • Awareness • Direct intervention • Domain-specific strategies • Emergent awareness
- Indirect intervention • Intellectual awareness • Metacognitive strategies • Strategy • Strategy training
- Task/habit training • Transfer of learning

Introduction

Cognitive challenges are prevalent across developmental (e.g., autism), injury-related (e.g., traumatic brain injury [TBI]), and acquired neurological (e.g., stroke, dementia) conditions. A wide array of systemic medical conditions (e.g., chronic obstructive pulmonary disease, cancer) also can directly or indirectly affect brain function and negatively influence a client's occupational performance and quality of life (Crichton et al., 2016; Nys et al., 2006). Occupational therapists are trained to administer assessments and provide interventions with the client and caregivers to help overcome or minimize the occupational performance deficits often associated with the functional impact of cognitive impairments.

This chapter describes how vital the choice of the appropriate intervention approach is to an occupational therapist's success in helping clients achieve their functional goals.

The discussions in the early sections of this text, related to Cognitive–Functional Evaluations (C–FEs; i.e., interview, occupational profile, performance-based testing) performed with the client, are instrumental in gathering the information occupational therapists need to determine the preferred intervention approach. This information, in conjunction with an understanding of the theoretical background and learning processes associated with each cognitive intervention approach discussed in this chapter, will help therapists in this decision-making process.

Cognitive Intervention Approaches: Theoretical Foundations and Concepts of Transfer

Learning Theory provides the conceptual foundation for the functional–cognitive intervention approaches that are most commonly used by occupational therapists (Clark-Wilson et al., 2014; Levy, 2018; McEwen et al., 2018; Toglia, 2018). Functional–cognitive intervention approaches can be classified into direct intervention approaches and indirect intervention approaches.

The **direct intervention** approaches are client-focused training approaches. They include both task/habit training (see Chapter 18, "The Neurofunctional Approach") and strategy training (see Chapter 19, "Cognitive Orientation to daily Occupational Performance," and Chapter 20, "The Multicontext Approach"). Direct intervention (i.e., client-focused training) approaches either train a specific task or habit (i.e., task/habit training approaches) or train a strategy (i.e., strategy training approaches; Haskins et al., 2012) to improve performance.

In contrast, **indirect intervention** approaches do not directly involve the client. These interventions are typically focused on environmental modifications, task adaptations, or caregiver training and education. Each approach, whether direct or indirect, is focused on the performance level and has the goal to improve the client's participation and quality of life (Clark-Wilson et al., 2014; Levy, 2018; McEwen et al., 2018; Toglia, 2018).

Direct Intervention

Task/Habit Training Approaches to Cognitive Intervention

Task/habit training in cognitive intervention involves the occupational therapist training a client in a specific task (Haskins et al., 2012). Using task/habit training approaches, therapists typically work with the same task in the same way using the same techniques until the client demonstrates consistent task mastery (Clark-Wilson et al., 2014; Trevena-Peters et al., 2018). The client is not expected to transfer the learning of the task to different tasks (or situations).

An example of the task/habit training approach is teaching a person who survived a TBI a morning self-care routine using a repetitive, systematic approach. The theoretical foundation of this approach is based on the learning theory known as *Behaviorism*—in particular, the science of applied behavior analysis. The science of applied behavior analysis seeks to apply the techniques in Behaviorism to effect change for clients but takes into account the environmental and behavioral interaction.

Learning that uses the Behaviorism approach occurs as part of an association between stimuli and responses (Bates, 2016). The end result is an acquisition of a new behavior or skill. Learning can be viewed as task mastery. Processes that facilitate learning in Behaviorism include repetition, practice, routines, rules, and sometimes rewards. The occupational therapist's role is to focus on the client learning a task through repetition and practice. Routine in performing the task is important to establish.

Task/habit training approaches based on Behaviorism are intended to be used with clients with more profound cognitive loss, who are unable to rely on high-level cognitive processes to develop goals and modify behavior. In essence, the cueing and feedback provided in these approaches is a compensatory method to overcome this cognitive loss. However, when a behavior is trained this way, the client does not develop the cognitive skills necessary to transfer the learned behavior to other activities or environments.

A common error in working with individuals with functional–cognitive deficits is that most of the time the intervention provided is behaviorally based, and therefore it is challenging for the client to transfer what they learn. If the person is able to effectively learn and use strategies, a strategy-based intervention is more appropriate to overcome this limitation of behaviorally based task/habit training approaches.

Strategy Training Approaches to Cognitive Intervention

When using **strategy training** approaches, the occupational therapist assists the client in learning strategies to overcome existing cognitive challenges (Haskins et al., 2012). In strategy training approaches, the concept of a client being able to transfer the strategy to a new activity or situation is viewed as an important goal. A **strategy** is a tool or method used to help facilitate action toward a goal.

There are 2 primary types of strategies used in strategy-training programs:

1. **Metacognitive strategies,** which focus on teaching a global strategy that the client can use in any context to overcome cognitive limitations that affect occupational performance generally

2. **Domain-specific strategies,** which the client can use to compensate for specific cognitive limitations that affect occupational performance across similar tasks (e.g., taking notes to remember appointments and important information).

Strategy training approaches to intervention are rooted in a division of Learning Theory known as *Cognitivism*.

Cognitivism. Cognitivism focuses on the client as an active learner who learns by recognizing how new information may compare with previously learned information (Bates, 2016). Cognitivism is built on the theory that clients process and interpret the information they receive. Behaviorism, conversely, is more of a response-oriented approach. For learning to occur, the client must have prior knowledge with which to associate the new information. These connections start the process of transferring learned information to novel contexts and problems and are how strategy development occurs.

Cognitive processes (e.g., memory, insight, information processing, perception) play an important role in learning and strategy transfer ability. Strategies that facilitate learning in cognitivism approaches include internal strategies (e.g., classifying or chunking information, linking related concepts, using visual imagery) and external strategies (e.g., taking notes, using checklists, using various types of calendar systems). The occupational therapist's role is to help the client identify the strategies that facilitate their occupational performance and to apply these strategies across daily life activities. The goal is for the client to be able to apply strategies in different situations and activities as needed.

Many theories have stemmed from Cognitivism and are sometimes considered extensions of Cognitivism (Bates, 2016). Many of these related theories (e.g., Insight Theory, Constructivism, Reception Learning Theory, Discovery Theory) include learning processes that have been incorporated into cognitive intervention approaches used by occupational therapists.

For example, Insight Theory is focused on creating optimal conditions for learning to occur. This involves encouraging new ideas, learning from mistakes, evaluating errors, and continuing to find solutions. An occupational therapist may provide education and guidance to help the client learn a problem-solving process to develop potential solutions to their unique functional challenges, test the solutions in daily life, and revise them as appropriate.

Engaging in learning new tasks using metacognitive strategy–based approaches helps the client learn general strategies that are more easily transferred to different activities and contexts. This aligns with our understanding of transfer and generalization. *Transfer of learning* (i.e., generalization) is the ability to reproduce a learned behavior in another context or environment other than the learned environment. It also encompasses the ability to transfer learned behavior to another skill or task.

Concept of transfer: Key points. Six criteria for fostering transfer and generalization have been identified in the literature (Geusgens et al., 2007):

1. The learner must first know what transfer is and how it occurs.

2. The learner must have a certain level of awareness of their capabilities before implementing strategies to improve performance.

3. The learner must be able to realize when and where transfer may be applied.

4. The teaching of general knowledge, as opposed to overly detailed knowledge, supports ease of transfer.

5. Contextual interference, or variation in the task demands and environment, should be introduced during learning.

6. Transfer must be directly addressed during learning, because it does not occur spontaneously.

These concepts require the use of strategies and emphasize the need to allow for trial-and-error learning, 2 components that are largely absent from current behavioral training approaches. Recent evidence suggests that for clients who are able to use strategy-based learning, allowing for errors not only helps promote generalization but also is a more efficient way to learn an activity, which could reduce the client's length of stay in rehabilitation (Ownsworth et al., 2013). These findings highlight the importance of not using behavioral approaches if the client is able to engage in trial-and-error learning.

Indirect Intervention

Indirect intervention approaches are focused on providing caregiver education and training, environmental modifications, and task adaptations, with the goal to improve the client's participation and quality of life. Indirect approaches do not involve direct client training and therefore are not focused on helping the client "learn" a task or a strategy. When these approaches are used, the client is dependent on an external person or source to help them function in some way. Indirect approaches are commonly used with persons with dementia or other profound cognitive loss.

Indirect approaches have their foundation in Learning Theory, which uses applied behavior analysis to manage antecedent events in the environment to modify the behavior. For example, if a client is prone to wandering, placing door alarms on points of exit to alert caregivers is an appropriate environmental modification. The occupational therapist's role in this process is supportive, educational, and often environment and caregiver focused (Levy, 2018).

Person, Environment, and Occupation Considerations in Intervention Selection

The occupational therapist begins consideration of the person, environment, and occupation factors by examining the results of an interview with the client and significant others or caregiver, the C–FE, and the resulting occupational profile. Intervention selection is an integrative process that combines knowledge in theory and cognitive intervention approaches with clinical reasoning. The person, environment, and occupation factors contain the information the therapist requires to select the appropriate cognitive intervention approach.

Person (P) Factors

The C–FE process provides the necessary information to determine key person factors involved in intervention selection. Key person factors include

- The narrative that clients construct about themselves in relation to their cognitive deficits and the type and severity of cognitive deficits that are limiting functioning,

- Their level of awareness of their cognitive deficits, and

- What their functional goals are.

Particularly with clients with cognitive impairment, it is helpful to gather information from significant others to corroborate information provided by the client (given awareness deficits the client may be experiencing). Other person factors the occupational therapist needs to consider include the client's

- Age;

- Education level;

- Premorbid functioning;

- Current medical and psychiatric comorbidities; and

- Psychological, social, and cultural background.

When the clinician is determining the intervention approach, it is important that they not expect more of the client than the client is neurologically, educationally, or psychologically capable of achieving. Self-awareness of cognitive deficits has been identified as the key factor to be considered in decisions about which cognitive intervention approach is best suited to the client (Haskins et al., 2012). *Awareness* (also known as *metacognition*) is a person's knowledge of their cognitive strengths and weaknesses and the resulting ability to monitor and adapt behavior and use strategies accordingly. There are varying levels and types of awareness, which include intellectual, emergent, and anticipatory awareness.

Levels of Self-Awareness of Cognitive Deficits

It is common for persons with cognitive challenges to lack awareness of their cognitive deficits (Barco et al., 1991; Crosson et al., 1989; Fleming & Ownsworth, 2006; Haskins et al., 2012; Toglia & Kirk, 2000). The etiology for awareness deficits includes difficulties due to neurocognitive deficits, psychological issues, social and environmental factors, and lack of education about the current cognitive difficulties (Fleming & Ownsworth, 2006; Toglia & Maeir, 2018). Occupational therapists can choose different approaches to intervene to address awareness deficits, dependent on etiology. It is important to use the information obtained in the occupational profile, client and significant-other interviews, and C–FE to determine whether the client is aware of their cognitive challenges and implications related to their daily functioning.

Awareness of cognitive deficits, particularly when the cause is related to neurocognitive mechanisms (e.g., as may occur after TBI), is not an all-or-none phenomenon (Crosson et al., 1989; Haskins et al., 2012). A client may have no awareness, partial awareness, or full awareness of cognitive challenges. They may have awareness of some cognitive deficits but not others. Self-awareness of cognitive functioning is a crucial factor in determining the client's willingness to participate in therapy as well as their potential for benefiting from various occupational therapy intervention approaches.

Although terminology surrounding awareness deficits can vary in the literature, it is generally agreed that there are at least 3 major types of awareness deficits (intellectual awareness, emergent awareness, anticipatory awareness) that can occur after a brain injury (Crosson et al., 1989; Haskins et al., 2012). The Awareness Pyramid Model (Barco et al., 1991; Crosson et al., 1989) describes the levels of awareness, how to facilitate awareness at each level, and appropriate treatment interventions. Although the topic is beyond the scope of this chapter, it is important to try to improve self-awareness and adjust treatment approaches as awareness increases (Barco et al., 1991; Doig et al., 2017; Fleming & Ownsworth, 2006; Toglia et al., 2011; Toglia & Kirk, 2000).

Intellectual Awareness. **Intellectual awareness** of a cognitive deficit is the most basic awareness that the cognitive deficit exists, also referred to as *awareness knowledge*. A client with only intellectual awareness is able to verbally state that a cognitive deficit exists (e.g., "I have trouble paying attention") but likely does not realize how the cognitive deficit actually affects their daily functioning. Intellectual awareness is necessary for higher levels of awareness to exist. It is known as the base of the pyramid that supports the other levels of awareness.

Without intellectual awareness, the client does not realize a difficulty exists, so they perceive no need for therapy or strategies. Severe cognitive deficits that impair learning often are present, which may be why the client's intellectual awareness is compromised.

Lack of intellectual awareness is most common with severe memory and learning impairment or severe receptive aphasia. Clients may not be able to retain information long enough (or understand information sufficiently) for intellectual awareness to be established. If the client's lack of awareness of cognitive deficits is injury related, lack of education provided acutely by health care providers should be ruled out as a reason.

Emergent Awareness. **Emergent awareness,** otherwise known as *online awareness* (Toglia & Kirk, 2000), is the next level of the awareness pyramid. It is present when a client is able to recognize a cognitive difficulty while it is actually hindering their performance in a functional activity. The client must be aware that a difficulty exists (i.e., intellectual awareness) before they can have emergent awareness. Thus, when a client can state they have a cognitive deficit indicating intellectual awareness (e.g., "I have a memory deficit") but is not able to recognize when it is currently hindering them in real time (e.g., the client is not aware they have repeated the story several times to the same person), emergent awareness difficulties exist. Conversely, a person who has emergent awareness may realize that they are not processing the content of a conversation and ask the person speaking to slow down, repeat key points, or move the conversation to a quiet environment.

Thus, in situations in which emergent awareness is absent, the client is unable to have the awareness in the moment to identify that they are having difficulties and need to implement a strategy. Conversely, if the client could recognize they are experiencing difficulties due to a cognitive impairment, they would be able to implement the strategy as needed. Lack of emergent awareness exists when a client has difficulty accurately perceiving the relationship between their actions and the environment. This can be due to a variety of types and severities of cognitive impairment.

Anticipatory Awareness. **Anticipatory awareness** is the most advanced level of awareness. This level of awareness involves a client being able to plan and anticipate that a cognitive deficit may affect their performance on a functional task before performing the task. Clients must have intellectual and emergent awareness to support the presence of anticipatory awareness.

With anticipatory awareness, the client can plan and implement learned strategies in advance to avoid functional difficulties that may result from cognitive challenges. For example, a person who is living with attention deficits might anticipate difficulties grocery shopping because of the stimulating environment and plan to shop at an "off time," such as 6:00 p.m. on a Friday, when there are fewer distractions.

Lack of anticipatory awareness is most common with clients who have difficulties in executive function. Such clients have challenges in the ability to anticipate, plan, problem solve, and make decisions. Thus, being able to anticipate, plan, and implement a strategy to overcome a cognitive challenge before performing the functional task is difficult.

Environment (E) Factors

The environment surrounding the client often includes their current environment and future environments. The current environment may be a medical intensive care unit, acute care hospital, rehabilitation center, or community-based treatment or health and wellness facility. The future environment could include home, work, school, or social and community surroundings. It is important for the occupational therapist to be attuned to these environments and any changes that may be likely to occur in them in the foreseeable future.

The client's support context is a critical factor, and it may change depending on the environment in which they are currently functioning. For example, family may be the client's support system at home, and an office manager may be their support system at work. Researchers consistently have found that 1 of the most important predictors of improvement for a client with cognitive challenges is a strong support system (Haskins et al., 2012). Some intervention approaches involve more follow-through with the client's support system than others, and they may include important home, work, or community modifications. It is important not to base a client's success on an intervention approach that is dependent on a support system that does not exist or on modifications that are unrealistic in the environment in which the client will be functioning.

A client's financial status and health insurance status are additional environmental considerations that can either support or impose limitations on the intervention. There is continued disparity in the United States in what providers of health care offer in terms of services when the client does or does not have health insurance benefits (Fang et al., 2016; Johnson et al., 2017; Kim et al., 2017). Some intervention approaches require occupational therapy over more extended periods than others. Health insurance can be a strength or a barrier to the rehabilitation process and, unfortunately, can constrain the choice of an intervention approach.

Occupation (O) Factors

Clients may have very similar or very different occupations from one another. For example, most adult clients have a focus on ADLs and IADLs. ADL needs are similar among individuals. IADL needs, conversely, can be highly varied across individuals.

For example, not all individuals clean their own home, manage their own finances, or have child care responsibilities.

The occupational therapist also needs to understand the tasks related to the client's occupation, in terms of whether these tasks are more *procedural* (i.e., tasks that are routine and automatic to the client) or *novel* (i.e., tasks that the client rarely has performed, that have intrinsic variability, or that are less predictable). It is important to remember that tasks that were premorbidly procedural (e.g., dressing) may in fact be more novel after injury or illness (e.g., 1-handed dressing after stroke).

Different cognitive processes are responsible for novel tasks in comparison with more automatic, procedural tasks. Tasks that are associated with occupations that are routine and procedural (e.g., brushing teeth, drinking out of a cup, combing hair, tying shoes) involve different demands on learning than tasks that are new or less frequently performed (e.g., holding a pencil with a nondominant hand, entering a phone number into a new cell phone, writing a check for the first time, balancing a bank statement). Thus, the occupational therapist needs to consider the type of task (e.g., routine, procedural, novel) in relationship to the client's person factors (e.g., disease severity, diagnosis) when selecting the cognitive intervention approach.

It is most important for the occupational therapist to know what occupations the client has been doing, can no longer do, but wants to do. When awareness deficits exist, it is important to recognize that a client's goal to return to certain occupations may not always be realistic. This can be challenging for the therapist, because the focus of occupational therapy is to be client centered. Therapists can often find ways to show clients how using task grading of different functional activities addressed in therapy relates to their personal long-term goals (Lenze et al., 2013) without confronting the low likelihood that the client's ultimate goal is achievable.

Guidelines: Selection of a Cognitive Intervention Approach

Choosing an intervention approach is an integrative process that includes person, environment, and occupation factors. Clinical reasoning involves weighing and considering how each factor affects treatment choices. Insight and the ability to learn and transfer are key factors in deciding whether a task/habit training, strategy training, or indirect approach is indicated. Intervention approaches are rooted in theory; however, occupational therapists know frames of references as the mechanisms that link theory to practice (Zoltan, 2007). Frames of references for cognitive intervention can be categorized into those that emphasize task/habit training (Clark-Wilson et al., 2014; Giles, 2018), strategy training (McEwen et al., 2018; Toglia, 2018), or indirect approaches (Levy, 2018; see Table 17.1).

Significant awareness deficits (often seen among clients with more severe cases of learning and memory impairments) respond better to task/habit training and indirect approaches. Clients who lack intellectual or emergent awareness do not see the reason to use a cognitive strategy (lack of intellectual awareness) or are unable to know when to implement the strategy (lack of emergent awareness; Clark-Wilson et al., 2014). These clients typically have more severe cognitive impairment, which makes learning and transferring skills learned in 1 setting or context to another setting or context challenging. Conscious session-to-session retention is extremely difficult or absent. The client may be unable to recall that they had difficulties in activities performed during therapy, which has a negative impact on their ability to gain intellectual awareness.

Continued lack of intellectual and emergent awareness in combination with severe learning challenges is a clear indicator that the preferred approach should be task/habit training or an indirect approach to improving occupational performance. When task/habit training is the chosen approach, the occupational therapist needs to carefully prioritize and choose very specific tasks for client training. The skill training needs to be repetitive, rote, and heavily practiced (see Chapter 18 on the Neurofunctional Approach). Transfer of learning to new situations or tasks is not a realistic goal with clients who require this type of intervention (see Case Example 17.1 later in this chapter).

Clients who have more awareness of their cognitive deficits (i.e., emergent or anticipatory awareness) are a good fit for strategy training approaches to cognitive interventions (see Figures 17.1 and 17.2). Clients at these levels of awareness generally have less-severe cognitive and learning challenges. They have the potential to learn different strategies and to transfer strategy use to new situations or tasks. Strategy training approaches can use a variety of occupational tasks and can incorporate internal strategies (e.g., verbal rehearsal, visual imagery) and external strategies (e.g., taking notes, choosing to work in quiet environments, rephrasing instructions, using problem-solving frameworks; see Case Example 17.2 at the end of this chapter).

TABLE 17.1. Cognitive Intervention Approaches: Associated Theory and Frames of Reference

COGNITIVE INTERVENTION APPROACH	LEARNING THEORY	FRAME(S) OF REFERENCE
Task/habit training (direct approach)	Behaviorism Applied behavior analysis	Neurofunctional Approach (see Chapter 18)
Strategy training (direct approach)	Cognitivism	Multicontext Approach (see Chapter 20) Cognitive Orientation to daily Occupational Performance (see Chapter 19)
Environmental modifications, caregiver education (indirect approach)	Behaviorism Applied behavior analysis	Cognitive Disabilities Model (see Chapter 21)

FIGURE 17.1. Choosing a cognitive intervention approach on the basis of awareness and potential to transfer skills.

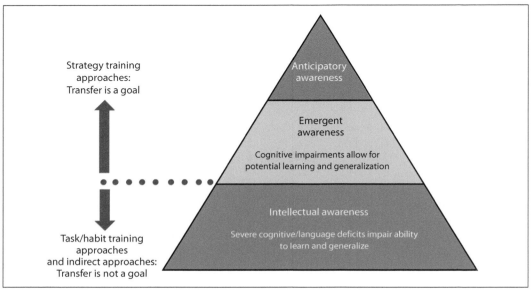

Source. From "Occupational Therapy for People With Stroke in the Outpatient Rehabilitation Setting," by P. P. Barco and M. S. Dappen, in *Stroke: Interventions to Support Occupational Performance* (Neurorehabilitation in Occupational Therapy Series, Vol. 2, p. 279), by T. J. Wolf (Ed.), 2014, Bethesda, MD: AOTA Press. Copyright © 2014 by the American Occupational Therapy Association. Adapted with permission.

FIGURE 17.2. Frames of reference: Decision tree for choosing a cognitive intervention approach.

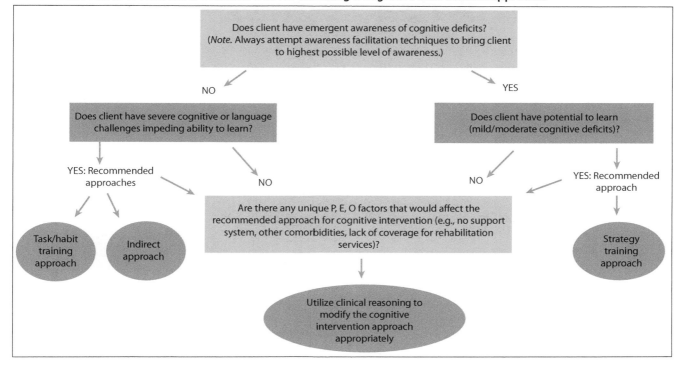

Note. P = person; E = environment; O = occupation.

Approaches to identifying and using these strategies in cognitive intervention sessions vary depending on the frame of reference. In practice, if an occupational therapist is in doubt of the client's abilities, it is common to first default to task/habit training approaches, when in fact therapists should first default to strategy-based approaches, because of their advantages in terms of generalization. It will become evident in the treatment session whether the client is unable to learn new strategies or apply strategies, and the therapist can then modify to a task/habit training approach.

Application

This chapter has provided critical information that occupational therapists can use to guide how they select interventions. Each client has a unique combination of both strengths and challenges across person, environment, and occupation factors that need to be weighed and considered carefully. Although level of awareness and severity of learning challenges are typically prioritized in the process of selecting interventions, in some instances, particular person, environment, and occupation factors make the more straightforward intervention approach unrealistic. Consider the following examples:

- A client has severe learning challenges and lacks intellectual awareness. This client requires indirect support yet is homeless. How would your cognitive intervention approach be altered? *Answer: Determine whether an area that is a priority can be addressed in*

therapy with a task/habit training approach, and work to determine a placement for the client that will be beneficial in the long term. This may involve working with community resources and social services.

- A client has recently had a stroke. The client has mild cognitive impairment and good learning potential. She has recently improved and now has emergent awareness of her cognitive deficits. She does not have outpatient rehabilitation benefits and qualifies for 3 charity visits. The client is an excellent candidate for strategy training, which usually takes more visits. Does your cognitive intervention approach (i.e., strategy training) change? *Answer: You might shift your intervention to include both a strategy training approach and an indirect approach. Education and work with significant others to facilitate the continuation and transfer of skills into the community will be important until the client has sufficiently learned the strategies. Planning the best way to use the limited therapy visits is also important. For example, it might be best to spread the 3 therapy visits over time (to continue to provide therapeutic guidance to the client and significant others over a longer time span).*

- A client with a TBI and spinal cord injury has moderate memory impairment, good learning potential, and signs of emergent awareness. From a cognitive perspective, strategy training is indicated. However, the client has expressive aphasia and does not have functional use of his upper extremities because of spasticity and motor

---

CASE EXAMPLE 17.1. Task/Habit Training Approach to Cognitive Intervention

Tom, age 17, has had a severe TBI and is at a Rancho Los Amigos Scale of Cognitive Functioning (Hagen, 1997) Level V (confused, inappropriate but not agitated) to Level VI (confused but appropriate). He was in a motor vehicle accident 2 weeks ago and is currently in posttraumatic amnesia (Trevena-Peters et al., 2018). Before the accident, Tom was in his senior year of high school; he has a grade point average of 3.8 and was planning to go to college to major in engineering.

Tom currently is in acute care. He is confused, is not oriented to place or time (he seems to know his name), and has difficulty learning new information. He responds to simple commands and is starting to attend to highly familiar tasks.

The **occupational therapist** introduces herself, but Tom is not focused and keeps asking where his cat is. The therapist asks whether he knows where he is or what has happened to him. He has no awareness that he has any cognitive challenges or that he has sustained a TBI. The therapist discerns that Tom does not have intellectual awareness at this time. His ability to learn is severely impaired, as indicated by his current cognitive challenges and stage of recovery.

Tom's lack of intellectual awareness of his cognitive deficits is evidenced by his confusion and disorientation. His severe learning impairment is evidenced by his lack of orientation and his Rancho level of functioning.

For a cognitive intervention, the occupational therapist selects a task/habit training approach to work with Tom on ADLs. She hands him a toothbrush and asks whether he can brush his teeth. The therapist observes that Tom does not seem to know what to do with the toothbrush; he starts trying to comb his hair with it, and then throws it down on the bedside table. Continuing to work with task/habit training, the therapist focuses on guiding Tom through brushing his teeth using techniques that are part of the frame of reference known as the Neurofunctional Approach (this approach is discussed further in Chapter 18). As Tom hopefully improves in his insight and makes cognitive gains, the intervention approach may evolve into a strategy training approach.

---

impairment. Does your cognitive intervention approach (i.e., strategy training) change? *Answer: Unfortunately, because of the client's language and motor impairment, many of the strategies to assist with the memory impairment (e.g., tape recorders, note taking, computer use) might not be useful. It is important to be realistic in these situations. The occupational therapist should do an exhaustive search of any new technology that may be available while considering the financial resources available to the client. It is important to use indirect approaches that inform the caregiver how to assist the client—while still allowing the client some independent decision making and control. It is also important to include the client in the decision-making process, because they have adequate awareness of the situation. Task/habit training in adaptive equipment will be most useful. The therapist and caregivers need to monitor the client's frustration and depression, which may result from their awareness.*

These are examples of difficult but not uncommon situations that occupational therapists may encounter. These situations involve clinical reasoning, and there are not always clearly right or wrong choices. The therapist needs to more closely assess the different person, environment, and occupation factors of the client and then choose the intervention approach that will most improve occupational performance. In some cases, the intervention approach may be the same approach that would be recommended on the basis of awareness level and cognitive severity. In other cases, the approach may differ because of the client's unique circumstances. The goal is to work toward improved function and quality of life, building on individual client strengths to overcome the challenges.

Conclusion

Occupational therapists recognize the individuality of each client and are encouraged by their training and by the ethos of the profession to view individuals holistically. This chapter serves as a guide to help therapists choose the cognitive intervention approach best suited for the individual client. Understanding the person, environment, and occupation factors is integral to choosing the appropriate intervention approach. Level of client awareness and ability to learn and transfer skills are key determinants in the choice of the cognitive intervention approach best suited for each client. Whether the functional–cognitive intervention is task/habit training, strategy training, or an indirect approach, common goals are improving occupational engagement, function, and quality of life.

CASE EXAMPLE 17.2. Strategy Training Approach to Cognitive Intervention

Mary, age 50, had a stroke approximately a month ago. She is receiving outpatient therapy and is oriented to person, place, and time. When the occupational therapist asks her what her difficulties are since the stroke, Mary explains that she notices she has trouble with her memory and has difficulty multitasking. The **occupational therapist** confirms this information as accurate through spouse report and through the C–FE.

The therapist observes that Mary not only is intellectually aware of her deficits but was able to notice that she was becoming distracted and forgetful during a meal-planning task (which indicates the presence of emergent, or online, awareness). The therapist determines Mary's level of cognitive deficits (mild to moderate) on the basis of the results of her C–FE.

The therapist determines that a strategy training approach is appropriate for Mary to address her memory and attention difficulties. The therapist has several choices of strategy training frames of reference she could begin to implement with Mary, which include the Cognitive Orientation to daily Occupational Performance and the Multi-context Approach. These frames of reference are described in detail in Chapters 19 and 20, respectively.

Mary's goals are to return to work as a legal assistant and to resume driving. She is also having difficulty managing some of the IADLs that she used to do independently at home before her stroke (e.g., meal preparation, money management). Using the Multicontext Approach, Mary and the therapist decide to work on a strategy focused on limiting distractions during functional activities. The strategy is to complete the functional task once started and monitor distractions by noting the distraction (and addressing it later). They begin to work with this approach with a simple functional cooking task (which involves a short, distracting conversation) to practice it. Because Mary is able to use the strategy successfully, the therapist guides Mary in transferring the strategy to new situations and tasks.

Working with clients with cognitive challenges and developing intervention plans can be a challenging but rewarding career focus for occupational therapists. It involves creativity, problem solving, and the ability to modify treatment interventions as the client changes or additional client information becomes available. Cognitive intervention involves an ongoing and dynamic process of evaluating, teaching, training, modifying, educating, and reevaluating until realistic goals are developed and achieved. Once an occupational therapist becomes comfortable appropriately using the various intervention approaches, they might find that a combination of approaches is indicated. The chapters that follow provide detailed information about each of the intervention approaches discussed in this chapter (see Table 17.1) and how these approaches are used with clients.

References

Barco, P. P., Crosson, B., Bolesta, M. M., Werts, D., & Stout, R. (1991). Training awareness and compensation in postacute head injury rehabilitation. In J. S. Kreutzer & P. H. Wehman (Eds.), *Cognitive rehabilitation for persons with traumatic brain injury* (pp. 129–146). Baltimore: Brookes.

Barco, P. P., and Dappen, M. S. (2014). Occupational therapy for people with stroke in the outpatient rehabilitation setting. In T. J. Wolf (Ed.), *Stroke: Interventions to support occupational performance* (Neurorehabilitation in Occupational Therapy Series, Vol. 2, pp. 275–309). Bethesda, MD: AOTA Press.

Bates, B. (2016). *Learning theories simplified*. Thousand Oaks, CA: Sage.

Clark-Wilson, J., Giles, G. M., & Baxter, D. M. (2014). Revisiting the Neurofunctional Approach: Conceptualizing the core components for the rehabilitation of everyday living skills. *Brain Injury, 28,* 1646–1656. https://doi.org/10.3109/02699052.2014.946449

Crichton, S. L., Bray, B. D., McKevitt, C., Rudd, A. G., & Wolfe, C. D. A. (2016). Patient outcomes up to 15 years after stroke: Survival, disability, quality of life, cognition and mental health. *Journal of Neurology, Neurosurgery and Psychiatry, 87,* 1091–1098. https://doi.org/10.1136/jnnp-2016-313361

Crosson, B. C., Barco, P. P., Velozo, C. A., Bolesta, M. M., Cooper, P. V., Werts, D., & Brobeck, T. C. (1989). Awareness and compensation in postacute head injury rehabilitation. *Journal of Head Trauma Rehabilitation, 4,* 46–54. https://doi.org/10.1097/00001199-198909000-00008

Doig, E., Fleming, J., Ownsworth, T., & Fletcher, S. (2017). An occupation-based, metacognitive approach to assessing error performance and online awareness. *Australian Occupational Therapy Journal, 64,* 137–148. https://doi.org/10.1111/1440-1630.12322

Fang, J., Zhao, G., Wang, G., Ayala, C., & Loustalot, F. (2016). Insurance status among adults with hypertension: The impact of underinsurance. *Journal of the American Heart Association, 5,* e004313. https://doi.org/10.1161/JAHA.116.004313

Fleming, J. M., & Ownsworth, T. (2006). A review of awareness interventions in brain injury rehabilitation. *Neuropsychological Rehabilitation, 16,* 474–500. https://doi.org/10.1080/09602010500505518

Geusgens, C. A. V., Van Heugten, C. M., Cooijmans, J. P. J., Jolles, J., & Van den Heuvel, W. J. A. (2007). Transfer effects of a cognitive strategy training for stroke patients with apraxia. *Journal of Clinical and Experimental Neuropsychology, 29,* 831–841. https://doi.org/10.1080/13803390601125971

Giles, G. M. (2018). Neurofunctional Approach to rehabilitation after brain injury. In N. Katz & J. Toglia (Eds.), *Cognition, occupation, and participation across the lifespan: Neuroscience, neurorehabilitation, and models of intervention in occupational therapy* (4th ed., pp. 419–442). Bethesda, MD: AOTA Press.

Hagen, C. (1997). *Rancho Los Amigos Scale of Cognitive Functioning.* Bakersfield, CA: Centre for Neuro Skills.

Haskins, E. C., Cicerone, K., Dams-O'Connor, K., Eberle, R., Langenbahn, D., & Shapiro-Rosenbaum, A. (2012). *Cognitive rehabilitation manual: Translating evidence-based recommendations into practice.* Reston, VA: ACRM Publishing.

Johnson, N. X., Marquine, M. J., Flores, I., Umlauf, A., Baum, C. M., Wong, A. W. K., . . . Heaton, R. K. (2017). Racial differences in neurocognitive outcomes post-stroke: The impact of healthcare variables. *Journal of the International Neuropsychological Society, 23,* 640–652. https://doi.org/10.1017/S1355617717000480

Kim, M. J., Lee, H., Kim, E. H., Cho, M. H., Shin, D. W., Yun, J. M., & Shin, J. H. (2017). Disparity in health screening and health utilization according to economic status. *Korean Journal of Family Medicine, 38,* 220–225. https://doi.org/10.4082/kjfm.2017.38.4.220

Lenze, E. J., Host, H. H., Hildebrand, M., Morrow-Howell, N., Carpenter, B., Freedland, K. E., . . . Binder, E. F. (2013). Enhanced medical rehabilitation is feasible in a skilled nursing facility: Preliminary data on a novel treatment for older adults with depression. *American Journal of Geriatric Psychiatry, 21,* 307. https://doi.org/10.1016/j.jagp.2012.11.006

Levy, L. L. (2018). Neurocognition and function: Intervention in dementia based on the Cognitive Disabilities Model. In N. Katz & J. Toglia (Eds.), *Cognition, occupation, and participation across the lifespan: Neuroscience, neurorehabilitation, and models of intervention in occupational therapy* (4th ed., pp. 499–522). Bethesda, MD: AOTA Press.

McEwen, S., Mandich, A., & Poloatajko, H. (2018). CO–OP Approach: A cognitive-based intervention for children and adults. In N. Katz & J. Toglia (Eds.), *Cognition, occupation, and participation across the lifespan: Neuroscience, neurorehabilitation, and models of intervention in occupational therapy* (4th ed., pp. 315–334). Bethesda, MD: AOTA Press.

Nys, G. M. S., Van Zandvoort, M. J. E., Van der Worp, H. B., De Haan, E. H. F., De Kort, P. L. M., Jansen, B. P. W., & Kappelle, L. J. (2006). Early cognitive impairment predicts long-term depressive symptoms and quality of life after stroke. *Journal of the Neurological Sciences, 247,* 149–156. https://doi.org/10.1016/j.jns.2006.04.005

Ownsworth, T., Fleming, J., Tate, R., Shum, D. H., Griffin, J., Schmidt, J., . . . Chevignard, M. (2013). Comparison of error-based and errorless learning for people with severe traumatic brain injury: Study protocol for a randomized control trial. *Trials, 14,* 369. https://doi.org/10.1186/1745-6215-14-369

Toglia, J. (2018). The Dynamic Interactional Model and the Multicontext Approach. In N. Katz & J. Toglia (Eds.), *Cognition, occupation, and participation across the lifespan: Neuroscience, neurorehabilitation, and models of intervention in occupational therapy* (4th ed., pp. 355–386). Bethesda, MD: AOTA Press.

Toglia, J., Goverover, Y., Johnston, M. V., & Dain, B. (2011). Application of the multicontextual approach in promoting learning and transfer of strategy use in an individual with TBI and executive dysfunction. *OTJR: Occupation, Participation and Health, 31*(Suppl.), S53–S60. https://doi.org/10.3928/15394492-20101108-09

Toglia, J., & Kirk, U. (2000). Understanding awareness deficits following brain injury. *NeuroRehabilitation, 15,* 57–70.

Toglia, J., & Maeir, A. (2018). Self-awareness and metacognition: Effect on occupational performance and outcome across the lifespan. In N. Katz & J. Toglia (Eds.), *Cognition, occupation, and participation across the lifespan: Neuroscience, neurorehabilitation, and models of intervention in occupational therapy* (4th ed., pp. 143–164). Bethesda, MD: AOTA Press.

Trevena-Peters, J., McKay, A., Spitz, G., Suda, R., Renison, B., & Ponsford, J. (2018). Efficacy of activities of daily living retraining during posttraumatic amnesia: A randomized controlled trial. *Archives of Physical Medicine and Rehabilitation, 99,* 329–337. https://doi.org/10.1016/j.apmr.2017.08.486

Zoltan, B. (2007). *Vision, perception, and cognition* (4th ed.). Thorofare, NJ: Slack.

The Neurofunctional Approach

GORDON MUIR GILES, PhD, OTR/L, FAOTA

LEARNING OBJECTIVES

After completing this chapter, readers should be able to

- Describe the theoretical background of the Neurofunctional Approach (NFA);
- Describe the target population of the NFA in terms of diagnoses and severity of occupational performance deficits;
- Explain the NFA intervention and describe its clinical applications to clients in different stages of recovery and with different severities of functional impairment;
- Describe the process of observational assessment, intervention planning, task analysis, and errorless skill training using the NFA;
- Describe techniques such as antecedent control, errorless learning, self-generation, and overlearning and how they contribute to the development of implicit knowledge structures (habits and routines) that support independent function.

KEY TERMS AND CONCEPTS

- Errorless learning • Habits and routines • Overlearning • Practice • Self-generation effect • Task analysis
- Therapeutic alliance

Background to the Neurofunctional Approach

This chapter provides an outline of the practical application of the Neurofunctional Approach (NFA) to the rehabilitation of clients with acquired neurological impairment and neurobehavioral disability (Clark-Wilson et al., 2014; Giles & Clark-Wilson, 1993). The NFA is a task/habit training approach in which the occupational therapist

1. Identifies an area of dysfunction, then

2. Designs a procedure that allows the client to accomplish needed ADL and simple IADL tasks, then

3. Facilitates the client's ***practice*** of the procedure (i.e., repetition of the behavior) until they can perform it automatically.

This approach is therefore the polar opposite of *metacognitive strategy training,* in which the client is taught an internal thinking routine intended to facilitate their own problem solving (see, e.g., Dawson et al., 2017; Toglia, 2018). For a further discussion of the difference between task/habit training approaches and metacognitive approaches, see Clark-Wilson et al. (2014) as well as Chapter 17, "Intervention Selection," in this text.

I developed the NFA with Jo Clark-Wilson in the late 1980s and early 1990s (Clark-Wilson et al., 2014; Giles & Clark-Wilson, 1993; Trevena-Peters, McKay, Spitz, et al., 2018). The theoretical foundations of the NFA are Learning Theory, Motor Learning Theory, and social psychology. In the early 1980s there was little evidence regarding how to rehabilitate individuals with severe traumatic brain injury (TBI). However, Miller (1980) showed that even individuals who had sustained a severe TBI could learn and, if given sufficient practice, could reach skill levels that approximated those of individuals who were neurologically healthy (Giles, 2018).

On the basis of these observations, we developed the skill-training methods of the NFA. These methods have been

189

applied successfully to the retraining of clients who had profound impairments of attention, memory, and executive functioning (EF) and who lacked insight into their impairments. In many cases, improvements were achieved many years postinjury, allowing clients to live in less restrictive care settings (Parish & Oddy, 2007).

Central to the NFA is the provision of highly structured retraining programs designed to develop **habits and routines** (i.e., behaviors and behavior sequences that people engage in without conscious deliberation) that obviate the need for online problem solving for individuals who have impaired planning and decision-making ability. The goal of these programs is to train specific ADLs and simple IADLs in which the client can be independent. Improvements are achieved through the use of highly structured training methods that engage the client's relatively less impaired implicit learning systems (Reber, 2013; Wood & Rünger, 2016).

The development of appropriate skill–habit structures is regarded as central to addressing the impaired functional cognition that contributes to ADL and simple IADL skill deficits. These skill–habit structures also assist in the management of impaired impulse control, which is a cardinal feature of neurobehavioral disability that may follow many neurological insults, including severe TBI. As learning progresses, chained actions, which are cued by the preceding actions in the sequence, are chunked together and increasingly can be executed as a unit (Healy et al., 2012; Wood & Rünger, 2016; Yin & Knowlton, 2006). Once acquired, the trained activities

*   Are activated by cues in the environment,

*   Can often be executed rapidly, and

*   Require limited decision making (Wood & Rünger, 2016; i.e., they are dependent on implicit memory and are largely independent of the impaired executive control system).

The selection of which ADL or simple IADL to address is person centered, but in the acute care setting therapists may initially focus on the most essential ADLs that are impaired, such as transfers or self-feeding. If the client is or becomes independent in these tasks, the therapist then can move on to bathing; dressing; self-care; and simple IADLs, such as making a hot drink or a sandwich (Giles et al., 2019; Trevena-Peters, McKay, & Ponsford, 2018). Habits, once developed, are also resistant to changes in reinforcement contingencies, which makes them robust to extinction (Wood & Rünger, 2016). The NFA provides a framework for assessment and intervention (it comprises a set of principles) rather than a collection of specific measures and interventions, and as a result it is highly adaptable to clients' individual needs.

Target Population

In the World Health Organization's classification of impairment, abilities, and participation (WHO, 2001), the NFA emphasizes the enhancement of abilities and participation, not the restitution of impaired cognitive processes (i.e., it is directed at the performance level; American Occupational Therapy Association [AOTA], 2014; WHO, 2001). The NFA has been used primarily with clients in the acute or postacute stage of recovery from TBI or cerebrovascular accident. The approach is also applicable to clients with anoxic damage, metabolic imbalances or poisonings causing neurological damage (e.g., diabetic coma, carbon monoxide poisoning), or infections (e.g., encephalitis, meningitis).

Similar approaches have been demonstrated to improve occupational performance among persons with various progressive major neurocognitive disorder diagnoses. However, the applicability of the NFA is determined primarily by the needs of the client, not by the underlying pathology (Turner-Stokes, 2008).

As an experientially based treatment, the NFA was conceptualized as being effective during any period of recovery when learning is possible. In the 1980s and 1990s, the initial proof-of-concept studies were conducted with postacute clients (more than 1 year postinjury from TBI, when spontaneous neurological recovery was considered to have only a limited impact), with the goal of isolating the specific effects of the intervention (Whyte et al., 2009). More recently, the NFA has been shown to be effective when applied early in recovery (i.e., during posttraumatic amnesia [PTA]) and during post-PTA acute rehabilitation (Trevena-Peters, McKay, Spitz, et al., 2018; Vanderploeg et al., 2006, 2008), and other studies have suggested that this type of intervention is possible in acute neurosurgical settings (Kelly & Nikopoulis, 2010).

The target populations for the NFA are

*   Individuals during PTA;

*   Individuals with moderate to severe impairment of attention and episodic memory;

*   Individuals with severely impaired EF; and

*   Individuals who have mild to moderate impairments of attention, memory, or EF in combination with severely impaired self-awareness.

Such individuals may not be able to make use of or tolerate strategy-based approaches but may respond to task/habit training–based approaches.

Additionally, individuals with mild impairments who have retained self-awareness and can make use of trial-and-error learning and strategy training (Ownsworth, 2018) may wish to develop specific routines using NFA principles as an adjunct to other primary modes of intervention. Individuals who can recognize task-performance errors, correct the errors on subsequent task trials, and retain those corrections over time are most likely to be able to make use of trial-and-error learning and strategy-based approaches (see Chapter 17, "Intervention Selection").

For many clients for whom the NFA is appropriate, severe deficits become rapidly evident on ADL assessment (e.g., during PTA or after severe TBI). For those clients without obvious ADL deficits, screening measures can be used. Clients for whom use of the NFA is appropriate show marked deficits on cognitive screening measures such as the Montreal Cognitive Assessment (MoCA; Nasreddine et al., 2005) and are impaired on measures of functional cognition or are unable to recognize or adequately correct errors. For example, on the Executive Function Performance Test (Baum et al., 2003) and the Performance Assessment of Self-Care Skills (Rogers et al., 2016), these individuals make errors, do not recognize their errors, and require direct cueing or physical assist to complete tasks safely.

Clients in the early phase of recovery from TBI are appropriate for NFA intervention if they have emerged from coma and are able to respond to cueing (i.e., if they have sufficient arousal and attentional skills to respond to 1-step cueing). Clients can respond to NFA intervention despite profound deficits in memory. The NFA is the only approach that has been demonstrated to be effective in improving ADL and simple IADL skills in a randomized controlled trial among participants in PTA from moderate to severe TBI (Trevena-Peters, McKay, Spitz, et al., 2018). The NFA has also been demonstrated to be as effective as a cognitive approach among individuals in the acute state of recovery from TBI (Vanderploeg et al., 2008).

Administration

There are no NFA training courses that are approved by the authors. Occupational therapists who have adopted the NFA have typically relied on the original book from 1993 (Giles & Clark-Wilson, 1993), the descriptions of specific applications of the approach in the literature by the original authors and others (Giles et al., 1997; Parish & Oddy, 2007; Trevena-Peters, McKay, Spitz, et al., 2018), and a restatement of the basic principles of the approach (Clark-Wilson et al., 2014).

The NFA is a collection of intervention principles, some of which may be more or less central to the approach, depending on the specific needs of the client. (Amnesia-based confusion must be managed during PTA, whereas complete rejection of the therapeutic process absent severe memory impairment may occur in later stages of rehabilitation, and other individuals may be highly motivated by their therapeutic gains.) Some background in applied behavioral analysis or motor learning theory and in motivational interviewing (Miller & Rollnick, 2013) is helpful but not required.

Application of the NFA requires a degree of flexibility during program development, and in later stages (during the training intervention) it requires very specific behaviors from the therapist, so therapists must structure their own behaviors in ways with which they may be unfamiliar. Trevena-Peters, McKay, and Ponsford (2018) reported that therapists described, in addition to enhancing client skills, that use of the NFA promoted the therapeutic alliance and meaningful use of therapy time without elevating client agitation.

In this chapter, the application of the NFA is described as a series of steps (see Exhibit 18.1). In describing the application of the approach, different authors have emphasized different elements of the approach (Parish & Oddy, 2007; Rotenberg-Shpigelman et al., 2012; Trevena-Peters, McKay, Spitz, et al., 2018). The importance of each step and its actual application depend on the specific circumstances under which intervention is to be provided.

Step 1: Develop a Positive Therapeutic Alliance

The first step of the NFA is development of a positive *therapeutic alliance,* focused on clients' perspective, their values and goals, and what they want to do (i.e., person centered). In an acute care setting, family and friends will provide information about the client's preferred behaviors and habits that can assist the occupational therapist in designing retraining programs and finding ways to engage clients who are in PTA. Trevena-Peters, McKay, and Ponsford (2018) reported that therapists using the NFA described engaging with the clients during PTA as challenging and that therapists looked for something unique that resonated with the individual. This was particularly important in rapport building, the specific language used with the client, and how to describe the goals of intervention.

When clients have emerged from PTA, it is most important to engage with them, to listen to their perspective, and to

---

EXHIBIT 18.1. The Neurofunctional Approach as a Series of Steps

1. Develop a positive therapeutic alliance focused on the client's perspectives, values, and goals and what the client wants to do (i.e., person centered).
2. Gather and assimilate relevant information to understand the client's current functioning in their natural environment and identify their likely responses to intervention.
3. Create a case formulation of the client's goals, and reconcile these with available resources and current constraints.
4. Develop operational performance goals that can be translated into retraining programs (i.e., goals stated in behaviorally explicit terms).
5. Observe performance in everyday situations, with reference to the nature of the task, client characteristics, environmental resources, and constraints.
6. Create skill-retraining programs (incorporating aids or environmental supports where appropriate), developed from an analysis of the person, activity, and environment.
7. Develop automaticity, generalization, and the maintenance of skills in the client's everyday life.
8. Provide feedback, appropriate to the client, to encourage progress and engagement.

understand the dynamics of clients in their family context. This is consistent with the person-centered principle of occupational therapy and with the occupational therapy therapeutic process (AOTA, 2014).

Principles of motivational interviewing allow the therapist to accept that the client has a particular perspective, and in an outpatient or home health environment, working in the context of that perspective is central to the therapist's ability to render intervention (Miller & Rollnick, 2013). Understanding the client's and the family's experiences with therapy may also be central to the therapist's ability to address the client's needs. Prioritizing the client's perceived needs allows the development of trust and therapeutic engagement and is especially important in the context of lack of insight.

Step 2: Gather and Assimilate Relevant Information

Step 2 involves gathering and assimilating relevant information to understand clients' current functioning in their natural environment, as well as identifying their likely responses to intervention. Although it is listed here as the 2nd step in the process, the occupational therapist should gather and assimilate relevant information before engaging with the client and family. It is important that the therapist learn from nursing staff and medical records the nature and severity of the injury and the client's current physical, cognitive, behavioral, and functional status (considerations relevant to length of treatment and likely treatment response) and contraindications for intervention. Especially in an acute care setting, family members expect that the therapist will be knowledgeable about the background of the injury or neurological insult before engaging with the client—and these first encounters are central to developing a therapeutic relationship with the family.

Step 3: Determine the Client's Goals and Available Resources

In Step 3, the occupational therapist must determine the client's goals and reconcile these with the available resources and current constraints. Depending on the client's position in the trajectory of recovery, the therapist may need to generate a case formulation to guide intervention. The formulation will influence both the goals that are set and how the therapist chooses to interact with the client. Do clients understand their situation? Are they naturally compliant with instructions? Do they attempt to defer activities?

In early recovery, such as during PTA, or among clients with severe neurocognitive deficits, it is important to identify whether clients know that they have had a brain injury and need therapy. How activities are introduced is important for client engagement. Therapists may attempt to avoid asking questions that might overwhelm the client (e.g., "Are you ready for a shower?"). Some confused clients may respond positively to the therapist presenting simple orienting information (e.g., "You are in a hospital after having had a brain injury, and I am here to help you get more independent in bathing and dressing"); others respond better to antecedent control (e.g., "I am

here to assist you to take a shower," "I have your shower running"). When clients are amnestic, the therapist can experiment with the best ways to engage with them.

Clients who are later in the recovery process and who are not confused, but who are ambivalently engaged in the therapy process, can be assisted by a nonconfrontational approach that relies on motivational interviewing techniques. In these circumstances, establishing a positive therapeutic relationship is a prerequisite for therapeutic engagement.

Step 4: Set Operational Performance Goals

Step 4 in the NFA process is to set operational performance goals that can be translated into retraining programs (i.e., goals stated in behaviorally explicit terms). During PTA, if the client is independent in an area of functioning with a single prompt, the therapist can move to the next area to assess. If assistance is required, document the functional level and implement a retraining program.

In the postacute period if a client is not independent in an ADL or IADL skill, the therapist must make a decision as to whether the client can respond to the therapist's heightening the client's awareness of an area of functioning or whether a retraining program is warranted. For example, if the therapist observes potentially unsafe behavior in the kitchen, does the cue, "This time when making tea, I would like you to pay special attention to safety," lead to behavior change, and is that behavior change sustained? If a client is unable to recognize or to consciously attend to an area of deficit, they are unlikely to respond to anything but a task/habit training retraining approach.

In the postacute stage clients may have general goals, and it is the task of the therapist to prioritize these in a way that is acceptable to the client. This is often most problematic for clients who lack insight into their need for assistance. It may be necessary to begin with goals that the therapist thinks are of less urgency, to obtain the client's acceptance of the rehabilitative endeavor. Sometimes clients will reject a goal if it is presented directly but can accept one if it is relabeled in a way that does not suggest deficits (e.g., the client rejects a street-crossing training but accepts walking to the local convenience store, which includes crossing the street safely).

Step 5: Observe Performance

Step 5 consists of observation of performance, with reference to the nature of the task, the client characteristics, environmental resources, and constraints. How baseline task performance is established varies depending on the circumstances of clients and their point in the trajectory of recovery. In community settings naturalistic observation is often possible, whereas in acute or inpatient settings by necessity the observations are cued. Whenever possible, only minimal cues should be used to get clients to initiate the task (e.g., "Show me what you would normally do to get up and dressed . . . take a shower . . . make toast . . . cross the street"). If the client is not able to generate a relevant behavior chain to a single cue, additional cues are provided as needed in an attempt to promote independent performance (see the initial segment of the washing and dressing example in Video 18.1).

If the client is not independent, the therapist's task is to observe for spontaneously generated behaviors that can be incorporated into a retraining program (i.e., part of an ADL or IADL that the client does automatically, without cueing, that can be "built" into the retraining program). Doing so reduces the amount of new learning required of the client. For example, clients may be able to brush their teeth in response to a single cue and may do this automatically after face washing.

The therapist should be cognizant of how clients order activities and incorporate this overlearned activity order into the program. They should observe whether the client can generate "islands of competency" (i.e., sequences of adequate performance) but intervene to ensure the client's safety and to promote feelings of success. Clients should be provided with the opportunity to complete task components before the therapist provides assistance. Observation of occupational performance normally occurs over several days. Also during the observation, the therapist is performing an individualized *task analysis* (i.e., the process of identifying the essential behaviors required for the completion of a task) so as to be able to develop a chain of activities that, when performed in sequence, result in independent task performance for the targeted ADL or simple IADL.

Therapists can also score performance on standardized measures (e.g., the FIM®; Keith et al., 1987). To participate in NFA interventions, a client needs to be able to follow a single-stage command (i.e., comprehend a command and generate behaviors consistent with it). For clients early in recovery from neurological insult, inconsistency in this ability is not necessarily a barrier to treatment, because both the progress of recovery and the development of the routine will likely make cued commands easier to follow. During the observational period, the therapist generates hypotheses about the amount and type of cueing that will be required in a retraining program, but detailed observation of how the client responds to specific cues is reserved for Step 6.

Step 6: Create Skill-Retraining Programs

Step 6 takes place once client goals have been determined and the therapist has established how the client attempts to address the area of functioning spontaneously or when minimally prompted. This step involves creation of a skill-retraining program (incorporating aids or environmental supports when appropriate), developed from the analysis of the person, activity, and environment. After establishing a baseline, the therapist focuses on areas where the client needs cueing and engages in the process of "cue experimentation," in which the therapist observes the client's response to specific cues to establish the specific behaviors that are reliably generated from the cues and the detail with which behaviors need to be cued (e.g., "Wash your face" vs. "Pick up the washcloth . . ."). Handwritten notes of client performance can be taken, and charting of preestablished subroutines can be rated as independent, cued (number of cues), or performed with physical assistance. There is, however, often variability in client performance over presentations of the programs. The therapist's task is to engage in "cue experimentation" to ensure that the cue is adequate to achieve functionally equivalent performance of the activity step whenever the cue is presented. The therapist may have to alter the wording of a cue or use more cues to reliably elicit a multistep behavior (e.g., "Wash your face" may not be adequate, and more-detailed cueing may be necessary: "Pick up the washcloth, put soap on the washcloth, wash your face").

The cueing must be provided so as to prevent errors (errorless learning), because once an error is established, it may be very difficult to override for clients with severe impairments. Cueing is therefore concrete and directive regarding the tasks, and abstract cueing (e.g., "What should you do next?") and the system of least prompts are avoided (Wolery et al., 1990). The NFA employs a whole-task method in which the client is cued through the entire activity, so that they are successful in achieving the task each time the program is enacted (see Exhibit 18.2 and Case Example 18.1). The shortest possible chain of cues should be employed that results in the client's consistent task performance.

For clients with both cognitive and physical impairments, early in the program physical assistance may be required, but the therapist must judge that the client will be able to learn to perform the activity independently given the likely trajectory of recovery. For example, if during the likely rehabilitation time frame independent transfers seem achievable but independent ambulation does not, the retraining program should be geared toward functional independence with a wheelchair.

Some clients may require physical guidance (hand-over-hand assistance) for some program steps, but the goal is to develop a physical routine that the client can accomplish independently. By employing physical guidance, the therapist provides physical support for the client to perform the task (rather than doing the task for the client) and provides the verbal cues at the same time as guiding the movement to foster the client's learning of the task sequence. The client learns by performing the task with or without physical guidance.

The environment can also be altered to assist in learning; for example, personal hygiene products can be placed strategically and may also be used to cue activities. Once a stable pattern of client responses to cues is established (i.e., the client responds consistently to the cues), the occupational therapist formalizes the cueing program kept electronically or on a clipboard with a recording form so that it can be performed by non–occupational therapy staff who have appropriate training. Task analyses and the retraining programs are by necessity individualized, because the nature of the deficits (combination of motor and cognitive deficits affect the activity demands) of retained performance skills and the environment in which the occupational performance is to occur all influence the structure of the retraining program.

EXHIBIT 18.2. Steps in a Neurofunctional Approach Program Applied to the Goal of Walking to the Café

1. Establish program goals with client. Select methods to engage the client and enhance buy-in to the program goals.
2. Establish an observational baseline to determine what the client does unprompted and with minimal prompting. Focus on street safety in the specific intersections and navigations. Does the client need a directions check-off sheet or map?
3. Note the order in which the client attempts the tasks and sequences of behaviors that are effective so that these attributes can be incorporated into the retraining program to minimize new learning. How does the provision of a check-off sheet or map assist the client?
4. Conduct individualized task analysis, accounting for physical and motor disorders and the environment in which the retraining program is to take place. Cues should be made specific to the route.
5. Engage in cue experimentation to determine the most effective cueing system. Here a system of least prompts may be used, but only until the most effective level of cueing is established. Then cueing should be concrete and specific. Remember that safety is the first priority.
6. Develop a formal, written cueing system that can be used to record the cues provided.
7. Implement whole-task retraining methods with identical prompts, and record prompts or physical assistance that is rendered each day. Staff need to be trained in the cueing system and how to provide the program so that consistency is maintained.
8. Provide feedback to the client to show progress.

Note. In a program that incorporates street crossing, safety is paramount. Get agreement from the interdisciplinary team before starting the program. Do not train street crossing with clients who are unpredictable or impulsive or who do not follow commands. Initially, be at arm's length and be ready to stop the client if they are unsafe. As the client is approaching independence, walk with them but behind them and outside their visual field to reduce your presence as a cue to safe performance. For the final assessment, have someone other than the treating therapist assess the client's safety, because the treating therapist may be a cue to safe street crossing. Therapists must use their own judgment and expertise as to whether to recommend that the client cross the street without supervision.

Step 7: Develop Automaticity, Generalization, and Skill Maintenance

Step 7 encompasses development of automaticity, generalization, and skill maintenance in the client's everyday life. Once the cueing system for the functional retraining program is complete, the client must enact it on multiple occasions to benefit from the program (i.e., for learning to take place and for the skill to be acquired; Healy et al., 2012; Wood & Rünger, 2016). Learning is incremental, and researchers have hypothesized that with each repetition of the program, gradual changes occur in the neural mechanisms that underlie procedural learning (Wood & Rünger, 2016).

Cueing is provided to prevent errors (errorless learning; Haslam & Kessels, 2018). Learning in the NFA is experiential, and, as stated earlier, errors must be avoided. It may be particularly important to avoid errors early in learning. Our experience is that the majority of (but not all) clients can benefit from this type of skills training; we have had the least success with clients who cannot follow cues and those clients with profound deficits in initiation. Other than in instances in which the therapist is teaching physical movements to help the client overcome motor-skill problems, the physical movements do not need to be identical. Rather, the ordering of conceptually distinct actions is important (Wood & Rünger, 2016).

The occupational therapist should maintain daily records of the client's response to the cue. A staff checklist that parallels the cueing system, kept electronically or on a clipboard, lets the team record the client's response to each step on a daily basis. The therapist can assess whether learning is taking place by slightly increasing the time delay between the end of the last activity and provision of the next cue in the sequence. If the client seems to be initiating an incorrect step, then the therapist is ready to interrupt the error before it occurs and to cue the correct behavior. Clients' learning will become apparent if they transition uncued correctly to the next step in the sequence.

Clients may also develop subroutines of behaviors that initially needed multiple cues (e.g., for the face-washing task, "Pick up the washcloth," "Put soap on the washcloth," "Rub your face with the washcloth . . . right ear . . . left ear . . ." is consolidated to "Wash your face"). A program that began with 50 cues might be progressively consolidated, becoming shorter as the complexity of the behavior that the client produces to a single cue increases (Wood & Rünger, 2016). Each day the intervention is provided, the therapist records the client's need for cues and so can chart progress on a daily basis. When the program is executed by non–occupational therapy staff, the therapist needs to perform regular audits to assess learning and to consolidate cues when appropriate.

There is evidence from neurologically healthy people that learning follows an asymptotic curve (Lally et al., 2010). As a result, the early days of the program may be the most important, but therapists should not expect to see immediate reductions in cueing, because learning may be evident only once it has passed a threshold. In our clinical experience, some learning is evident among individuals with severe TBI within 10 days, and often much sooner. However, we do not believe that this has ever been formally assessed in regard to ADL retraining of neurologically impaired clients at any stage in the recovery process.

Trevena-Peters et al. (Trevena-Peters, McKay, Spitz, et al., 2018; Trevena-Peters, Ponsford, & McKay, 2017) were able to show the superiority of the NFA over treatment-as-usual during PTA (average duration = 44.31 days), with an average of 3 to 4 weeks of treatment (*M* = 15.39 days, with daily 60-minute treatment sessions; Trevena-Peters, McKay, & Ponsford, 2018;

CASE EXAMPLE 18.1. Client With Severe TBI and ADL Impairment

Client 1 was a 20-year-old, right-handed man who had sustained a severe closed brain injury with right frontal contusion from an automobile accident. His Glasgow Coma Scale score (Teasdale & Jennett, 1974) was 3 on acute hospital admission, and he had a coma duration of approximately 4 weeks, followed by gradual emergence from coma over 5 weeks. Acute hospital care was followed by 5 months of rehabilitation services.

On admission to the postacute treatment center 8 months postinjury, Client 1 was independent in wheelchair mobility indoors and had a severe left-sided hemiparesis, which was more pronounced in the lower extremity. Right-elbow extension was limited by 10% by heterotopic ossification.

On admission to the program, Client 1's memory was severely impaired; reproduction of a complex figure was nonexistent at 20 minutes, and immediate recall of a paragraph-length story was very poor, with delayed recall nonexistent. The client's performance on the Trail Making Test A (Reynolds, 2002) was below the first percentile, and he was unable to complete the Trail Making Test B. Observation over 3 days showed that the client was unable to bathe and dress himself, which was an important therapy goal for his parents, who were unable to physically assist him with transfers. A 22-item morning hygiene program was developed, with which he was cued for 20 days (see Exhibit 18.3).

EXHIBIT 18.3. Morning Hygiene Program

In advance: Staff to lay out today's clothes by the side of the sink

1. Push back the covers.
2. Swing legs off the side of the bed.
3. Push up to sit on the edge of the bed.
4. Put on shoes.
5. Position feet flat on the floor.
6. Reach for the wheelchair (both arms).
7. Get into wheelchair.
8. Go to sink (sit directly in front of sink).
9. Take off undershirt.
10. Brush teeth.
11. Fill sink.
12. Wash face (wash, rinse, dry).
13. Wash underarms (wash, rinse, dry).
14. Push wheelchair back from the sink, apply wheel locks, place hands on armrests, make a good hip bend, stand up, push down underwear, and sit down.
15. Wash groin (wash, rinse, dry).
16. Dress top half.
17. Take off shoes.
18. Put on socks.
19. Put on underwear and pants over feet.
20. Put on shoes.
21. Place hands on armrests, make a good hip bend, stand up, pull up underwear and trousers, and sit down.
22. Comb hair.
23. Well done, you have gotten yourself washed and dressed!

A reduced need for cueing was evident by Day 6. Physical assistance was no longer needed by Day 8, and by Day 20 Client 1 had achieved full independence in the program, which was maintained at a 3-month follow-up.

Trevena-Peters, McKay, Spitz, et al., 2018). Ehlhardt et al. (2008), in their evidence-based practice guidelines for individuals with neurogenic memory impairment, suggested that more practice opportunities lead to more-durable learning. Of the 16 studies that targeted multistep procedures that the authors reviewed, 14 reported positive treatment outcomes,

and all but 1 prescribed treatment dosages ranging from 6 to 30 or more sessions. The 2 studies that Ehlhardt et al. reviewed that did not report clear positive results involved a treatment dosage of fewer than 4 training sessions.

Concerns may be raised regarding the ability to administer the program with this level of frequency and on a daily basis.

In some specialized TBI rehabilitation centers, staff of other disciplines or auxiliary staff can be trained to administer the program developed by the occupational therapist, but in most settings the program is not executed 7 days per week. Evidence from neurologically healthy learners suggests that missing days even early in the course of learning does not pose a major obstacle to learning, and in our clinical practice we have never been able to guarantee daily intervention. However, when the program addresses an activity that has to occur daily—transfers, toileting, bathing, dressing, eating, and so forth—we have attempted to get as much consistency as possible. When we are not able to provide the program, we encourage staff to carry out the task for the client rather than have the client perform the task in an alternative way.

With some postacute clients who have memory impairment but adequate initiation ability, written instructions with check-off sheets can be substituted for the therapist cueing each performance of the program. For community-dwelling individuals, electronic cueing systems have been shown to help some clients learn and then have become unnecessary as learning takes place (Wilson et al., 2005).

Step 8: Provide Feedback

The last step in the NFA process is provision of feedback, appropriate to the client, to encourage progress and engagement. The type of feedback to provide to client learners depends on their awareness of impairment and attitude to the training that is taking place. As learning takes place and independence increases, some clients may find the graphing of their learning encouraging. For other clients, any reminder that they are not regarded as independent is dispiriting. There is evidence that reinforcement maximizes long-term retention, so the addition of tangible reinforcement may assist in retention (Abe et al., 2011). Parish and Oddy (2007) suggested that review of prior learning success may increase motivation to engage in further programs.

Documentation

Good record keeping is an essential part of the NFA, because it is essential for program consistency. Therapists should be able to know the number of prompts or steps that required physical assistance, that needed cueing, or that were performed independently on any particular day of program administration. Because there is some variation in client performance from day to day, weekly averages are superior in documenting learning. Progress can therefore be charted in terms of reduced need for cueing and for physical assistance.

SOAP (i.e., *Subjective, Objective, Assessment, Plan*) notes offer an ideal method of documenting case information clearly and succinctly for all staff who might treat the client. The following sections give examples of SOAP notes documenting different stages of client learning using the NFA. (Notes correspond to the 2 stages of NFA application demonstrated in Video 18.1.)

SOAP Note 1
October 15, 2018

S: The patient's mother stated, "We just can't handle him at home if he can't take care of himself."

O: Patient seen for 60 minutes to promote self-initiation and ability to participate in ADLs. Patient responded "yes" but did not initiate activities to a verbal cue of "Do what you would normally do to get washed and dressed in the morning." He did not initiate behavior to simple 1-step cues but did so with combined 1-step cues and tactile cueing. He required standby assist with verbal and tactile cueing for bed–wheelchair transfer. Patient required 1-step cues to engage in personal hygiene behaviors 100% of the time.

A: Patient demonstrated limitations in initiation of ADLs but was able to follow simple 1-step commands combined with tactile cues.

P: Continue skilled occupational therapy to develop (1–2 sessions) and implement (10–15 sessions) ADL retraining program according to the evidence-based practice NFA approach.

Soap Note 2
October 21, 2018

S: No relevant subjective report.

O: Patient seen for 60 minutes to promote bathing and dressing independence. Patient cued through an individualized 22-step ADL program that addresses his cognitive and physical impairments. Patient required 14 verbal cues and required no physical assistance to perform the washing and dressing routine. He spontaneously and accurately positioned his feet prior to transfer and required contact guard for bed–wheelchair transfer.

A: Patient is demonstrating learning and has increased his ADL independence. Over the 4 days of program implementation, patient has reduced the number of cues required for performance of the washing and dressing routine from 30 on Day 1 (he required multiple cues for some steps initially) to 14 today. Initially requiring physical assist for 6 program steps, he required no physical assistance today.

P: Patient requires continued skilled occupational therapy daily × 10 days to reduce cueing while minimizing errors during ADLs. Goals will be updated once ADL independence is consolidated.

Intervention Considerations

In a series of publications based on a randomized controlled trial, Trevena-Peters and colleagues (Mortimer et al., 2019; Trevena-Peters, McKay, & Ponsford, 2018; Trevena-Peters, McKay, Spitz, et al., 2018; Trevena-Peters et al., 2017) have greatly expanded the field's understanding of the effect of the application of the NFA to individuals in PTA. The additional cost of ADL retraining with the NFA, including training and supervision, amounted to 2.5% of the total per-patient cost but resulted in significant per-patient cost savings over treatment as usual (Mortimer et al., 2019).

In the postacute period, when moderate cognitive deficits coexist with physical problems, the client's occupational performance problems are frequently the result of the client's inability to independently develop an appropriate strategy to achieve independence. In these circumstances, the occupational therapist provides the strategy and then trains the client to use it. The combination of the strategy developed by the therapist and the client's only moderately impaired learning ability can result in very rapid improvement (Giles et al., 2019).

Elsewhere we have provided evidence that in the postacute TBI population, ADLs and IADLs are hierarchically related in terms of the client's ability to perform them (Giles et al., 2019). The NFA can address difficulties in ADLs and simple IADLs (see Exhibit 18.4) but cannot adequately address complex IADLs that cannot be fully routinized and that require the client to manage novelty.

Some clients reject the rehabilitative endeavor because they lack awareness of their deficits. According to the developers of these approaches, awareness of deficit is a prerequisite for some metacognitive strategy instruction–based interventions (e.g., Cognitive Orientation to daily Occupational Performance, Multicontext Approach) in which the client needs to learn to apply novel "thinking routines" to develop ways to address daily-life problems (Dawson et al., 2017; Toglia, 2018). Although there is some evidence that awareness can be improved in specific areas of functioning (Toglia et al., 2010), there are reasons to doubt that interventions of this type can be effective for persons with severe lack of insight and neurobehavioral impairments (Clark-Wilson et al., 2014; Crosson et al., 1989; Ergh et al., 2002). To use metacognitive strategies, clients need to

- Be aware of limitations in their functioning,

- Acknowledge the validity of such strategies (Ergh et al., 2002), and

- Have the cognitive capacity to learn the strategies.

Insight is less critical in the application of the NFA. Many clients deny that they have had any cognitive loss but nonetheless recognize that their performance could be improved as long as this discussion is not linked to an acknowledgment of cognitive impairment. Training can in many cases be unobtrusive, because it simply involves having the client perform the same behaviors in the same way over an extended period. Recognition of having had a TBI or stroke and resulting deficits is unnecessary.

In the postacute period, when the client can read and has adequate initiation skills, therapists can make the learning process less labor intensive for themselves by using a check-off sheet (see Exhibit 18.5). During the initial sessions (Sessions 3–4), the therapist uses cue experimentation to ensure that the written instructions are adequate to guide the behavior (i.e., the therapist observes the client's behavior to the written cue to make sure that the cue is adequate to reliably guide the necessary behaviors). The client can then follow the instructions and check off each step as they go independently. For many clients, after a period of following the check-off sheet, the steps will be internalized, and the check-off sheet is no longer necessary.

Box 18.1 describes elements that facilitate client learning of retraining programs.

EXHIBIT 18.4. Examples of ADLs and Simple IADLs Amenable to the Development of Retraining Programs

- Bathing
- Dressing
- Oral hygiene
- Street crossing
- Traveling to a local store, café, or gym
- Shopping in a grocery store
- Riding the bus
- Doing laundry
- Making a hot drink
- Preparing a light meal
- Managing and paying bills
- Managing medications

EXHIBIT 18.5. Checklist Program for Making Instant Hot Cocoa

In advance: Cup, teaspoon, hot cocoa mix, and kettle are on a tray by the side of the sink.

1. Fill the electric kettle up to the line marked 0.1 L with cold water from the faucet.
2. Press switch on handle so that the red light comes on. (If it does not come on, make sure it is plugged in and the wall switch is on.)
3. Put 2 teaspoons of the hot cocoa mix in the bottom of your cup with half an inch of water from the faucet and make a paste.
4. When the kettle boils (the kettle will click off, and the light will go out), pour hot water slowly into the cup, leaving an inch of space at the top, and stir with the teaspoon.
5. Go to the refrigerator and get milk.
6. Fill the cup up to a half inch from the top with milk.
7. Put the milk back in the refrigerator.
8. Carry the cup carefully and put it down on the kitchen table.
9. Sit at the table and enjoy your hot cocoa!

BOX 18.1. Elements of the Retraining Program

- **Chaining:** Functional tasks can be thought of as complex stimulus–response chains in which the completion of each activity acts as the stimulus for the next step in the chain (Kazdin, 2012). Three chaining options are available:
  1. Backward chaining
  2. Forward chaining
  3. The whole-task method.

  In the Neurofunctional Approach, the whole-task method is adopted whenever possible because of its practical advantages and the natural reinforcing effect of task achievement (Martin et al., 2000; McDonnell & Laughlin, 1989; Spooner, 1984).

- **Cueing:** Events that facilitate the production of a behavior are called *cues* (or *prompts*). In many instances, cues are available in the environment but are no longer sufficient to guide behavior or have lost their meaning entirely (e.g., arriving at a busy intersection no longer cues safe street-crossing routines). The therapist adds additional cues to those already available in the environment (e.g., saying, "Stop," when the client arrives at the curbside). Therapists can facilitate the learning of skills with differing types of cues.

- **Errorless learning:** Sufficient cueing "scaffolding" is provided to ensure correct performance. As learning takes place, that scaffolding is gradually withdrawn, but only at the rate at which correct performance is maintained (Haslam & Kessels, 2018).

- **Overlearning:** Overlearning is the practice of a skill beyond the point of mastery, such that no more performance improvements are observed with continued practice (Driskell et al., 1992; Krueger, 1929; Postman, 1962). Overlearning increases the chances that a skill will be consolidated in the individual's repertoire of skills and reduces the effort required for performance of the skill (Clark-Wilson et al., 2014; Giles & Clark-Wilson, 1993).

- **Practice:** Practice is the repetition of a behavior: A functionally identical response is provided to functionally identical stimuli. The development of performance skills results from practice (Healy et al., 2012; Newell & Rosenbloom, 1981).

- **Reinforcement:** A reinforcer is an event that increases the likelihood that a behavior that preceded it will be repeated. There is some evidence that reinforcement aids immediate learning (Dolan, 1979; Lahey & Drabman, 1974; O'Doherty, 2004; O'Doherty et al., 2001). Long-term retention is more effective under conditions of anticipated reward than under neutral or punishment conditions, and the effect extends to social reward (Fischer & Born, 2009; Sugawara et al., 2012), an effect that seems to be associated with offline, sleep-related consolidation (Abe et al., 2011).

- **Self-generation effect:** The self-generation effect is the learning advantage provided by clients initiating the activity themselves. The use of a combined self-generation and errorless approach has been shown in some studies to further enhance learning over errorless learning alone (Goverover et al., 2010; Haslam & Kessels, 2018; Haslam et al., 2017).

- **Task analysis:** Task analysis is a process of identifying the essential behaviors required for the completion of a task.

- **Therapeutic alliance:** Three components of the alliance have been identified:
  1. The emotional bond between client and therapist
  2. Mutual agreement on goals
  3. Mutual agreement on the tasks that form the substance of the intervention (Bordin, 1979).

Conclusion

Studies by independent research groups suggest that the NFA has a wider applicability than was originally envisaged, is practical and cost effective, can improve client–therapist relationships, and improves outcomes (Giles, 2010; Trevena-Peters, McKay, & Ponsford, 2018; Trevena-Peters, McKay, Spitz, et al., 2018; Trevena-Peters et al., 2017; Vanderploeg et al., 2008). Despite accumulating evidence of the efficacy of the NFA, further research is required to define more precisely the clients who are most assisted by it, as well as the optimal duration and intensity of its application.

References

Abe, M., Schambra, H., Wassermann, E. M., Luckenbaugh, D., Schweighofer, N., & Cohen, L. G. (2011). Reward improves long-term retention of a motor memory through induction of offline memory gains. *Current Biology, 21,* 557–562. https://doi.org/10.1016/j.cub.2011.02.030

American Occupational Therapy Association. (2014). Occupational therapy practice framework: Domain and process (3rd ed.). *American Journal of Occupational Therapy, 68*(Suppl. 1), S1–S48. https://doi.org/10.5014/ajot.2014.682006

Baum, C. M., Morrison, M. T., Hahn, M., & Edwards, D. F. (2003). *Test manual: Executive Function Performance Test.* St. Louis: Washington University in St. Louis.

Bordin, E. S. (1979). The generalizability of the psychoanalytic concept of the working alliance. *Psychotherapy, 16,* 252–260. https://doi.org/10.1037/h0085885

Clark-Wilson, J., Giles, G. M., & Baxter, D. M. (2014). Revisiting the Neurofunctional Approach: Conceptualizing the core components for the rehabilitation of everyday living skills. *Brain Injury, 28,* 1646–1656. https://doi.org/10.3109/02699052.2014.946449

Crosson, B., Barco, P., Velozo, C., Bolesta, M., Cooper, P., Werts, D., & Brobeck, T. C. (1989). Awareness and compensation in postacute head injury rehabilitation. *Journal of Head Trauma Rehabilitation, 4,* 46–54. https://doi.org/10.1097/00001199-198909000-00008

Dawson, D., McEwen, S. E., & Polatajko, H. (2017). *Cognitive Orientation to daily Occupational Performance in occupational therapy: Using the CO–OP Approach™ to enable participation across the lifespan.* Bethesda, MD: AOTA Press.

Dolan, M. P. (1979). The use of contingent reinforcement for improving the personal appearance and hygiene of chronic psychiatric inpatients. *Journal of Clinical Psychology, 35,* 140–144.

Driskell, J. E., Willis, R. P., & Copper, C. (1992). Effect of overlearning on retention. *Journal of Applied Psychology, 77,* 615–622. https://doi.org/10.1037/0021-9010.77.5.615

Ehlhardt, L. A., Sohlberg, M. M., Kennedy, M., Coelho, C., Ylvisaker, M., Turkstra, L., & Yorkston, K. (2008). Evidence-based practice guidelines for instructing individuals with neurogenic memory impairments: What have we learned in the past 20 years? *Neuropsychological Rehabilitation, 18,* 300–342. https://doi.org/10.1080/09602010701733190

Ergh, T. C., Rapport, L. J., Coleman, R. D., & Hanks, R. A. (2002). Predictors of caregiver and family functioning following traumatic brain injury: Social support moderates caregiver distress. *Journal of Head Trauma Rehabilitation, 17,* 155–174. https://doi.org/10.1097/00001199-200204000-00006

Fischer, S., & Born, J. (2009). Anticipated reward enhances offline learning during sleep. *Journal of Experimental Psychology: Learning, Memory, and Cognition, 35,* 1586–1593. https://doi.org/10.1037/a0017256

Giles, G. M. (2010). Cognitive versus functional approaches to rehabilitation after traumatic brain injury: Commentary on a randomized controlled trial. *American Journal of Occupational Therapy, 64,* 182–185. https://doi.org/10.5014/ajot.64.1.182

Giles, G. M. (2018). Neurocognitive rehabilitation: Skills or strategies? (Eleanor Clarke Slagle Lecture). *American Journal of Occupational Therapy, 72,* 7206150010. https://doi.org/10.5014/ajot.2018.726001

Giles, G. M., & Clark-Wilson, J. (Eds.). (1993). *Brain injury rehabilitation: A Neurofunctional Approach.* San Diego: Singular.

Giles, G. M., Clark-Wilson, J., Baxter, D. M., Tasker, R., Holloway, M., & Seymour, S. (2019). The interrelationship of functional skills in individuals living in the community, following moderate to severe traumatic brain injury. *Brain Injury, 33,* 129–136. https://doi.org/10.1080/02699052.2018.1539762

Giles, G. M., Ridley, J. E., Dill, A., & Frye, S. (1997). A consecutive series of adults with brain injury treated with a washing and dressing retraining program. *American Journal of Occupational Therapy, 51,* 256–266. https://doi.org/10.5014/ajot.51.4.256

Goverover, Y., Chiaravalloti, N., & DeLuca, J. (2010). Pilot study to examine the use of self-generation to improve learning and memory in people with traumatic brain injury. *American Journal of Occupational Therapy, 64,* 540–546. https://doi.org/10.5014/ajot.2010.09020

Haslam, C., & Kessels, R. P. C. (Eds.). (2018). *Errorless learning in neuropsychological rehabilitation: Mechanisms, efficacy, and application.* New York: Routledge. https://doi.org/10.4324/9781315660738

Haslam, C., Wagner, J., Wegener, S., & Malouf, T. (2017). Elaborative encoding through self-generation enhances outcomes with errorless learning: Findings from the Skypekids Memory Study. *Neuropsychological Rehabilitation, 27,* 60–79. https://doi.org/10.1080/09602011.2015.1053947

Healy, A. F., Schneider, V. I., & Bourne, L. E. (2012). Empirically valid principles of training. In A. F. Healy & L. E. Bourne (Eds.), *Training cognition: Optimizing efficiency, durability and generalizability* (pp. 13–39). New York: Psychology Press.

Kazdin, A. E. (2012). *Behavior modification in applied settings* (7th ed.). Long Grove, IL: Waveland Press.

Keith, R. A., Granger, C. V., Hamilton, B. B., & Sherwin, F. S. (1987). The Functional Independence Measure: A new tool for rehabilitation. *Advances in Clinical Rehabilitation, 1,* 6–18.

Kelly, F., & Nikopoulis, C. (2010). Facilitating independence in personal activities of daily living after a severe traumatic brain injury. *International Journal of Therapy and Rehabilitation, 17,* 474–482. https://doi.org/10.12968/ijtr.2010.17.9.78037

Krueger, W. C. F. (1929). The effect of overlearning on retention. *Journal of Experimental Psychology, 12,* 71–78. https://doi.org/10.1037/h0072036

Lahey, B. B., & Drabman, R. S. (1974). Facilitation of the acquisition and retention of sight-word vocabulary through token reinforcement. *Journal of Applied Behavior Analysis, 7,* 307–312.

Lally, P., Van Jaarsveld, C. H. M., Potts, H. W. W., & Wardle, J. (2010). How are habits formed: Modelling habit formation in the real world. *European Journal of Social Psychology, 40,* 998–1009. https://doi.org/10.1002/ejsp.674

Martin, D. J., Garske, J. P., & Davis, M. K. (2000). Relation of the therapeutic alliance with outcome and other variables: A meta-analytic review. *Journal of Consulting and Clinical Psychology, 68,* 438–450. https://doi.org/10.1037/0022-006X.68.3.438

McDonnell, J., & Laughlin, B. (1989). A comparison of backward and concurrent chaining strategies in teaching community skills. *Education and Training in Mental Retardation, 24,* 230–238.

Miller, E. (1980). The training characteristics of severely head-injured patients: A preliminary study. *Journal of Neurology, Neurosurgery, and Psychiatry, 43,* 525–528. https://doi.org/10.1136/jnnp.43.6.525

Miller, W. R., & Rollnick, S. (2013). *Motivational interviewing: Helping people change* (3rd ed.). New York: Guilford Press.

Mortimer, D., Trevena-Peters, J., McKay, A., & Ponsford, J. (2019). Economic evaluation of activities of daily living retraining during posttraumatic amnesia for inpatient rehabilitation following severe traumatic brain injury. *Archives of Physical Medicine and Rehabilitation, 100,* 648–655. https://doi.org/10.1016/j.apmr.2018.08.184

Nasreddine, Z. S., Phillips, N. A., Bédirian, V., Charbonneau, S., Whitehead, V., Collin, I., . . . Chertkow, H. (2005). The Montreal Cognitive Assessment, MoCA: A brief screening tool for mild cognitive impairment. *Journal of the American Geriatrics Society, 53,* 695–699. https://doi.org/10.1111/j.1532-5415.2005.53221.x

Newell, A., & Rosenbloom, P. S. (1981). Mechanisms of skill acquisition and the law of practice. In J. R. Anderson (Ed.), *Cognitive skills and their acquisition* (pp. 1–55). Hillsdale, NJ: Erlbaum.

O'Doherty, J. P. (2004). Reward representations and reward-related learning in the human brain: Insights from neuroimaging. *Current Opinion in Neurobiology, 14,* 769–776. https://doi.org/10.1016/j.conb.2004.10.016

O'Doherty, J., Kringelbach, M. L., Rolls, E. T., Hornak, J., & Andrews, C. (2001). Abstract reward and punishment representations in the human orbitofrontal cortex. *Nature Neuroscience, 4,* 95–102. https://doi.org/10.1038/82959

Ownsworth, T. (2018). Errors: Friend or foe? The theory and evidence base for error-based learning. In C. Haslam & R. P. C. Kessels (Eds.), *Errorless learning in neuropsychological rehabilitation* (pp. 164–179). New York: Routledge. https://doi.org/10.4324/9781315660738-11

Parish, L., & Oddy, M. (2007). Efficacy of rehabilitation for functional skills more than 10 years after extremely severe brain injury. *Neuropsychological Rehabilitation, 17,* 230–243. https://doi.org/10.1080/09602010600750675

Postman, L. (1962). Retention as a function of degree of overlearning. *Science, 135,* 666–667. https://doi.org/10.1126/science.135.3504.666

Reber, P. J. (2013). The neural basis of implicit learning and memory: A review of neuropsychological and neuroimaging research. *Neuropsychologia, 51,* 2026–2042. https://doi.org/10.1016/j.neuropsychologia.2013.06.019

Reynolds, C. R. (2002). *Comprehensive Trail-Making Test.* Austin, TX: Pro-Ed.

Rogers, J. C., Holm, M., & Chisholm, D. (2016). *Performance Assessment of Self-Care Skills* (Version 4.1). Pittsburgh: University of Pittsburgh.

Rotenberg-Shpigelman, S., Erez, A. B., Nahaloni, I., & Maeir, A. (2012). Neurofunctional treatment targeting participation among chronic stroke survivors: A pilot randomised controlled study. *Neuropsychological Rehabilitation, 22,* 532–549. https://doi.org/10.1080/09602011.2012.665610

Spooner, F. (1984). Comparison of backward chaining and total task presentation in training severely handicapped persons. *Education and Training of the Mentally Retarded, 19,* 15–22.

Sugawara, S. K., Tanaka, S., Okazaki, S., Watanabe, K., & Sadato, N. (2012). Social rewards enhance offline improvements in motor skill. *PLoS One, 7,* e48174. https://doi.org/10.1371/journal.pone.0048174

Teasdale, G., & Jennett, B. (1974). Assessment of coma and impaired consciousness: A practical scale. *Lancet, 304,* 81–84. https://doi.org/10.1016/S0140-6736(74)91639-0

Toglia, J. (2018). The Dynamic Interactional Model and the Multicontext Approach. In N. Katz & J. Toglia (Eds.), *Cognition, occupation, and participation across the lifespan: Neuroscience, neurorehabilitation,* *and models of intervention in occupational therapy* (4th ed., pp. 355–385). Bethesda, MD: AOTA Press.

Toglia, J., Johnston, M. V., Goverover, Y., & Dain, B. (2010). A multi-context approach to promoting transfer of strategy use and self regulation after brain injury: An exploratory study. *Brain Injury, 24,* 664–677. https://doi.org/10.3109/02699051003610474

Trevena-Peters, J., McKay, A., & Ponsford, J. (2018). Activities of daily living retraining and goal attainment during posttraumatic amnesia. *Neuropsychological Rehabilitation, 8,* 1–16. https://doi.org/10.1080/09602011.2018.1441033

Trevena-Peters, J., McKay, A., Spitz, G., Suda, R., Renison, B., & Ponsford, J. (2018). Efficacy of activities of daily living retraining during post-traumatic amnesia: A randomised controlled trial. *Archives of Physical Medicine and Rehabilitation, 99,* 329–337. https://doi.org/10.1016/j.apmr.2017.08.486

Trevena-Peters, J., Ponsford, J., & McKay, A. (2017). Agitated behavior and activities of daily living retraining during posttraumatic amnesia. *Journal of Head Trauma Rehabilitation.* Advance online publication. https://doi.org/10.1097/HTR.0000000000000363

Turner-Stokes, L. (2008). Evidence for the effectiveness of multidisciplinary rehabilitation following acquired brain injury: A synthesis of two systematic approaches. *Journal of Rehabilitation Medicine, 40,* 691–701. https://doi.org/10.2340/16501977-0265

Vanderploeg, R. D., Collins, R. C., Sigford, B., Date, E., Schwab, K., & Warden, D. (2006). Practical and theoretical considerations in designing rehabilitation trials: The DVBIC Cognitive–Didactic Versus Functional–Experiential Treatment Study experience. *Journal of Head Trauma Rehabilitation, 21,* 179–193. https://doi.org/10.1097/00001199-200603000-00010

Vanderploeg, R. D., Schwab, K., Walker, W. C., Fraser, J. A., Sigford, B. J., Date, E. S., . . . Warden, D. L. (2008). Rehabilitation of traumatic brain injury in active duty military personnel and veterans: Defense and Veterans Brain Injury Center randomized controlled trial of two rehabilitation approaches. *Archives of Physical Medicine and Rehabilitation, 89,* 2227–2238. https://doi.org/10.1016/j.apmr.2008.06.015

Whyte, J., Gordon, W., & Rothi, L. J. (2009). A phased developmental approach to neurorehabilitation research: The science of knowledge building. *Archives of Physical Medicine and Rehabilitation, 90*(Suppl.), S3–S10. https://doi.org/10.1016/j.apmr.2009.07.008

Wilson, B. A., Emslie, H., Quirk, K., Evans, J., & Watson, P. (2005). A randomized control trial to evaluate a paging system for people with traumatic brain injury. *Brain Injury, 19,* 891–894. https://doi.org/10.1080/02699050400002363

Wolery, M., Griffen, A. K., Ault, M. J., Gast, D. L., & Doyle, P. M. (1990). Comparison of constant time delay and the system of least prompts in teaching chained tasks. *Education and Training in Mental Retardation, 25,* 243–257.

Wood, W., & Rünger, D. (2016). Psychology of habit. *Annual Review of Psychology, 67,* 289–314. https://doi.org/10.1146/annurev-psych-122414-033417

World Health Organization. (2001). *International classification of functioning, disability and health.* Geneva: Author.

Yin, H. H., & Knowlton, B. J. (2006). The role of the basal ganglia in habit formation. *Nature Reviews Neuroscience, 7,* 464–476.

Cognitive Orientation to daily Occupational Performance

HORTENSIA GIMENO, DIP (OT), MSc, PhD; KATHERINE DITTMANN, BSc, MKin, MPT;
HELENE POLATAJKO, BOT, MED, PhD, OT Reg. (Ont.), OT(C), FCAOT, FCAHS;
AND SARA McEWEN, BSc (PT), MSc, PhD

LEARNING OBJECTIVES

After completing this chapter, readers should be able to

- Understand the background of the Cognitive Orientation to daily Occupational Performance (CO–OP) Approach,
- Discuss current evidence emerging from the use of CO–OP in different child and adult populations,
- Describe findings from published studies on transfer of learning with CO–OP among children and adults, and
- Discuss the chapter's case examples and video, which highlight key concepts of the CO–OP Approach.

KEY TERMS AND CONCEPTS

- Client-centered, occupation-focused goals • Cognitive strategy use • Dynamic performance analysis
- Enabling principles • Global cognitive strategy • Guided discovery

Background, Theory, and Development of the Approach

Background

The Cognitive Orientation to daily Occupational Performance (CO–OP) Approach™ was first developed in the 1990s, specifically to improve the occupational performance of children with developmental coordination disorder (DCD; Miller et al., 2001; Polatajko & Mandich, 2004). Children with DCD experience primarily motor coordination difficulties when performing daily activities (Blank et al., 2012), and their motor deficits are relatively mild compared with those of other populations.

However, other populations with more complex deficits, including cognitive impairments, have been shown to benefit from the approach as well. Researchers working with several populations of various ages and diagnoses have shown that CO–OP and its adaptations can enable both the acquisition of a variety of functional skills and the generalization and transfer of learning to other aspects of clients' life (Scammell et al., 2016).

CO–OP has demonstrated efficacy in populations with cognitive impairments, such as clients with acquired brain injury (Dawson et al., 2009; Dawson, Anderson, et al., 2013; Dawson, Binns, et al., 2013; Missiuna et al., 2010) or stroke (McEwen, 2009; McEwen, Donald, et al., 2015; McEwen, Huijbregts, et al., 2009; McEwen, Polatajko, et al., 2009, 2015; McEwen, Polatajko, Davis, et al., 2010; McEwen, Polatajko, Huijbregts, & Ryan, 2010; Poulin et al., 2017; Skidmore et al., 2017; Wolf et al., 2016) and older adults with subjective cognitive complaints (Dawson et al., 2014). However, CO–OP is not a cognitive rehabilitation technique that targets cognitive impairment reduction per se. Rather, it is an approach to rehabilitation that draws on functional cognition to facilitate the acquisition or reacquisition of functional skill.

The intervention is described as "a client-centered, performance-based, problem-solving approach that enables skill acquisition through a process of strategy use and guided discovery" (Polatajko & Mandich, 2004, p. 2). The 4 objectives of the intervention are

1. Skill acquisition,

2. Cognitive strategy use,

3. Generalization, and

4. Transfer of learning (Polatajko & Mandich, 2004).

These objectives are achieved through the application of CO–OP's 7 key features:

1. Client-centered, occupation-focused goals

2. Dynamic performance analysis

3. Cognitive strategy use

4. Guided discovery

5. Enabling principles

6. Parent or significant other involvement

7. Intervention format and structure.

Theoretical Framework

Several theoretical, evidence-based perspectives underpin the CO–OP Approach, including client centeredness and cognitive and motor learning theories. The approach uses a metacognitive framework to develop, apply, and generalize problem-solving strategies to everyday challenges. The CO–OP therapist actively engages the client in using a problem-solving framework to generate, test, and refine their own strategies to achieve their self-chosen goals. These aspects of CO–OP not only improve motivation and engagement but also support transfer and generalization to other goals, with benefits extending well beyond the duration of the therapy intervention.

Figure 19.1 provides a theoretical model of the mechanisms by which the CO–OP Approach works. Of the 7 key features just mentioned, 5 are considered essential elements:

1. ***Client-centered, occupation-focused goals*** are goals derived from a partnership between the therapist and the client as they identify priority occupational issues for intervention in light of assessment and evaluation results. In setting these goals, the therapist explicitly values the client's knowledge and experience and actively includes them in the process.

2. ***Dynamic performance analysis*** (DPA) is the process used to ascertain where the performance of the task or activity is breaking down and identify potential strategies.

3. ***Cognitive strategy use*** consists of problem-solving techniques to support skill acquisition, generalization, and transfer.

4. ***Guided discovery*** is a nondirective therapeutic process whereby the therapist prompts the client to develop and use the analysis and problem-solving skills to achieve their goal.

5. ***Enabling principles*** are principles related to facilitating, guiding, coaching, educating, promoting, listening, reflecting, encouraging, or otherwise collaborating with people to reach their goals (Skidmore et al., 2017; Townsend et al., 1997, p. 50).

These elements are displayed at the top of Figure 19.1. The remaining 2 key features, parent or significant other involvement and the intervention format, are considered structural

FIGURE 19.1. Theoretical model of the CO–OP Approach.

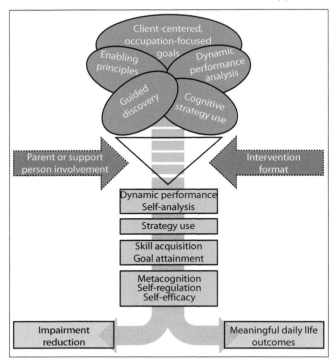

Source. From "Essential Elements and Key Features of the CO–OP Approach," by E. Skidmore, S. E. McEwen, D. Green, J. van den Houten, D. R. Dawson, and H. J. Polatajko, in *Cognitive Orientation to daily Occupational Performance in Occupational Therapy* (p. 17), by D. R. Dawson, S. E. McEwen, and H. J. Polatajko (Eds.), 2017, Bethesda, MD: AOTA Press. Copyright © 2017 by the American Occupational Therapy Association. Reprinted with permission.

elements; they support the essential elements but are not essential to producing the intervention effects. The 5 essential elements supported by the structural elements teach clients dynamic performance self-analysis skills and how to use cognitive strategies, which in turn leads to skill acquisition and goal attainment. Those successes lead to improvements in metacognition, self-efficacy, and self-regulation. Through those mechanisms, clients experience impairment reduction and improvements in meaningful daily life participation.

Development

Polatajko and colleagues (Miller et al., 2001; Polatajko & Mandich, 2004) designed CO–OP on the basis of Meichenbaum's (1977) self-instructional problem-solving approach, which uses Goal–Plan–Do–Check (GPDC) to improve cognitive-based performance. GPDC is based on the ***global cognitive strategy*** (i.e., a global problem-solving strategy used as a metacognitive strategy) so that participants learn to apply this global concept in their daily routine.

GPDC is at the core of CO–OP and is augmented with domain-specific strategies and the inclusion of DPA, guided discovery, and enabling principles, all framed in a client-centered philosophy. These methods help the client elucidate the "Plan" and check the "Do." Together, they form a framework that enables the client to identify solutions to occupational performance problems that encompass cognitive, motor, and affective domains.

CO–OP is a top-down approach; in other words, it is a task-oriented approach that focuses treatment on the performance of whole functional tasks or occupations rather than performance components. Performance components (i.e., memory, attention, core stability, bilateral integration) move to the background, and the direct acquisition of functional skills becomes the foreground. In line with current theories of skill acquisition and neuroplasticity (Cramer et al., 2011; Dayan & Cohen, 2011; Diaz Heijtz & Forssberg, 2015; Friel et al., 2016; Hallett, 2005; Ismail et al., 2017; Kirton, 2013; Kolb & Muhammad, 2014; Nahum et al., 2013; Nava & Röder, 2011), CO–OP challenges the traditional view of a hierarchy of skill acquisition wherein skill components must be learned first, before the acquisition of functional skills.

CO–OP is not a cognitive rehabilitation approach aiming to reduce cognitive impairment but rather is a holistic approach that addresses functional skills in a variety of populations, including those with cognitive impairment. Research has shown that CO–OP does this effectively in a range of pediatric and adult populations with a variety of diagnoses; these studies are discussed next. Two case examples are given to illustrate the use of the CO–OP Approach in pediatric and adult populations.

Target Population

Because CO–OP is a learning-based approach to rehabilitation, the populations for whom it is effective and the settings in which it may be used are broad. A 2016 scoping review identified 27 peer-reviewed research articles examining the application of CO–OP with 7 different child and adult populations (Scammell et al., 2016). Subsequent studies have added to the list of populations with whom CO–OP has yielded positive results. Certain populations, such as children with DCD and adults with stroke, have a significant body of evidence supporting the use of CO–OP, whereas some have only limited evidence to date. In this section, we

- Outline the populations with published evidence supporting treatment with CO–OP, emphasizing those with cognitive impairments;

- Describe the CO–OP treatment contexts; and

- Recommend client prerequisites that occupational therapists should consider before initiating CO–OP treatment.

Scammell et al. (2016) reported that CO–OP has been investigated for use with children with DCD, autism spectrum disorder (i.e., pervasive development disorder and Asperger syndrome), and acquired brain injury. Studies published since have tested the approach with children with cerebral palsy (CP; Cameron et al., 2017; Ghorbani et al., 2017; Gimeno et al., 2018a, 2018b,

2019; Jackman et al., 2014, 2017), Down syndrome (Halayko et al., 2016), attention deficit hyperactivity disorder (Gharebaghy et al., 2015), and dystonia (Gimeno et al., 2018a, 2018b, 2019). Improvement on chosen goals has been reported across these populations, as have generalization and transfer, where assessed. These findings have been reported for populations with known motor and cognitive deficits—for example, participants with CP and dystonia (Aarnoudse-Moens et al., 2009; Coenen et al., 2018; Crajé et al., 2010; Kirkpatrick et al., 2013; Pirila et al., 2011; Steenbergen et al., 2013).

CO–OP has been investigated for use with adults with stroke, adults with traumatic brain injury (TBI), and older adults with subjective cognitive complaints (Ahn et al., 2017; Dawson et al., 2009; Dawson, Anderson, et al., 2013; Dawson, Binns, et al., 2013; Henshaw et al., 2011; McEwen, 2009; McEwen, Donald, et al., 2015; McEwen, Huijbregts, et al., 2009; McEwen, Polatajko, et al., 2009, 2015; McEwen, Polatajko, Davis, et al., 2010; McEwen, Polatajko, Huijbregts, & Ryan, 2010; Polatajko et al., 2012; Poulin et al., 2017; Skidmore, 2014, 2015; Skidmore et al., 2011, 2014; Wolf et al., 2016). Most of the adult studies included participants with cognitive impairment, and many specifically studied those with cognitive impairment (Dawson et al., 2009, 2014; Dawson, Anderson, et al., 2013; Dawson, Binns, et al., 2013; Skidmore, 2014; Skidmore et al., 2011, 2014).

Cumulatively, the findings indicate that CO–OP has a large and maintained effect, compared with control conditions, on generalization and transfer to untrained goals (Ahn et al., 2017; Houldin et al., 2018; McEwen, Polatajko, et al., 2015) and on functional independence (Skidmore, 2015) among people with stroke. Compared with control conditions, CO–OP or CO–OP-derived treatment has also demonstrated an effect on apathy, cognitive flexibility, participation, quality of life, self-awareness, self-efficacy, and upper extremity function (Skidmore et al., 2018; Skidmore, Dawson, et al., 2015; Skidmore, Whyte, et al., 2015; Wolf et al., 2016).

CO–OP has been delivered in several treatment contexts and with modifications to the initial CO–OP intervention format. For the most part, studies with children have taken place in an outpatient clinical setting or in the child's home. The studies with adults with stroke have included

- Acute rehabilitation (i.e., inpatient setting, 1–2 weeks poststroke; Skidmore et al., 2018; Skidmore, Dawson, et al., 2015; Skidmore, Whyte, et al., 2015),

- Subacute rehabilitation (outpatient setting, less than 3 months poststroke; McEwen, Polatajko, et al., 2015; Wolf et al., 2016), and

- Chronic stroke (more than 6 months poststroke; Henshaw et al., 2011; McEwen, Polatajko, et al., 2009; McEwen, Polatajko, Huijbregts, & Ryan, 2010).

A single case study has demonstrated that it is feasible to deliver CO–OP with a telerehabilitation model to adults living in the community after TBI (Ng et al., 2013). For clients with executive functioning (EF) impairments, Dawson and colleagues (2009) expanded the number of treatment sessions from the original 10 to 20. CO–OP has also been delivered through an interprofessional model (McEwen et al., 2017).

Polatajko and Mandich (2004) provided client prerequisites for an occupational therapist to consider before using the CO–OP Approach with a particular client. Clients should have

- Skills they want to acquire or improve,

- Sufficient cognitive and communication skills to engage with the therapist, and

- Sufficient behavioral responsiveness to be able to learn with therapist support.

Because the primary objective of CO–OP is skill acquisition, it is imperative that the client have at least 1 functional skill to learn that will become the focus of therapy. It is highly preferable that this is a skill that the client has chosen, so that it is meaningful and important to them. There are exceptions to that rule, such as in the case of children who are required by their teachers and parents to devote some time to improving their handwriting. When that occurs, the CO–OP therapist uses enabling skills to ensure engagement in the intervention. They also may negotiate with the client and significant others to ensure that the additional skills to be addressed in CO–OP are those that are most important to the client.

For the client prerequisites related to cognition, communication, and behavioral responsiveness, the degree required is a sufficient amount to allow client–therapist engagement. Specific levels based on standardized tests have not been suggested, because the definition of "a sufficient amount" may vary depending on the specific client–therapist dyad. Furthermore, surprising successes with clients with very low cognition, intellectual capacity, and communication have been published or reported anecdotally, which makes us hesitant to set strict limits; much is dependent on the therapists' expertise.

For example, Halayko and colleagues (2016) used an adaptation of the CO–OP Approach to enable children with Down syndrome to learn to ride 2-wheeled bikes. Gimeno and colleagues (2016) included 1 nonverbal young person and 2 people with moderate learning disability in their study. Therapists often question whether clients with low self-awareness of their deficits are appropriate for CO–OP; research suggests that people with poor awareness benefit from CO–OP-derived cognitive strategy training to improve functional independence, in comparison with control participants (Skidmore et al., 2018).

Administration

As mentioned previously, the CO–OP Approach has 7 key features, 5 of which are considered essential elements for adequate administration, and 2 of which are considered structural elements that may vary depending on context. Polatajko and Mandich (2004) described administration of CO–OP through skillful integration of the key features. Updates, nuances, and advances in the administration related to specific populations and treatment contexts are outlined in a more recent book edited by Dawson et al. (2017).

Although the books are excellent support materials for learning to use the CO–OP Approach, therapists who wish to implement CO–OP in their clinical or research practices should take a workshop led by a certified CO–OP instructor. Instructors are certified by the International CO–OP Academy, and a list of certified instructors may be found at http://co-opacademy. ca/education-and-workshops/co-op-workshops/finding-a-certified-instructor/.

Currently, the standard CO–OP workshop consists of 3 days in 2 parts, led by certified instructors. Part 1 is 2 days of instruction and practice in the CO–OP key features. Part 2 is a 3rd day designed for consolidation of learning, which occurs a few months after Part 1. Therapists are asked to practice using CO–OP in the intervening time and to return for the consolidation day with a short case study prepared. The cases are presented in small groups, and therapists discuss their successes and challenges with using CO–OP in their clinical contexts. Further opportunities for practice of reportedly challenging scenarios are provided.

Therapists who have participated in a 3-day CO–OP workshop or demonstrated equivalency may undertake an additional step and become a certified CO–OP therapist. This involves demonstrating competency in administering CO–OP's 7 key features through case presentation (including a video clip of the candidate using CO–OP with a client) and questions, responses, and discussion among candidates in the small-group-format course. Please contact the CO–OP Academy (www.co-op academy.ca) for more information about the instructor certification process.

Step-by-Step Administration

CO–OP is an iterative rather than a linear process and thus does not lend itself well to step-by-step instructions. Figure 19.2 displays the process, which is grounded in GPDC and begins with the establishment of a client-centered, occupation-based goal. After establishing the *goal*, the occupational therapist and client work together to develop a *plan* to meet the goal.

Developing the plan is an iterative subprocess of its own, beginning with having the client perform the goal if it is doable in the clinical setting or describe how to do the goal if performance is not possible in the clinical setting. If the goal cannot be performed in the clinical setting because of space or time limitations or the nature of the task (e.g., taking the city bus to go grocery shopping), the client should describe to the therapist how the goal would be accomplished.

During this initial performance (or description), the therapist begins DPA to discover performance breakdown points. The therapist then guides the client to discover potential domain-specific strategies to overcome the specific performance breakdowns. Once the client has decided on a plan, they *do* the plan and then are guided to *check* whether the plan worked.

FIGURE 19.2. The CO–OP global strategy use process.

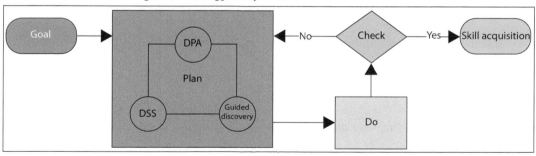

Note. CO–OP = Cognitive Orientation to daily Occupational Performance; DPA = dynamic performance analysis; DSS = domain-specific strategies.

If the plan was performed, the goal was attained, and the skill is acquired, the process is over. What is more likely in the first few iterations is that the plan was either not successful or only partially successful, in which case the client learns that the plan needs modification. The client and therapist return to the planning process, using DPA, and the therapist guides the client to come up with a new plan and reiterate the process as often as is necessary (see Video 19.1, which shows how CO–OP is used). The 2 case examples in this chapter also provide detailed examples of CO–OP administration.

Other Administration Considerations

The CO–OP is always administered with consideration of the individual client, their life context, and the clinical context. The latest CO–OP book (Dawson et al., 2017) provides information about goal-setting in the CO–OP context, using CO–OP with several populations, involving parents and significant others, using CO–OP in a group format, interprofessional application of CO–OP, and CO–OP's place in e-health. In addition, both CO–OP books provide numerous, diverse examples of paper-based tools that may help with administration (Dawson et al., 2017; Polatajko & Mandich, 2004).

Those who use CO–OP in research should ensure treatment fidelity through careful, independent application of the *CO–OP Fidelity Checklist* (McEwen et al., 2018). They should also contact the International CO–OP Academy for support.

Case Example 19.1 (a youth with a childhood-onset movement disorder) and Case Example 19.2 (an adult poststroke) illustrate the use of the CO–OP Approach in pediatric and adult populations.

Goals and Documentation

CO–OP uses a collaborative approach to goal setting, establishing a partnership between the clinician and the client in identifying client-centered performance issues. Client-centered goal setting is critical in CO–OP, because these goals become the focus of the intervention. Moreover, working toward personally meaningful goals promotes skill acquisition, generalization, and transfer, which are objectives of CO–OP.

The goal-setting steps in CO–OP include

- Providing context,

- Identifying occupational performance issues, and

- Translating performance issues into goals.

To involve the client (and family, as appropriate), it is important to include them in the process and start by providing context. That is, explain the process that will be used to develop goals, how the goals will be used, and any limitations to goals (i.e., it should be a goal that can be worked on in the specific practice setting, be that hospital, clinic, home, or community). The Canadian Occupational Performance Measure (COPM; Law et al., 2014) provides structure for documentation of performance issues and as a preintervention and postintervention outcome measure for client-perceived goal performance. The COPM is a semistructured interview to identify performance issues in ADLs and is the preferred tool of CO–OP to enable patients to identify and prioritize everyday issues that limit or affect their performance in everyday living.

Some examples of CO–OP therapy goals include

- Picking up a 2-year-old grandson,

- Getting dishes from the top shelf on the tips of toes,

- Climbing the stairs at a social club to get to the bathroom with 1 rail and no cane,

- Walking from the subway station to work on a busy city street without having to think about it or having to "hop,"

- Carrying a casserole dish to the dining room for family without dropping it,

- Getting up from the floor without support,

- Putting on eyeliner,

- Riding a normal bike without stabilizers,

- Making a sandwich, and

- Carrying a cup of tea and a bowl of cereal.

CASE EXAMPLE 19.1. Carol, a Young Person With Genetic Dystonia

Carol is an 18-year-old who has a 4-limb movement disorder related to a diagnosis of benign hereditary chorea. She also has diagnoses of obsessive–compulsive disorder, anxiety, and EF deficit. In terms of motor severity, Carol is able to walk independently, and dystonia does not affect her lower limbs. She is able to walk in most settings even though she avoids certain environments, such as mechanical escalators, because she is not able to hold on to the rail to go up and down. Dystonia affects mainly her upper limbs and trunk.

In terms of manual function, Carol handles some objects with difficulty, needs help with food preparation, and makes adaptations to chosen ingredients so that the tasks are easier (e.g., using soft margarine rather than butter). As with other clients with dystonia–myoclonus, certain tasks are provocative and trigger dystonia, such as tasks requiring handling liquids, sharp knives, or hot contents from the oven or grill.

Carol's degree of independence therefore is related to the supportiveness of the environmental context. She lives at home with her parents and siblings and is planning to attend university next year, where she will be required to complete activities such as carrying a cup of coffee and making herself simple meals. Carol's functional ability is summarized in Figure 19.3, on the basis of the *International Classification of Functioning, Disability and Health* framework from the World Health Organization (2001).

FIGURE 19.3. Carol's impairments and functional abilities classified by the *ICF* framework.

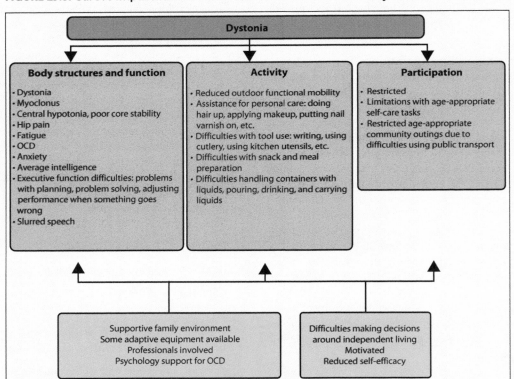

Note. ICF = International Classification of Functioning, Disability and Health (World Health Organization, 2001); OCD = obsessive–compulsive disorder.

(Continued)

CASE EXAMPLE 19.1. Carol, a Young Person With Genetic Dystonia *(Cont.)*

Carol took great care in choosing her intervention goals and offered a rationale for each. Carol wanted to be able to

1. Apply eyeliner and mascara,
2. Carry a cup of coffee and a plate of cookies to her room upstairs,
3. Turn bacon on the grill to make herself a sandwich,
4. Do her hair in a "messy bun," and
5. Pick up a drink and take it to her mouth with 1 hand without spilling.

The first 3 goals were addressed directly in the CO–OP sessions, and the last 2 goals (messy bun and drinking) were used to evaluate transfer and generalization. The COPM and the Performance Quality Rating Scale (PQRS; Martini et al., 2015) were used to establish baseline and postintervention performance levels.

The CO–OP Approach was used with Carol as part of a research project (Gimeno et al., 2018a, 2018b, 2019). Before entering this study, Carol had had considerable experience with cognitive–behavioral therapy. She had received occupational therapy and physical therapy when she was a young child, because she had a diagnosis of CP (which was later disregarded when a genetic cause for her dystonia was discovered).

Given her genetic diagnosis of dystonia, Carol underwent deep brain stimulation surgery to reduce her involuntary movements. Despite the success of the surgery, Carol continued to have performance difficulties and entered the CO–OP study.

All CO–OP intervention sessions took place at Carol's home, with her mother present for most of them. The sessions typically lasted around 1 hour and were held once or twice a week, depending on Carol's and her family's schedules. As per the CO–OP Approach format, the intervention was delivered across 10 treatment sessions, with Session 1 devoted to introducing the GPDC global strategy. The global strategy was used throughout the sessions, as was DPA. In line with the CO–OP Approach's classic format of delivery, goals were introduced 1 at a time. Exhibit 19.1 shows the time spent in each session and the goals Carol and the therapist worked on in each session.

For Carol, the first 4 sessions were dedicated exclusively to her first goal, putting on eyeliner. Even though it is suggested that therapists delivering the CO–OP Approach introduce Goal 2 at about Session 2 or 3, Carol decided it was important for her to achieve Goal 1 before she moved on to her other goals. Because CO–OP is a client-centered approach, Carol and her therapist dedicated more time to working on this goal.

To describe the intervention, Exhibit 19.2 presents an excerpt from Session 5, the first time Carol attempted her goal of carrying a cup of coffee and a plate of cookies. The exhibit outlines the session with verbatim dialogue; the key CO–OP features shown during the session are listed as well.

The excerpt from Session 5 with Carol shows how guided discovery and DPA were used throughout the intervention. At times, guided discovery included a question with 2 possible options (e.g., "Are we looking at the water level inside the cup? Or the position of your hand in relation to the cup?"), and sometimes the question was more general (e.g., "What else could you try?"). The plans were named, and strategy generation happened throughout the session, with plans becoming more sophisticated as they were tried (i.e., the "Do" step of GPDC) and then checked to see whether they worked.

The approach worked well for Carol, and she improved on all her trained goals. Her COPM and PQRS scores, as rated by a blind independent rater, changed greatly over the course of the intervention (see Table 19.1).

The untrained goals (doing a messy hair bun and drinking) did not change significantly when measured objectively, which indicates that generalization and transfer did not take place. However, Carol's performance scores (on the COPM) did achieve clinical significance. The reasons for the lack of an objective improvement in untrained goals are likely multifactorial and may include something as basic as the difficulty in coming up with effective strategies for the magnitude of the performance issues Carol experienced.

(Continued)

CASE EXAMPLE 19.1. Carol, a Young Person With Genetic Dystonia *(Cont.)*

EXHIBIT 19.1. Carol's Goals and Time Spent in CO–OP Sessions

Review of goals postintervention

SESSION	1	2	3	4	5	6	7	8	9	10
	45:12	69:27	57:39	50:23	68:22	71:03	60:08	78:25	48:39	45:46
	Introduction of GPDC	Homework revision	Homework revision	Homework revision	Homework revision	Homework revision	Homework revision	Homework revision	Homework revision	Homework revision
	Eyeliner	Eyeliner	Eyeliner	Eyeliner	Eyeliner	Eyeliner		Eyeliner		
					Carrying a cup of coffee and cookies	Carrying a cup of coffee and cookies	Carrying a cup of coffee and cookies	Carrying a cup of coffee and cookies	Carrying a cup of coffee and cookies	Carrying a cup of coffee and cookies
							Turning bacon and making sandwich	Turning bacon and making sandwich	Turning bacon and making sandwich	
	Homework setup	Homework setup	Homework setup	Homework setup	Homework setup	Homework setup	Homework setup	Homework setup	Homework setup	

Baseline assessments preintervention

Note. Values indicate session duration (in minutes:seconds). CO–OP = Cognitive Orientation to daily Occupational Performance; GPDC = Goal–Plan–Do–Check.

(Continued)

EXHIBIT 19.2. Example of a CO–OP Session and Key Features Used to Work on Goal to Carry Coffee

DIALOGUE	KEY CO–OP FEATURE
Therapist: What do you think is the main problem when carrying a cup of coffee?	Guided discovery
Carol: The way I hold it.	DPA
T: Right, let's think about that. What do you think happens with the way you hold it?	Guided discovery
C: It digs in [handle of the mug on her finger].	DPA
T: Okay, it digs in. So, how many ways can you hold it [the mug]?	Guided discovery
C: I can hold it like this, or like that, or like this [shows therapist ways of holding the mug].	Strategy generation
T: Okay, could we try and hold it in each different way and walk with the mug to see?	Plan generation
C: Yes, let's do that.	Do
T: So, when we try these new plans, what are you going to focus on first?	Check generation
C: The way I hold it.	Guided discovery
T: Okay, we are going to focus on the way you hold it. Are you going to fill the mug to the top with water?	Guided discovery
C: Do I need to?	
T: It is up to you. Are you worried about the hot water?	Guided discovery
C: Yep.	DPA
T: We could try it with cold water first if you want.	Guided discovery
C: [Fills the mug with cold water.]	Do
T: I notice that you picked up the mug with your hand and kept it there to fill it up, but if it would have been hot water, you would have placed it in the sink—is this right?	Guided discovery
C: Yes, the hot water will bring on my jerks and I would spill it, but I don't know why I jerk more if it is hot.	DPA
T: That is what I want us to work on and notice. What happened when you were focusing on your jerk movements when you were doing the mascara?	Guided discovery
C: It was worse.	DPA
T: What happened when you focused on the jerk movements when doing your eyeliner?	Guided discovery
C: That was also worse.	DPA
T: What would happen if you were to focus on the jerky movements when carrying the water?	Guided discovery
C: The movements will be worse.	Transfer
T: What did you think when you just opened that tap to fill the mug now?	Guided discovery
C: Nothing.	

(Continued)

CASE EXAMPLE 19.1. Carol, a Young Person With Genetic Dystonia *(Cont.)*

EXHIBIT 19.2. Example of a CO–OP Session and Key Features Used to Work on Goal to Carry Coffee *(Cont.)*

DIALOGUE	KEY CO–OP FEATURE
T: And your performance was good?	Guided discovery
C: Yes.	Check
T: Did you get water on your hands?	Guided discovery
C: No.	Check
T: Were you worried about getting water on your hands?	Guided discovery
C: Not really . . . because it doesn't matter.	DPA
T: Okay, let's think about how you hold that cup.	Guided discovery
C: Two fingers.	Naming plans
T: We are calling this plan "2 fingers"?	
C: Yes, this is the 2-finger plan [holding mug handle with two fingers].	Do
C: [Performs activity.]	
T: Is it digging in much?	Guided check
C: Yes [shows the therapist].	DPA
T: Why do you think it digs in so much?	Guided DPA
C: I am putting a lot of pressure on it. I am holding it tight.	DPA
T: Okay, so how else can you hold it then?	Guided discovery
C: With the 3-finger plan.	Naming plan
C: [Performs activity.]	Do
C: It does not dig in.	Check
T: Okay, so with the 3-finger plan you did spill it a little bit more, and I notice you were intensely looking at the cup while you were carrying it; what were you thinking?	Guided discovery
C: That I didn't want to spill it. Maybe that is why I did spill it.	DPA
T: Were you thinking, "I don't want to spill it?" Or were you thinking, "The therapist is looking at me"? Or were you not aware of what was going on around you?	Guided discovery
C: I think I was thinking, "I don't want to spill it." Actually, I was thinking, "I am going to spill it."	DPA
T: Right, so you were actually telling yourself, "I am going to spill it, I am going to spill it"?	Affirming DPA
C: Yes.	Affirming DPA

Note. CO–OP = Cognitive Orientation to daily Occupational Performance; DPA = dynamic performance analysis.

(Continued)

CASE EXAMPLE 19.1. Carol, a Young Person With Genetic Dystonia *(Cont.)*

TABLE 19.1. COPM and PQRS Pretest and Posttest Scores for Carol

	SCORE				
	PERFORMANCE			SATISFACTION	
GOAL	PRETEST	POSTTEST		PRETEST	POSTTEST
COPM					
(T) Applying eyeliner	1	5		1	5
(T) Carrying a cup of coffee and cookies	3	6		2	5
(T) Turning bacon on the grill	2	6		2	6
(UT) Doing a messy hair bun	3	5		3	4
(UT) Picking up a drink and drinking	2	4		2	4

	PRETEST		POSTTEST	
GOAL	*M*	*SD*	*M*	*SD*
PQRS				
(T) Applying eyeliner	4.50	1.25	8.17	1.60
(T) Carrying a cup of coffee and cookies	3.03	1.87	6.5	0.55
(T) Turning bacon on the grill	7.62	2.12	8.17	1.33
(UT) Doing a messy hair bun	6.29	0.85	6.5	1.22
(UT) Picking up a drink and drinking	7.48	2.08	8	1.55

Note. COPM = Canadian Occupational Performance Measure; M = mean; PQRS = Performance Quality Rating Scale; SD = standard deviation; (T) = trained; (UT) = untrained.

CASE EXAMPLE 19.2. Roger, a Senior Man With Left-Sided Hemorrhagic Stroke

Roger experienced a left-sided hemorrhagic stroke at 69 years old and presented with right-sided hemiparesis. His upper right extremity was more affected than his lower extremity, and his hand was more affected than his arm. He was walking independently with a single-point cane and was managing the stairs, in a step-to manner, using a railing or wall for support.

Roger had a Montreal Cognitive Assessment (Nasreddine et al., 2005) score of 20/30, suggestive of cognitive impairment, and exhibited decreased EF. Roger frequently gave unrelated answers, was distractible, and had difficulty staying focused on a task. He had difficulty with planning and organizing, sequencing, monitoring performance, exhibiting self-awareness, and concentrating and taking in information. He initially had difficulty in analyzing what was going wrong with a performance, and he had a tendency to be impulsive and try new plans without seeming to have thought them through beforehand.

Roger was 9 months poststroke at the time of entering the CO–OP study and had completed both inpatient and outpatient rehabilitation. He was a pleasant and talkative man. He often needed redirection to stay on topic and had difficulty remembering day-to-day details during his assessment. He described himself as a social person who frequented his local social club and enjoyed having coffee with friends. He lived with a roommate in an

(Continued)

apartment. English was his 2nd language, and he had a limited level of education. Roger did not seem to want to use written materials, possibly because of limited literacy or comprehension of written English.

Roger volunteered to participate in a research study that aimed at combining best evidence for mobility and gait for survivors of stroke using cognitive strategy training (an adaptation of CO–OP), run by a physical therapist and a physical therapy assistant. This program was run in a group setting but provided individualized goal practice and individualized exercise programs based on goals set by the participants. The 8-week active program consisted of 90-minute sessions twice per week.

Each week the participants had 1-on-1 time with the physical therapist for a goal practice session that was designed to work on a specific goal. During these sessions they used GPDC to develop strategies to attain the self-selected goals. Guided discovery instruction was used to support patient strategies and problem solving.

Introduction to Program and Assessment

For this CO–OP-based program, Roger attended 1 60- to 90-minute intervention preparation session with a registered physical therapist before the active intervention. During this session, Roger was taught to use GPDC, which was used throughout the program to support goal acquisition and future goals. After this education session, Roger and the physical therapist used the COPM to establish goals that were important to him. Roger set 3 goals, which he ranked in order of importance. His goals were to be able to

1. Walk around the block at his social club "straight, tall, look forward, confident and no toe catch" with his cane (at first; 10 importance on the COPM scores);
2. Go up the stairs at his local social club 1 foot at a time (reciprocal) without his cane to get to the bathroom upstairs (9 importance); and
3. Rest his head in his hand with his elbow on the table when talking with friends (10 importance).

Dynamic Performance Analysis

Using DPA, the therapist observed Roger's performance. Roger's plan was to go up the stairs reciprocally. His performance was not competent, in that he was not able to complete stair climbing in a reciprocal fashion. Roger reviewed his performance going up and down the stairs in a nonreciprocal pattern and was able to verbalize, "As I come up I put this [foot] then 'relax' a little bit, then put this [foot] up."

The therapist clarified with Roger that when he said "relax" he meant bend his knee, to which he replied, "Bend until I put force to straighten up." Roger named this domain-specific cognitive strategy "bend–relax" and continued to use it to practice stair climbing. He improved within the same 20-minute goal practice session, in particular in movement quality and confidence.

Once Roger had gained some confidence using his bend–relax strategy, the therapist guided him to discover that he was leaning to the left and depending heavily on the railing rather than transferring his weight over his right leg. The therapist asked, "Do you think you would be able to have more weight on your right leg if you used both railings for added support?" This is an example of direct guided discovery. The therapist used this approach because the client was having difficulty when less-leading questions were asked.

Roger agreed that this approach might help, and he agreed to try. After doing the task again using 2 railings, Roger was able to use this supplemental knowledge to get the feeling of a more equal distribution of weight. He was able to take this new knowledge ("this feeling") and attempt the stairs again without using the 2nd railing.

Continuing to use guided discovery for feedback purposes, the therapist asked, "How did that go?" Roger was able to identify that he wanted to be more "even." The therapist asked, "How will you know if you are 'even' or not?" Roger was able to identify that the distance from the railing provided him feedback. He often had to do the task multiple times before being able to respond to questions about his performance. (See Table 19.2 for an example of guided discovery and domain-specific strategies.)

(Continued)

TABLE 19.2. Example of Guided Discovery and Domain-Specific Strategies for Roger

GOAL: GO UPSTAIRS (AND DOWN)	DYNAMIC PERFORMANCE ANALYSIS	GUIDED DISCOVERY	DOMAIN-SPECIFIC STRATEGIES
First focus: to secure the knee before taking a step	Roger thought that it was okay but that it was not perfect. He established that if he practiced more he could get better. He had difficulty expressing specifically *what* would make it better with practice. Generally, he knew what to do and used his domain-specific strategies.		*Attention to doing:* To Roger, "bend–relax" meant to pay attention to the knee before taking the next step to make sure it was strong enough to hold him and then "put force to straighten it up" to get up the stair.
Second focus: to increase weight on right leg (lateral shift)	Roger was able to identify that he was leaning on the handrail quite a bit.	*Therapist:* "Do you think you are putting the same amount of weight over each leg?" *Roger:* "Let me try. [He needed to do the task again to assess.] No, I put more on this one [left]." *T:* "Is there a way you can tell if you are putting more—or less—weight on your right leg?" *R:* [After another attempt to assess] "Ah, [lean] less on the bar [railing]."	*Supplement task-knowledge strategy to establish "feeling the movement":* For lateral weight shifting, Roger was encouraged to use both railings to get a "feel" for having more weight on the right leg. Later he was able to use *body position* by paying attention to the distance between him and the railing.

In the early stages of Roger's occupational therapy work, he frequently requested validation for his performance from the therapist. He was encouraged to evaluate himself first (check), and then the therapist would use guided discovery to help Roger identify the difference between one attempt and another. The therapist would ask, "How did that feel?" or, "Did one attempt feel better than the other?" This would provoke a conversation about what made the attempts different from each other and could support strategy development and solidification for Roger.

Roger became much more confident in self-evaluation throughout the program and progressively needed less and less guidance. He later explained how he was able to use the same strategies in other actions: He used bend–relax when walking and used how close he was to the armrest on a chair to shift his weight when moving from sitting to standing. He was explaining skill transfer, which is 1 of the desired outcomes of the CO–OP Approach.

To track progress, the therapist used the COPM. This was tested before the intervention, after the intervention, and at follow-up but was also administered at the midpoint of the program. Although the therapist rated Roger's performance on walking as an 8/10 at follow-up, Roger was completely satisfied with his improvement on the stairs and rated his performance and satisfaction with performance as 10/10. His COPM scores for his 2 other goals also improved (see Table 19.3).

Objective measures showed that Roger improved his gait speed, endurance, and balance. He also improved on a measure intended to assess transfer of skill. Roger improved after the program and continued to improve at follow-up 1 month later (see Table 19.4).

(Continued)

CASE EXAMPLE 19.2. Roger, a Senior Man With Left-Sided Hemorrhagic Stroke *(Cont.)*

TABLE 19.3. Roger's COPM Scores for Each Goal

GOAL	COPM PERFORMANCE SCORE			COPM SATISFACTION SCORE		
	PRETEST	POSTTEST	FOLLOW-UP	PRETEST	POSTTEST	FOLLOW-UP
Walk	6.5	8	8	6.5	8	8
Stairs	7	9	10	8	9	10
Rest head in hand	6	8	10	8.5	8	10

Note. COPM = Canadian Occupational Performance Measure.

TABLE 19.4. Roger's Progress on 4 Standard Outcome Measures

OUTCOME	MCID OR MDC	PRETEST	POSTTEST	FOLLOW-UP
5-meter walk test (m/s)	MCID = 0.16	0.31	0.56[a]	0.53[b]
6-minute walk test (m)	MCID = 34.4	128.7	170[a]	175[b]
Berg Balance Scale (Berg et al., 1989)	MDC = 4.7	43/56	51/56[a]	51/56[b]
Community Balance and Mobility Scale (Howe et al., 2006)	MDC = 8	17/96	20/96	26/96[b]

Note. m = meters; MCID = minimal clinically important difference; MDC = minimal detectable change; m/s = meters per second.
[a]Change score was greater than or equal to the MCID or MDC from pretest to posttest. [b]Change score was greater than or equal to MCID from posttest to follow-up.

Highlighting Successes

Roger did not initially catch on to GPDC in a formal way—that is, he did not often use the specific words. However, GPDC is what he was doing. He would frequently say, "Let me do it again," and would check what he was doing and then make a plan to either adjust or think about the strategy that he came up with (bend–relax–bend–relax).

At first Roger needed a lot of validation from the therapist. He was unable to assess on his own and asked the therapist for feedback. The guided discovery did not just help with strategy development but also helped him learn how to self-evaluate—in other words, to use DPA.

A main objective of the CO–OP Approach is that clients learn to use the global cognitive strategy GPDC to establish and attain new goals in the future using problem-solving strategies. Short-term and long-term goals are not specifically outlined in CO–OP. Instead, clients set their main activity goals, usually 3, for the full CO–OP program after the COPM interview. Some of these goals may be accomplished relatively quickly, and others require a much longer time. In all cases, setting the performance plan involves establishing subgoals (possibly short-term goals); multiple such goals are set multiple times—often within a single session.

Because CO–OP is used in many different settings and with all types of clients, there is no standard for documentation at this time. We recommend that occupational therapists adhere to institutional standards. Nonetheless, we offer the following general guidelines, and we recommend that clinicians establish a method for documentation that is best suited to their specific setting (see Exhibit 19.3 for the documentation method that worked best for Roger, the patient in Case Example 19.2).

Components of CO–OP to consider when documenting are as follows:

- Clearly define client-centered, meaningful goals.

- Identify a specific intervention developed to achieve the client's chosen goals and goal-specific interventions.

- Outline how you will assess and monitor goal achievement (i.e., COPM or another tool?).

- Document baseline scores (COPM, PQRS, other), progress scores, and discharge scores.

EXHIBIT 19.3. Roger's Case Documentation Using the SOAP Format

CATEGORY	NOTE
Subjective The aim in the Subjective section is to clearly identify the goal of the intervention. This is also an opportunity to document the patient's strategy if one has been developed (e.g., "lift knee" or "step higher").	Patient goal: To walk without toe catching. Patient states he continues to do his walking program but is not thinking about how to improve his toe catch while walking.
Objective In the Objective section, the therapist can document the DPA from their own perspective. CO–OP discourages a primary impairment focus but recognizes that impairment issues may come into play during performance breakdowns. Potentially relevant impairment issues can be noted here. A notable variance from the traditional SOAP format is the inclusion of patient quotes and narrative in the treatment section. It is important to note that the discussions, planning, and guided discovery are all part of the problem-solving treatment approach to achieve generalization and transfer of skills as well as goal attainment. Thus, they should be included in the intervention section of documentation.	Patient is ambulating with a cane, right toe catches, heels touch with most steps, and right leg is in external rotation. Rx: Patient practiced stairs, was able to complete without rails. Identified that patient is capable to lift his leg and foot. Education provided around transfer of skill from stairs to walking as well as the concept of having to think about something while learning a new skill before it can become automatic. Patient has been struggling with, "This is how I always walked," "I didn't used to have to think about it." Patient identified *cognitive strategy* to "choose to lift my foot" with walking.
Assessment	Patient is reluctant to change, continually refers to therapist ("You tell me what to do"). Patient is able to lift his foot, will need to continue to develop strategies and task-specific practice to achieve goal to decrease toe catching, increase endurance with walking without toe catch.
Plan	Current focus is to develop self-evaluation skills. Homework is to focus on strategy to "choose to lift my foot" and continue with walking program.

Note. Rx = prescription; SOAP = Subjective, Objective, Assessment, Plan.

- Document strategies that worked well and those that have been abandoned.

- Document in the patient's own words whenever possible (because this is usually part of the strategy).

- Be descriptive in sharing successful strategies so others can replicate.

Intervention Considerations

CO–OP is an overarching approach to how occupational therapists interact with and empower clients to learn and develop independent problem-solving skills while acquiring a selected goal or skill, and it is therefore very broadly useful. As mentioned in the "Target Population" section, there are client prerequisites for CO–OP, in that clients must have sufficient cognition, communication, and behavioral responsiveness to benefit from CO–OP. If they do not meet these prerequisites, then another approach should be considered. A key feature of the CO–OP Approach is the DPA.

Using CO–OP's key feature, DPA, occupational therapists are able to identify what type of intervention would best address specific performance breakdown issues, whether they be motivational, cognitive, environmental, or capacity building.

CO–OP therapists intervene to increase motivation if the client does not want to do the task, by supplementing information if the client does not know how to do the task, by altering the occupational and environmental supports if they are insufficient, and by working to improve capacity if the client is not able to do the task.

Any of these interventions may involve using other approaches in conjunction with CO–OP. Even an impairment reduction or capacity-building intervention, such as strength training, can fall under the umbrella of the CO–OP Approach as long as it is evidence based and task specific. In addition, the therapist must ensure that the client understands that the conjunctional treatment or exercises are supporting their acquisition of personally meaningful goals and agrees to incorporate them into the plan.

Despite a growing body of evidence with different populations, there are several conditions for which no CO–OP studies are available. Although the theoretical framework underpinning CO–OP suggests it might be effective with diverse populations, it also suggests that there are populations for whom it may not be the most appropriate approach to use. For example, CO–OP is a highly verbally based intervention and therefore requires adaptations or may not be appropriate for use with clients who have no means of communicating. CO–OP requires the engagement of the client and may require adaptations or may not be appropriate for clients who cannot be engaged. Finally, CO–OP requires the use of cognition and may require adaptations or may not be appropriate for clients who have very low cognitive abilities.

References

Aarnoudse-Moens, C. S., Smidts, D. P., Oosterlaan, J., Duivenvoorden, H. J., & Weisglas-Kuperus, N. (2009). Executive function in very preterm children at early school age. *Journal of Abnormal Child Psychology, 37*, 981–993. https://doi.org/10.1007/s10802-009-9327-z.

Ahn, S. N., Yoo, E. Y., Jung, M. Y., Park, H. Y., Lee, J. Y., & Choi, Y. I. (2017). Comparison of Cognitive Orientation to daily Occupational Performance and conventional occupational therapy on occupational performance in individuals with stroke: A randomized controlled trial. *NeuroRehabilitation, 40*, 285–292. https://doi.org/10.3233/NRE-161416

Berg, K., Wood-Dauphine, S., Williams, J. I., & Gayton, D. (1989). Measuring balance in the elderly: Preliminary development of an instrument. *Physiotherapy Canada, 41*, 304–311. https://doi.org/10.3138/ptc.41.6.304

Blank, R., Smits-Engelsman, B., Polatajko, H., Wilson, P., & European Academy for Childhood Disability. (2012). European Academy for Childhood Disability (EACD): Recommendations on the definition, diagnosis and intervention of developmental coordination disorder (long version). *Developmental Medicine and Child Neurology, 54*, 54–93. https://doi.org/10.1111/j.1469-8749.2011.04171.x

Cameron, D., Craig, T., Edwards, B., Missiuna, C., Schwellnus, H., & Polatajko, H. J. (2017). Cognitive Orientation to daily Occupational Performance (CO–OP): A new approach for children with cerebral palsy. *Physical and Occupational Therapy in Pediatrics, 37*, 183–198. https://doi.org/10.1080/01942638.2016.1185500

Coenen, M. A., Eggink, H., Tijssen, M. A., & Spikman, J. M. (2018). Cognition in childhood dystonia: A systematic review. *Developmental Medicine and Child Neurology, 60*, 244–255. https://doi.org/10.1111/dmcn.13632

Crajé, C., Aarts, P., Nijhuis-van der Sanden, M., & Steenbergen, B. (2010). Action planning in typically and atypically developing children (unilateral cerebral palsy). *Research in Developmental Disabilities, 31*, 1039–1046. https://doi.org/10.1016/j.ridd.2010.04.007

Cramer, S. C., Sur, M., Dobkin, B. H., O'Brien, C., Sanger, T. D., Trojanowski, J. Q., . . . Vinogradov, S. (2011). Harnessing neuroplasticity for clinical applications. *Brain, 134*, 1591–1609. https://doi.org/10.1093/brain/awr039

Dawson, D. R., Anderson, N. D., Binns, M. A., Bottari, C., Damianakis, T., Hunt, A., . . . Zwarenstein, M. (2013). Managing executive dysfunction following acquired brain injury and stroke using an ecologically valid rehabilitation approach: A study protocol for a randomized, controlled trial. *Trials, 14*, 306. https://doi.org/10.1186/1745-6215-14-306

Dawson, D. R., Binns, M. A., Hunt, A., Lemsky, C., & Polatajko, H. J. (2013). Occupation-based strategy training for adults with traumatic brain injury: A pilot study. *Archives of Physical Medicine and Rehabilitation, 94*, 1959–1963. https://doi.org/10.1016/j.apmr.2013.05.021

Dawson, D. R., Gaya, A., Hunt, A., Levine, B., Lemsky, C., & Polatajko, H. J. (2009). Using the Cognitive Orientation to Occupational Performance (CO–OP) with adults with executive dysfunction following traumatic brain injury. *Canadian Journal of Occupational Therapy, 76*, 115–127. https://doi.org/10.1177/000841740907600209

Dawson, D. R., McEwen, S. E., & Polatajko, H. J. (Eds.). (2017). *Cognitive Orientation to daily Occupational Performance in occupational therapy*. Bethesda, MD: AOTA Press.

Dawson, D., Richardson, J., Troyer, A., Binns, M., Clark, A., Polatajko, H., . . . Bar, Y. (2014). An occupation-based strategy training approach to managing age-related executive changes: A pilot randomized controlled trial. *Clinical Rehabilitation, 28*, 118–127. https://doi.org/10.1177/0269215513492541

Dayan, E., & Cohen, L. G. (2011). Neuroplasticity subserving motor skill learning. *Neuron, 72*, 443–454. https://doi.org/10.1016/j.neuron.2011.10.008

Diaz Heijtz, R., & Forssberg, H. (2015). Translational studies exploring neuroplasticity associated with motor skill learning and the regulatory role of the dopamine system. *Developmental Medicine and Child Neurology, 57*(Suppl. 2), 10–14. https://doi.org/10.1111/dmcn.12692

Friel, K. M., Kuo, H. C., Fuller, J., Ferre, C. L., Brandão, M., Carmel, J. B., . . . Gordon, A. M. (2016). Skilled bimanual training drives motor cortex plasticity in children with unilateral cerebral palsy. *Neurorehabilitation and Neural Repair, 30*, 834–844. https://doi.org/10.1177/1545968315625838

Gharebaghy, S., Rassafiani, M., & Cameron, D. (2015). Effect of cognitive intervention on children with ADHD. *Physical and Occupational Therapy in Pediatrics, 35*, 13–23. https://doi.org/10.3109/01942638.2014.957428

Ghorbani, N., Rassafiani, M., Izadi-Najafabadi, S., Yazdani, F., Akbarfahimi, N., Havaei, N., & Gharebaghy, S. (2017). Effectiveness of Cognitive Orientation to (daily) Occupational Performance (CO–OP) on children with cerebral palsy: A mixed design. *Research in Developmental Disabilities, 71*, 24–34. https://doi.org/10.1016/j.ridd.2017.09.007

Gimeno, H., Brown, R. G., Lin, J.-P., Cornelius, V., & Polatajko, H. J. (2019). Cognitive approach to rehabilitation in children with hyperkinetic movement disorders post-DBS. *Neurology, 92*(11), e1212–e1224. http://doi.org/10.1212/WNL.0000000000007092

Gimeno, H., Brown, R., Lin, J. P., & Polatajko, H. (2016). Functional skills acquisition following cognitive based intervention after deep brain stimulation in children with hyperkinetic movement disorders: Results of 6 multiple baseline design experiments. *Developmental Medicine and Child Neurology, 58*(Suppl. 1), 2–18.

Gimeno, H., Polatajko, H., Cornelius, V., Lin, J. P., & Brown, G. B. (2018a). Protocol for N-of-1 trials proof of concept for rehabilitation of childhood-onset dystonia: Study 1. *Canadian Journal of Occupational Therapy, 85*, 242–254. https://doi.org/10.1177/0008417417707532

Gimeno, H., Polatajko, H., Cornelius, V., Lin, J. P., & Brown, G. B. (2018b). Protocol for N-of-1 trials with replications across therapists for childhood-onset dystonia rehabilitation: Study 2. *Canadian Journal of Occupational Therapy, 85*, 255–260. https://doi.org/10.1177/0008417417707734

Halayko, J., Magill-Evans, J., Smith, V., & Polatajko, H. (2016). Enabling 2-wheeled cycling for youth with Down syndrome. *Pediatric Physical Therapy, 28*, 224–230. https://doi.org/10.1097/PEP.0000000000000240

Hallett, M. (2005). Neuroplasticity and rehabilitation. *Journal of Rehabilitation Research and Development, 42*, xvii–xxii.

Henshaw, E., Polatajko, H., McEwen, S., Ryan, J. D., & Baum, C. M. (2011). Cognitive approach to improving participation after stroke: Two case studies. *American Journal of Occupational Therapy, 65*, 55–63. https://doi.org/10.5014/ajot.2011.09010

Houldin, A., McEwen, S. E., Howell, M. W., & Polatajko, H. (2018). The Cognitive Orientation to daily Occupational Performance approach and transfer: A scoping review. *OTJR: Occupation, Participation and Health, 38*, 157–172. https://doi.org/10.1177/1539449217736059

Howe, J. A., Inness, E. L., Venturini, A., Williams, J. I., & Verrier, M. C. (2006). The Community Balance and Mobility Scale: A balance measure for individuals with traumatic brain injury. *Clinical Rehabilitation, 20*(10), 885–895.

Ismail, F. Y., Fatemi, A., & Johnston, M. V. (2017). Cerebral plasticity: Windows of opportunity in the developing brain. *European Journal* of *Paediatric Neurology, 21,* 23–48. https://doi.org/10.1016/j.ejpn.2016.07.007

Jackman, M., Novak, I., & Lannin, N. (2014). Effectiveness of hand splints in children with cerebral palsy: A systematic review with meta-analysis. *Developmental Medicine and Child Neurology, 56,* 138–147. https://doi.org/10.1111/dmcn.12205

Jackman, M., Novak, I., Lannin, N., & Froude, E. (2017). Parents' experience of undertaking an intensive Cognitive Orientation to daily Occupational Performance (CO–OP) group for children with cerebral palsy. *Disability and Rehabilitation, 39,* 1018–1024. https://doi.org/10.1080/09638288.2016.1179350

Kirkpatrick, E. V., Pearse, J. E., Eyre, J. A., & Basu, A. P. (2013). Motor planning ability is not related to lesion side or functional manual ability in children with hemiplegic cerebral palsy. *Experimental Brain Research, 231,* 239–247. https://doi.org/10.1007/s00221-013-3687-x

Kirton, A. (2013). Modeling developmental plasticity after perinatal stroke: Defining central therapeutic targets in cerebral palsy. *Pediatric Neurology, 48,* 81–94. https://doi.org/10.1016/j.pediatrneurol.2012.08.001

Kolb, B., & Muhammad, A. (2014). Harnessing the power of neuroplasticity for intervention. *Frontiers in Human Neuroscience, 8,* 377. https://doi.org/10.3389/fnhum.2014.00377

Law, M., Baptiste, S., McColl, M. A., Opzoomer, A., Polatajko, H., & Pollock, N. (2014). *The Canadian Occupational Performance Measure.* Ottawa: CAOT Publications.

Martini, R., Rios, J., Polatajko, H., Wolf, T., & McEwen, S. (2015). The Performance Quality Rating Scale (PQRS): Reliability, convergent validity, and internal responsiveness for two scoring systems. *Disability and Rehabilitation, 37,* 231–238. https://doi.org/10.3109/09638288.2014.913702

McEwen, S. (2009). *Using the Cognitive Orientation to daily Occupational Performance (CO–OP) treatment approach with adults with stroke: Efficacy and adaptations.* Doctoral dissertation, University of Toronto.

McEwen, S., Cirone, D., & Lee, B. (2017). Incorporating a cognitive strategy approach into an outpatient stroke physiotherapy programme: Case report. *Physiotherapy Canada, 69,* 193–196. https://doi.org/10.3138/ptc.2016-13

McEwen, S. E., Donald, M., Dawson, D., Egan, M. Y., Hunt, A., Quant, S., . . . Linkewich, E. (2015). A multi-faceted knowledge translation approach to support persons with stroke and cognitive impairment: Evaluation protocol. *Implementation Science, 10,* 157. https://doi.org/10.1186/s13012-015-0346-6

McEwen, S. E., Huijbregts, M. P., Ryan, J. D., & Polatajko, H. J. (2009). Cognitive strategy use to enhance motor skill acquisition post-stroke: A critical review. *Brain Injury, 23,* 263–277. https://doi.org/10.1080/02699050902788493.

McEwen, S., Polatajko, H., Baum, C., Rios, J., Cirone, D., Doherty, M., & Wolf, T. (2015). Combined cognitive-strategy and task-specific training improve transfer to untrained activities in subacute stroke: An exploratory randomized controlled trial. *Neurorehabilitation and Neural Repair, 29,* 526–536. https://doi.org/10.1177/1545968314558602

McEwen, S. E., Polatajko, H. J., Davis, J. A., Huijbregts, M., & Ryan, J. D. (2010). "There's a real plan here, and I am responsible for that plan": Participant experiences with a novel cognitive-based treatment approach for adults living with chronic stroke. *Disability and Rehabilitation, 32,* 540–550. https://doi.org/10.3109/09638280903180189

McEwen, S. E., Polatajko, H. J., Huijbregts, M. P., & Ryan, J. D. (2009). Exploring a cognitive-based treatment approach to improve motor-based skill performance in chronic stroke: Results of three single case experiments. *Brain Injury, 23,* 1041–1053. https://doi.org/10.3109/02699050903421107

McEwen, S. E., Polatajko, H. J., Huijbregts, M. P., & Ryan, J. D. (2010). Inter-task transfer of meaningful, functional skills following a cognitive-based treatment: Results of three multiple baseline design experiments in adults with chronic stroke.

Neuropsychological Rehabilitation, 20, 541–561. https://doi.org/10.1080/09602011003638194

McEwen, S. E., Polatajko, H. J., Wolf, T., & Baum, C. (2018). CO–OP *Fidelity Checklist.* Retrieved from http://www.co-opacademy.ca/wp-content/uploads/2018/04/CO–OP-Fidelity-Checklist-Apr-4-2018.pdf

Meichenbaum, D. (1977). *Cognitive-behavior modification: An integrative approach.* New York: Plenum Press.

Miller, L. T., Polatajko, H. J., Missiuna, C., Mandich, A. D., & Macnab, J. J. (2001). A pilot trial of a cognitive treatment for children with developmental coordination disorder. *Human Movement Science, 20,* 183–210. https://doi.org/10.1016/S0167-9457(01)00034-3

Missiuna, C., DeMatteo, C., Hanna, S., Mandich, A., Law, M., Mahoney, W., & Scott, L. (2010). Exploring the use of cognitive intervention for children with acquired brain injury. *Physical and Occupational Therapy in Pediatrics, 30,* 205–219. https://doi.org/10.3109/01942631003761554

Nahum, M., Lee, H., & Merzenich, M. M. (2013). Principles of neuroplasticity-based rehabilitation. *Progress in Brain Research, 207,* 141–171. https://doi.org/10.1016/B978-0-444-63327-9.00009-6

Nasreddine, Z. S., Phillips, N. A., Bédirian, V., Charbonneau, S., Whitehead, V., Collin, I., . . . Chertkow, H. (2005). The Montreal Cognitive Assessment, MoCA: A brief screening tool for mild cognitive impairment. *Journal of the American Geriatrics Society, 53,* 695–699. https://doi.org/10.1111/j.1532-5415.2005.53221.x

Nava, E., & Röder, B. (2011). Adaptation and maladaptation insights from brain plasticity. *Progress in Brain Research, 191,* 177–194. https://doi.org/10.1016/B978-0-444-53752-2.00005-9

Ng, E. M., Polatajko, H. J., Marziali, E., Hunt, A., & Dawson, D. R. (2013). Telerehabilitation for addressing executive dysfunction after traumatic brain injury. *Brain Injury, 27,* 548–564. https://doi.org/10.3109/02699052.2013.766927

Pirila, S., Van der Meere, J. J., Rantanen, K., Jokiluoma, M., & Eriksson, K. (2011). Executive functions in youth with spastic cerebral palsy. *Journal of Child Neurology, 26,* 817–821. https://doi.org/10.1177/0883073810392584

Polatajko, H., & Mandich, A. (2004). *Enabling occupation in children: The Cognitive Orientation to daily Occupational Performance (CO–OP) Approach.* Ottawa: CAOT Publications.

Polatajko, H. J., McEwen, S. E., Ryan, J. D., & Baum, C. M. (2012). Pilot randomized controlled trial investigating cognitive strategy use to improve goal performance after stroke. *American Journal of Occupational Therapy, 66,* 104–109. https://doi.org/10.5014/ajot.2012.001784

Poulin, V., Korner-Bitensky, N., Bherer, L., Lussier, M., & Dawson, D. R. (2017). Comparison of two cognitive interventions for adults experiencing executive dysfunction post-stroke: A pilot study. *Disability and Rehabilitation, 39,* 1–13. https://doi.org/10.3109/09638288.2015.1123303

Scammell, E. M., Bates, S. V., Houldin, A., & Polatajko, H. J. (2016). The Cognitive Orientation to daily Occupational Performance (CO–OP): A scoping review. *Canadian Journal of Occupational Therapy, 83,* 216–225. https://doi.org/10.1177/0008417416651277

Skidmore, E. R. (2014). Activity interventions for cognitive problems. *Pediatric Blood and Cancer, 61,* 1743–1746. https://doi.org/10.1002/pbc.24781

Skidmore, E. R. (2015). Training to optimize learning after traumatic brain injury. *Current Physical Medicine and Rehabilitation Reports, 3,* 99–105. https://doi.org/10.1007/s40141-015-0081-6

Skidmore, E. R., Dawson, D. R., Butters, M. A., Grattan, E. S., Juengst, S. B., Whyte, E. M., . . . Becker, J. T. (2015). Strategy training shows promise for addressing disability in the first 6 months after stroke. *Neurorehabilitation and Neural Repair, 29,* 668–676. https://doi.org/10.1177/1545968314562113

Skidmore, E. R., Dawson, D. R., Whyte, E. M., Butters, M. A., Dew, M. A., Grattan, E. S., . . . Holm, M. B. (2014). Developing complex interventions: Lessons learned from a pilot study examining strategy training in acute stroke rehabilitation. *Clinical Rehabilitation, 28,* 378–387. https://doi.org/10.1177/0269215513502799

Skidmore, E. R., Holm, M. B., Whyte, E. M., Dew, M. A., Dawson, D., & Becker, J. T. (2011). The feasibility of meta-cognitive strategy training in acute inpatient stroke rehabilitation: Case report. *Neuropsychological Rehabilitation, 21,* 208–223. https://doi.org/10.1080/09602011.2011.552559

Skidmore, E. R., McEwen, S. E., Green, D., Van Den Houten, J., Dawson, D. R., & Polatajko, H. J. (2017). Essential elements and key features of the CO–OP Approach. In D. R. Dawson, S. E. McEwen, & H. J. Polatajko (Eds.), *Cognitive Orientation to daily Occupational Performance in occupational therapy: Using the CO–OP Approach to enable participation across the lifespan* (pp. 11–20). Bethesda, MD: AOTA Press.

Skidmore, E. R., Swafford, M., Juengst, S. B. & Terhorst, L. (2018). Self-awareness and recovery of independence with strategy training. *American Journal of Occupational Therapy, 72,* 7201345010. https://doi.org/10.5014/ajot.2018.023556

Skidmore, E. R., Whyte, E. M., Butters, M. A., Terhorst, L., & Reynolds, C. F., III. (2015). Strategy training during inpatient rehabilitation may prevent apathy symptoms after acute stroke. *PM&R, 7,* 562–570. https://doi.org/10.1016/j.pmrj.2014.12.010

Steenbergen, B., Jongbloed-Pereboom, M., Spruijt, S., & Gordon, A. M. (2013). Impaired motor planning and motor imagery in children with unilateral spastic cerebral palsy: Challenges for the future of pediatric rehabilitation. *Developmental Medicine and Child Neurology, 55*(Suppl. 4), 43–46. https://doi.org/10.1111/dmcn.12306

Townsend, E., Stanton, S., Law, M., Polatajko, H., Baptiste, S., Thompson-Franson, T., . . . Campanile, L. (1997). *Enabling occupation: An occupational therapy perspective.* Ottawa: CAOT Publications.

Wolf, T. J., Polatajko, H., Baum, C., Rios, J., Cirone, D., Doherty, M., & McEwen, S. (2016). Combined cognitive-strategy and task-specific training affects cognition and upper-extremity function in sub-acute stroke: An exploratory randomized controlled trial. *American Journal of Occupational Therapy, 70,* 7002290010. https://doi.org/10.5014/ajot.2016.017293

World Health Organization. (2001). *International classification of functioning, disability and health.* Geneva: Author.

20

The Multicontext Approach

CHELSEA J. STEINBERG, MS, OTR/L, AND SHARON ZLOTNIK, PhD, OTR/L

LEARNING OBJECTIVES

After completing this chapter, readers should be able to

- Describe the Multicontext (MC) Approach framework;
- Identify the MC treatment components, including the use of multiple environments, task analysis and establishment of criteria for transfer, metacognitive strategy training, processing strategies, and relation of new information to previously learned knowledge or skills;
- Understand guided questioning to promote client-directed strategy generation and transfer of strategies to control cognitive performance errors across a variety of contexts and activities;
- Apply, manipulate, and structure a wide range of functional–cognitive treatment activities to optimize clients' autonomy and efficiency with complex functional tasks; and
- Discuss mediation and pretask–posttask questioning to promote self-awareness and generalization of strategy use across all functional activities.

KEY TERMS AND CONCEPTS

- Metacognition • Self-awareness • Strategy training

Intervention Introduction

The Multicontext (MC) Approach is a strategy-based intervention using a metacognitive framework that was first described as an alternative to traditional remedial or deficit-specific approaches (Toglia, 1991). It is based on the Dynamic Interactional Model of cognition, in which therapists analyze and manipulate both external factors (e.g., environment, context, activity demands) and internal factors (e.g., the person's characteristics, processing strategies, metacognition) to optimize clients' learning and generalization of performance in various tasks and environments (Toglia, 1992, 2018).

The MC Approach provides the therapist with guidelines for facilitating and training strategy use, self-awareness, self-monitoring, and self-regulatory skills across everyday activities to treat a wide range of functional–cognitive lapses that interfere with daily life (Toglia, 2018). *Strategy training* reflects a treatment that involves helping a person recognize and manage cognitive performance errors by promoting use of effective strategies and self-monitoring skills in functional–cognitive

tasks and helping them to understand and manage their cognitive symptoms using general questions to guide self-discovery of strategies and problem solving (Toglia, 2017).

To facilitate clients' ability to transfer a learned strategy and eventually generalize it to real-life performance, the MC Approach begins training at the client's current level of functioning and progresses gradually along a 4-level transfer continuum (near transfer, intermediate, far, and very far). At each level of transfer, the treatment program progresses horizontally to enhance transfer of strategies to different activities that have the same or very similar cognitive demands. Movement from 1 level of transfer to another occurs when the client can independently apply the targeted strategy to a variety of tasks. Studies have shown that this approach is most successful when the client uses strategies at least 90% of the time during functional or structured activities and tasks (Toglia, 1991).

Treatment involves helping a person recognize and manage cognitive performance errors, such as omissions, skipped steps, unnecessary actions, or repetitions, by promoting use of effective strategies and self-monitoring skills in functional–cognitive tasks

(Toglia, 2017). The occupational therapist analyzes the performance errors observed during treatment with the client through guided questions or mediation, helping the client realize that the same error patterns interfere with performance across different situations. As awareness emerges, the client is encouraged to self-discover the appropriate strategy to overcome performance errors and to regulate, monitor, and control their performance (Toglia & Kirk, 2000; Toglia et al., 2012).

As treatment progresses and **self-awareness** (i.e., a dynamic relationship among knowledge about the task demands, the context of a situation, and beliefs about one's own ability) emerges, treatment activities become less structured. The client is also encouraged to identify similar treatment activities that mimic real-life functional activities. This has been shown to increase motivation and engagement, providing a closer resemblance to the client's daily life experiences. Toglia (2018) gives a detailed description of the MC concepts and theoretical basis.

Target Population

The MC Approach is suitable for adults, adolescents, and children with cognitive conditions that impede information processing, learning, and brain functioning. This includes spatial neglect (Toglia, 2011), visual–perceptual or object-recognition deficits (Perez et al., 1996; Toglia, 1989), executive function (EF) deficits, and memory deficits (Toglia et al., 2010). The literature has shown that an MC Approach can be used with clients who have a variety of neurological diagnoses and injuries, including

- Stroke (Toglia & Cermak, 2009),

- Traumatic brain injury (Toglia, 1991; Toglia et al., 2010, 2011; Zlotnik et al., 2009),

- Multiple sclerosis (Birnboim & Miller, 2004),

- Lupus (Harrison et al., 2005),

- Parkinson's disease (Foster et al., 2018),

- Mild cognitive impairment (Robnett & Toglia, 2015),

- Attention deficits (Cermak & Toglia, 2018), and

- Mental health conditions (Josman & Regev, 2018; So et al., 1997).

The MC Approach is particularly useful for clients with subtle or mild cognitive deficits. However, it has been successfully used with individuals who show moderate cognitive deficits as well.

Treatment can be conducted in a range of settings, including but not limited to inpatient, acute rehabilitation, and subacute settings as well as outpatient programs, community settings, and educational services. Waldman-Levi and Obermeyer (2018) recently described the use of the MC Approach in a school-based

setting for children with executive dysfunction. Literature also shows that the MC Approach has been integrated in group programs with various populations, including participants with mental health conditions (Josman & Regev, 2018) and women with lupus (Harrison et al., 2005).

Administration

Although specialized training or certification is not required, therapists need to have background knowledge in the Dynamic Interactional Model, cognition, and EF components. They must also be familiar with MC Approach guidelines, which focus on optimizing strategy use, self-awareness, and self-monitoring across functional activities. Implementation of the MC Approach requires the ability to

- Analyze functional–cognitive performance, including patterns of cognitive errors as well as task methods or strategies used;

- Understand the dimensions of **metacognition** (including self-monitoring and self-awareness), which involves a declarative knowledge about learning processes, the subjective assessments of ongoing cognitive activities, and the regulation of current activities (Roebers, 2017);

- Be proficient in the use of mediation or guided questions to facilitate performance; and

- Use a variety of cognitive–functional activities that are structured along a horizontal transfer continuum.

In addition, a key part of intervention is building self-efficacy and focusing on the methods that help the client understand and manage their cognitive symptoms. This requires skill in forming a close collaborative relationship and therapeutic alliance. Additional resources offer more in-depth theoretical explanation of the background, training, and administration of the MC Approach (Toglia, 2011, 2017, 2018). A manual with background and full intervention guidelines and worksheets is in progress (Toglia & Foster, in press).

Use of a Metacognitive Framework

A metacognitive framework that uses a preactivity discussion, mediation during performance, and a postactivity discussion is typically used across all treatment sessions. This framework is described elsewhere (Goverover et al., 2007; Toglia et al., 2010, 2018) and is illustrated in the case example in this chapter.

The metacognitive framework requires skill in use of mediation and guided questions. Ideally, an occupational therapist should first practice guided questioning with a colleague or peer before implementing it in treatment. This can be easily done through a simulation in which the "treating" therapist leads the "client" through a series of guided questions that assess the client's awareness of cognitive performance errors and ideas about possible strategy solutions to manage these errors.

Video 20.1 outlines examples of preactivity and postactivity guided questions that can be used. There is a technique and an art to leading a successful mediation that does not involve direct cueing or instruction. Mediation in an MC Approach requires more general, rather than task-specific, questions to guide self-discovery and problem solving.

As we have recommended, the treating therapist should set up a "client–therapist" simulated interaction (with a colleague, friend, or family member) and practice leading an interview. Videos and review during practice or during treatment of a client are ideal in providing the therapist with the opportunity to reflect on and analyze their own performance. This kind of practice emphasizes a semistructured flow of more generalized questions and limits direct verbal cues. Practicing using open-ended questions that are not task or symptom specific can be difficult at first, because most therapists are used to providing direct verbal or gestural cues, as with a cognitive remediation approach.

Toglia (2017) provided an outline of pre- and posttask semistructured questions, with suggestions for various probes or prompts that therapists can use during treatment to optimize clients' self-awareness and strategy generation. This guide helps to structure a proper flow in the pre- or posttask discussion. Exhibit 20.1 provides examples of questions therapists can use before the task to promote strategy generation. Similar questions are used immediately after the task.

The MC guidelines (Toglia & Foster, in press) include

- Detailed guidelines about how to use metacognitive techniques to enhance clients' self-awareness and self-monitoring,

- Recommendations for guided questioning, and

- Extensive case examples.

Ideally, providing clients with suggestions or choice for strategies is the last option, but in some cases, early on in treatment when self-awareness is not present yet or is only minimally emergent, the client may require more-structured guidance.

Use of Multiple Tasks and Environments and the Horizontal Continuum

Transfer of information is facilitated when a client is required to apply the newly learned skill or strategy to multiple situations or environments. This ensures that a specific strategy will not be associated with only 1 type of task or environment but can be generalized across functional tasks (Toglia, 1992, 2018). Occupational therapists should combine task grading and practice in multiple types of contexts and situations with other aspects of the MC Approach for optimal results.

Functional–cognitive treatment activities are structured in a sideways or horizontal manner, with tasks that display decreasing degrees of physical and conceptual similarity to the original learning situation (Toglia, 1991). Video 20.1 illustrates various levels of transfer, along with examples that demonstrate how a task can gradually be changed so that eventually the final task is completely different in physical appearance from the initial task. This approach allows a client to effortlessly implement learned strategies in all types of functional situations.

Repeated exposure and practice in a variety of conditions provides clients the opportunity to understand a strategy's significance and infer some of the properties of situations in which that strategy is applicable (Toglia, 1991). Once the client has practiced and successfully applied the same strategy across different activities (horizontally), treatment activities are graded up in complexity or difficulty (vertically). This process is outlined in Exhibit 20.2 as well as in Video 20.1.

Structured Activities

The use of similarly structured tasks and activities in the initial stages of MC treatment is instrumental in facilitating self-awareness and strategy use, as we have described. Structured

EXHIBIT 20.1. Sample Strategy Generation Questions

- "Before we start, let's think of the best way to go about doing this . . ."
Sample general mediation
- "Can you think of some special methods or strategies that you could use to help you to complete everything you need to do?"
Sample symptom-specific mediation (related to general cognitive symptoms; therapist chooses symptom they observe)
- "What can you do to help keep track of which step is next? . . . Locate everything? . . . Identify which part comes first?"
- "What can you do to help pay attention to details?"
Sample task-specific mediation (i.e., related to task components)
- "What can you do to help remind you when to take the cookies out of the oven?"
- "What can you do to help you keep track of which bills you have already paid?"
Provide strategy suggestion or choice
- "There may be some methods that can help. Do you think it would be better to write a list or keep track of things in your head?"

Source. From Schedule Activity Module: Functional Cognitive Rehabilitation Activities and Strategy-Based Intervention (p. 25), by J. Toglia, 2017, Hastings on Hudson, NY: MC CogRehab Resources. Copyright © 2017 by J. Toglia. Reprinted with permission.

EXHIBIT 20.2. Sample Multicontext Horizontal Activities Across Treatment Sessions: Basic (Search and Locate)

All activities require: finding and locating information from a 10-item list
Typical performance error: loses track of information on the list (e.g., forgets items or loses place)
Sample strategy to control performance error across all activities: verbal rehearsal of key words during searching (talking aloud, whispering, or using internal dialogue)
Sample directions across activities: "Remember the first 3 items from the list and see whether they are in or on the . . ."

Schedule module	Schedule module	Menu module	Schedule module supplementary activities	Everyday activities
Class and activity weekly schedule	Television program schedule	Picture menu Written menu	Kitchen cabinets	Keeps track of day, time, and pill that needs to be put into medication organizer slot
Sightseeing activities and events schedule	Things to do schedule or calendar	**Business card module** Business cards or name lists	Bathroom Office supply closet	Keeps track of first 3 items from packing list when packing to go home for weekend

Initial task	⟶	Similar	⟶	Different
	Near transfer	Intermediate	Far transfer	

Source. From *Schedule Activity Module: Functional Cognitive Rehabilitation Activities and Strategy-Based Intervention* (p. 4), by J. Toglia, 2017, Hastings on Hudson, NY: MC CogRehab Resources. Copyright © 2018 by J. Toglia. Adapted with permission.

activities introduce elements of novelty and challenge that can be tailored to the client's cognitive abilities. Such activities also can address specific performance errors that have been observed across activities. Treatment activities that closely resemble functional day-to-day tasks provide an opportunity for the client to explore their current level of ability and identify task challenges while enhancing engagement and motivation in treatment. Also, functionally relevant activities that share similarities with everyday situations can facilitate the expectation that strategies should be used and thus increase the likelihood of transfer of strategies to real-life functioning (Toglia, 2017, 2018).

There are structured functional–cognitive activity sets available for use that involve everyday materials and are designed to be used in an MC treatment program. Occupational therapists can use the activities in a variety of ways to place demands on different cognitive performance areas (Toglia, 2017). Using prepackaged activity sets can optimize setup time, increase efficiency with treatment sessions, and provide consistency with task demands so strategies are better generalized.

Similar cognitive demands across activities provide opportunity for repeated practice in self-monitoring performance and in generating or using the same strategies. For example, a series of tasks that repeatedly place similar demands on the person's ability to recall items from a list lets clients explore and generate strategies to help keep track of information. A client might select the strategy of verbal rehearsal and apply it across activities. They might then further generalize that strategy to other tasks in everyday life, such as keeping track of grocery items or keeping track of pills when setting up a pill organizer.

Structured functional activity sets and additional modules can be found on www.multicontext.net and are available for purchase. The Schedules functional activity set provides a wide range of flexible activities that revolve around 4 types

of schedules (i.e., class and activities, sightseeing, television schedule, things to do), with a variety of activity themes and instructions to choose from (Toglia, 2017). There is also an additional Menu module that uses menus, lists, and cards in a parallel way to the Schedules kit.

Themes found in the activity sets and modules include searching and locating, creating lists, shifting directions, finding information, and answering complex questions. The modules provide varying levels of task complexity to allow the therapist to match task difficulty to the client's level of cognitive abilities. Easier levels target more basic cognitive perceptual skills, including tasks that involve using immediate recall, matching, pacing speed, following simple instructions, and shifting between different instructions or task components. More challenging levels require multitasking, simultaneous shifting, mentally keeping track of multiple criteria, and higher levels of organization.

Once self-awareness emerges during treatment, structured activities are gradually faded, and clients play a greater role in choosing treatment activities themselves. It is useful to also structure more-challenging and meaningful activities chosen by the client in a format similar to those found in the structured activities, so that transfer and generalization of strategies are promoted.

Alternative Methods and Considerations

Alternative methods and techniques that therapists can use as part of a structured MC Approach to facilitate self-awareness and strategy use include

- Role reversal,
- Video feedback,

- Goal attainment scales, and

- Goal-mapping techniques (Toglia, 2018).

Administration of the MC Approach requires practice and planning. A wide range of activities and materials need to be available and accessible.

Assessment Considerations

The MC Approach requires performance analysis that focuses on the process of how someone goes about doing a task, including

- Methods used,

- Types of errors that occur,

- Detection or self-correction of performance errors, and

- The ability to adjust performance to challenges (Toglia, 2018).

Information on strategy use and self-awareness, both inside and outside the context of activities, provides a foundation for MC treatment. For example, the Weekly Calendar Planning Activity (WCPA; Toglia, 2015) and the Contextual Memory Test (CMT; Toglia, 1993) are both standardized tools that provide information on strategy use and awareness in the context of an activity. These tools can be supplemented by other measures, which can include the Self-Awareness Deficits Interview (Fleming et al., 1996), Self-Regulation Skills Interview (SRSI; Goverover et al., 2007; Ownsworth et al., 2000; Toglia et al., 2011), Daily Living Questionnaire (DLQ; Rosenblum et al., 2017), and Cognitive Self-Efficacy Questionnaire (Toglia & Johnston, 2017). These additional awareness questionnaires and assessment resources can also be found at the Multicontext website (www.multicontext.net).

Setup of Tools and Materials in Treatment

To ensure that treatment activities require little planning and can be easily administered, therapists should organize and set up structured activity sets and prewritten discussion guidelines ahead of time. Having structured activity sets readily available in the beginning stages of treatment can be instrumental in facilitating a standardized approach to treatment that will best facilitate self-awareness and strategy generation and use across the remainder of treatment. Clients may make more meaningful connections to specific targeted strategies if activities are structured and executed with similar materials and tools.

Documentation

As per American Occupational Therapy Association (2018) guidelines, short-term and long-term goals should be measurable, meaningful, and occupation based and should directly relate to a client's ability and need to engage in desired occupations. When the occupational therapist is documenting goals in an MC Approach, goals should also

- Reflect the client's awareness capacity and recognition of performance errors,

- Indicate their generation and use of strategies, and

- Demonstrate how their strategy use improves functional performance.

This method of documentation is illustrated in Case Example 20.1. In this case example, awareness and strategy use are incorporated into goals as prerequisites for independence in functional activities.

The metacognitive framework used in the MC Approach can also be used to structure progress notes. For example, progress notes can have subheadings such as "Prior to Task," "During Task," and "After Task" (Toglia & Foster, in press). Prior to the task, the therapist comments on the client's ability to identify and anticipate challenges and generate strategies to enhance performance and reduce the risk for performance errors. During the task, the therapist comments on the frequency of strategy use, the effectiveness of strategies, and the client's ability to manage and correct performance errors if they occur. After the task, the therapist comments on the client's awareness of their performance and strategy use, their ability to identify alternative strategies to use the next time, and how they generalize successful strategies to contexts and tasks they engage in on a daily basis.

Intervention Considerations

The MC Approach relies heavily on verbal mediation; therefore, clients with major language impairments may not fully benefit from verbal mediation or guided questions. Thus, the MC principles may have limited application for such clients, and the therapist would need to adapt treatment techniques to tactile, kinesthetic, or visual prompts and feedback (Toglia, 2011).

The MC Approach is also not appropriate for

- Clients with moderate to severe dementia or severe cognitive deficits;

- Clients who show limited responsiveness to cues, resist guided questions, exhibit defensive denial, or refuse suggestions of strategy use; or

- Clients who have limited potential for learning or change in awareness.

In these cases, because awareness of cognitive performance deficits is a crucial aspect of the MC Approach, the occupational therapist should conduct treatment progressively, with caution, or consider other approaches (Fleming & Ownsworth, 2006; Katz et al., 2002; Toglia & Kirk, 2000).

Acknowledging performance difficulties could be a threatening experience for some individuals, especially those who are more prone to denial, have a highly defensive personality style, have difficulty admitting mistakes or failures, have difficulty asking for help, or are inflexible. Therefore, when a client tends to blame external sources for their errors or shows hostility and anger when errors are recognized, approaches that focus on task-specific training or modifications of the task or environment to promote success may be more effective in increasing safety and function (Toglia & Kirk, 2000).

Other approaches should also be considered for clients who display high levels of unawareness, impaired judgment, or denial; they are more likely to be at risk for unsafe behaviors (e.g., when driving or handling finances). To ensure that a client is safe, the therapist may need to use external compensation, such as modifying the environment or the client's responsibilities and using behavioral management methods (Katz et al., 2002; Sohlberg, 2000). In situations in which tasks are critical for function, a task-specific approach that involves repetitive practice with fading cues, such as the Neurofunctional Approach (Giles, 2018; see Chapter 18), could be used.

The MC Approach provides broad guidelines for using a range of strategies. Thus, other approaches that use strategies, including goal management (Levine et al., 2011), can be used in conjunction with this approach. Technology, such as automatic text messages to cue self-checking or encourage strategy use, can support strategy use in the MC Approach. Caregiver interventions involving collaborative problem solving focused on occupational performance issues can also supplement the MC Approach.

Case Example

Case Example 20.1 demonstrates how a therapist can carry out and progress treatment using an MC Approach. The case involves a 70-year-old man with a new diagnosis of multiple brain tumors, recently resected, who showed little insight and awareness of cognitive performance and minimal strategy use on initial evaluation. The therapist in the case example

- Uses functional and skill-based assessments;

- Evaluates self-awareness and strategy use both in and out of context;

- Gradually progresses treatment activities along a horizontal and vertical continuum; and

- Facilitates self-awareness with guided mediation before, during, and after the task.

In addition, the case describes the use of self-rating and prediction opportunities and strategy discussions regarding implementation and effectiveness of methods used. Sample goals that illustrate the focus on self-awareness and strategy use are included. Documentation of progress is also illustrated.

CASE EXAMPLE 20.1. Brian, a Client With Multiple Brain Tumors

Background and Occupational Profile

Brian is a 70-year-old man who was diagnosed with multiple frontal brain tumors 2 months ago. He was referred by his physician for an outpatient occupational therapy functional evaluation after surgery and discharge from the hospital to manage new limitations in both motor and cognitive function.

Brian is a retired portfolio manager who worked for a large finance firm for more than 40 years. He lives in a metropolitan city, in an elevator apartment, with his wife. He travels frequently to France, where he has a 2nd home.

Before surgery, Brian was independent in all ADLs, managed the household finances, managed his daily medications, and was able to complete all community errands and tasks without assistance. He had an avid passion for cooking and had recently begun to learn French to be able to communicate with locals when staying in France. Brian also endorsed being very social among same-age peers, frequently going to dinner parties and events with his wife. Brian, along with his wife, reported that their goals for therapy were to decrease overall burden of care and maximize Brian's independence and participation in basic self-care; to take on more complex household management tasks, such as keeping track of daily medications; and to enjoy more social engagement.

Initial Assessment and Evaluation of Cognitive Performance

The **therapist** performed a standard occupational profile and interview, followed by administration of skill- and function-based performance assessments, including the CMT and the WCPA. Both assessments provided information directly relevant to MC treatment planning on self-awareness and strategy use. In addition to

(Continued)

performance-based assessments, the therapist evaluated awareness outside the context of a task using the SRSI. Self-reported participation and activity limitations were evaluated with the DLQ.

Table 20.1 summarizes the key results, interpretations, and synthesis of Brian's initial assessments and highlights functional concerns, cognitive strengths and challenges, awareness, and strategy use. Table 20.2 summarizes Brian's results on the WCPA, including observed strategies, performance errors and patterns, and posttask awareness.

Overall, the initial assessment suggested the following cognitive error performance patterns: lack of preplanning, and difficulty with recall and keeping track of information. Brian's self-awareness in interviews and during

TABLE 20.1. Initial Assessment Overview for Brian

EVALUATION CONSIDERATIONS	SUMMARY OF ASSESSMENT

Client's functional–cognitive concerns and observations	• Independent with all basic self-care
	• Wife assisting with
	  o Preparing meals
	  o Managing and reminding Brian to take his medications
	  o Scheduling and keeping track of all appointments
	• With further probing, Brian reported
	  o Trouble "concentrating on things" and "remembering things"
	  o Difficulty keeping track of day-to-day items and tasks
	• As per DLQ, Brian endorsed minimal to no difficulty in various complex tasks and cognitive domains, despite his wife's concern.

Spouse's functional–cognitive concerns	• Decreased ability to keep track of information; forgets something told to him just 5 minutes prior (instructions, date, social conversations) • Unable to schedule and keep track of medical appointments • Difficulty recalling events that happened the day before • Difficulty keeping track of basic instructions, such as to take medication or to drink a glass of water to keep up with daily water intake, as recommended by his doctor • Difficulty engaging in daily self-care, such as regular bathing • Resistant to being social with friends ("too tired") Per Brian's wife, this lack of initiation and motivation was a change from his prior level of functioning.
Cognitive strengths	• Shifting attention • Sustained attention for up to 30 minutes during WCPA, ignores distracters • Working memory with very few items, could keep track of 2–3 words or items or 3–4 rules on the WCPA • Strong visualization skills and association when recalling contextually related items on the CMT • Emergent self-awareness, able to self-correct errors when they became evident (e.g., on WCPA, correcting placement of 2 errands because of an overlap in errand times). • During the WCPA, Brian also was able to ignore the therapist's deliberate distractions and was able to effectively solve a problem and add hours to the table when needed.
Cognitive challenges	• Scored 24/30 on the MoCA, indicating mild cognitive limitations, mostly in the areas of immediate and delayed recall as well as orientation and EF • Suspected impairment in immediate and delayed recall, as evidenced by CMT results • Decreased preplanning skills and task efficiency, as evidenced by performance on WCPA • Lacked effective insight and anticipatory awareness of cognitive performance • Showed poor correlation between cognitive challenges he faced and participation in basic self-care and IADLs

(Continued)

(Continued)

CASE EXAMPLE 20.1. Brian, a Client With Multiple Brain Tumors *(Cont.)*

TABLE 20.1. Initial Assessment Overview for Brian *(Cont.)*

EVALUATION CONSIDERATIONS	SUMMARY OF ASSESSMENT
Awareness	General self-awareness • Demonstrated an average self-regulation skills score of 7.166, which indicates moderate to low awareness, strategy knowledge, or use of strategies • Reported, "I'm not using specific strategies. I just try to take my time." Task-specific awareness • *Pretask mediation:* On the CMT, Brian demonstrated accurate anticipation of recall before administration, not under- or overestimating performance (anticipated recall of 12 items). • *During-task awareness:* Brian self-corrected 2 errors during WCPA in situ; however, he made additional timing errors that were not corrected and showed limited insight regarding ability to keep track of multiple pieces of information and conceptualize instructions. • *Posttask interview:* Brian showed good posttask awareness on the WCPA, endorsing a strategy of "preplanning" for next time and reading through his list before jumping right into the task. He had good insight into which strategies worked well for him on the CMT (associations, grouping, storytelling).

Strategy use	• Self-generated pretask
	  ○ No strategies were identified in interviews or pre-assessments.
	• Strategy execution within task
	  ○ Used self-talk during CMT; however, his total strategy score of 6 was below age-related norms, and he demonstrated low, ineffective strategy use
	  ○ During WCPA, Brian was partially efficient with check mark use (only used halfway through WCPA)
	  ○ Decreased frequency of self-checking work
	  ○ Poor preplanning and prioritization; seemed to have no plan to execute tasks but rather aimed to correct errors once they occurred
	• After task:
	  ○ After CMT, Brian reported use of associations, storytelling, and grouping to keep track of items
	  ○ No additional strategies reported after WCPA, but partially aware of the strategies that were observed

Note. CMT = Contextual Memory Test; DLQ = Daily Living Questionnaire; EF = executive functioning; MoCA = Montreal Cognitive Assessment (Nasreddine et al., 2005); WCPA = Weekly Calendar Planning Activity.

activities was limited; however, he generally acknowledged difficulties immediately after tasks. His strategy use was also limited; however, he demonstrated the ability to generate strategies.

Treatment Goals

Brian indicated that he would like to be more independent at home, especially taking back responsibility for managing his medications, managing his daily schedule, and being autonomous with his daily self-care routine without needing his wife to "nag him." Brian also expressed that returning to cooking and socializing with friends would improve his self-esteem and overall quality of life. Ultimately Brian endorsed a long-term goal of being "well enough" to travel to his 2nd home in Paris.

Brian's wife agreed that she would like Brian to be completely autonomous with his daily schedule, initiating his morning self-care routine, keeping track of his water intake, and taking his medications. She also hoped that

(Continued)

TABLE 20.2. WCPA Initial Scores, Observations, and After-Task Interview Reponses

ASSESSMENT CONSTRUCTS	SCORE	AFTER-TASK INTERVIEW
Planning time (min:sec)	0:35	***Awareness of task challenges:*** Brian demonstrated minimal insight into task challenges and required probing to elicit awareness of performance. He reported he was aware that flexible appointments were entered first, which "appeared to be [his] downfall." Brian's overall awareness of error-free performance was low, given that he anticipated he accurately placed 8 of 10 appointments. He rated the task as "somewhat easy" for him despite making numerous errors, and he thought that he mostly used efficient methods.
Total time (min:sec)	12:25	
No. rules followed (0–5)	4	
Total no. strategies used (observed + reported)	3 (3 + 0)	
No. appointments entered (0–10)	10	***Strategy generation:*** Brian demonstrated use of 3 strategies during the task (circling key words, pausing and self-checking, crossing out entered appointments). He reported no additional strategies; however, once that task was completed and he was aware of errors made, he further generated the strategy of "preplanning" and "prereading" instructions and lists of appointments for next time.
No. accurate appointments (0–10)	4	
No. appointments missing	0	
Location errors	5	***Observations:*** Brian began the task without adequate planning; he did not read his list of appointments beforehand to best organize and schedule flexible appointments to prevent conflicts. Instead, he entered listed appointments in order from top to bottom. When he made an error with a flexible appointment placement, he sighed and then attempted to correct the error by using an alternative time allotted. He seldom looked at the instruction sheet, had no issue with Saturday–Sunday reversal, and followed all rules except for stating the correct time indicated. He did not check his work when he finished.
Time errors	2	
Repetition errors	1	
Incomplete errors	0	
Total no. errors	8	
Self-recognition of errors	2	

Note. min:sec = minutes:seconds; no. = number of; WCPA = Weekly Calendar Planning Activity.

she could decrease her role as Brian's caregiver, because it was putting unwanted strain on their marriage and relationship dynamic.

On the basis of the Dynamic Interactional Model and using an MC Approach, the therapist focused treatment on the following:

- Increase Brian's overall self-awareness of performance and insight with challenges
- Improve his self-monitoring so he could better correct and avoid errors
- Promote strategy generation and use during more complex tasks with similar task demands
- Enable him to carry strategies across a variety of activities to increase autonomy and safety.

Brian's short-term goals were as follows:

- As a prerequisite to independence with medication management, Brian will be able to recognize errors during performance 80% of the time without additional mediation or cueing from his therapist or spouse.
- As a prerequisite to independence with 5-step meal-prep activity, Brian will be able to generate at least 2 strategies pretask (e.g., making and following a list or verbal rehearsal), more than 1 time, to optimize keeping track of information and steps accurately.
- As a prerequisite to independence with managing his daily schedule and activities, Brian will independently implement a predetermined strategy (e.g., list, external reminder, verbal rehearsal) at least 80% of the time without any additional meditation or guided questioning.

(Continued)

Consistent with the MC Approach, Brian's short-term goals emphasized self-awareness, strategy generation, and strategy implementation. Ultimately, these goals were stepping-stones used to build on and achieve his long-term goals:

- Brian will independently identify, create, and use a self-cueing system across activities (e.g., repeated rehearsal of mantra or list making), 100% of the time, to increase success and autonomy with IADL performance.
- Brian will independently identify and use at least 2 cognitive–perceptual strategies before preparing a multiple-step, novel meal to optimize initiation and participation in meaningful IADLs.
- Brian will demonstrate independent and effective self-awareness by actively initiating, monitoring, and managing his daily water intake, without assistance from his spouse, 100% of the time.

To achieve these goals, Brian would require cognitive, structural support, such as temporary external prompting and reminders from the therapist and his wife, as well as external cognitive aids for schedules, initiation, and reminders. For example, Google Calendar and designated free smartphone applications (e.g., Aida Reminder, Water Tracker, and Can Plan) could support him with initiating and sequencing his morning routine and novel, complex tasks. These tools could also help him keep track of his daily water intake and remind him to follow treatment goals.

Description of the Treatment Program
The outpatient MC treatment program consisted of a 45-minute session 2 times a week for a total of 6 weeks (see Table 20.3 for details of the program). Table 20.3 illustrates the focus of 12 treatment sessions and includes sample activities, techniques used, and a summary of observed outcomes in each treatment session. Sessions were structured on a horizontal continuum of tasks, in which the client completed 2 to 3 therapeutic activities with similar cognitive demands. These activities were chosen to facilitate the practice of strategy use as well as performance exploration aimed at facilitating self-awareness. The initial focus of sessions was on helping Brian recognize that, across different activities, he tended to lose track of information and jump into activities too quickly.

In Sessions 1–3, Brian practiced detecting errors and correcting them both in and out of treatment. The therapist supervised as he organized his list of daily morning routine activities as well as supervised his setup of his pill caddy once a week after he made his list of medications. Pretask and posttask guided questioning during these sessions focused on promoting self-awareness. Mediation throughout all treatment sessions involved prompts such as, "Tell me about the parts of the task that were easy and the parts that were more challenging," and, "How can you be sure you don't miss information?"

As self-awareness emerged over Sessions 1–3, the therapist emphasized guiding Brian to generate and use effective strategies. Treatment was directed at helping Brian recognize that his performance was more successful if he took the time to plan ahead and if he created and used systems to help him keep track of information during a task. Brian began self-generating lists on his own by Session 4.

At this time, probing was gradually faded, because Brian spontaneously recognized patterns of performance errors. He knew that the difficulties he experienced represented the same types of difficulties that had occurred in previous activities. By Session 6, Brian was partially able to recognize that he needed his wife to encourage him not to ignore the smartphone reminders (i.e., to take medications, to start his self-care routine, and to check his calendar).

During Sessions 4–6, Brian's wife also reinforced the use of guided questioning to facilitate his self-awareness and independence for initiation of various IADL tasks. In situations when Brian failed to initiate specific ADL and IADL tasks, his wife was trained to use questions such as, "How will you go about this?" and, "Are there any special strategies or methods you have been using that could be helpful here?"

During Sessions 7–9, the therapist used guided questions to facilitate discovery of appropriate strategies for different tasks, such as breaking more complex IADLs into smaller steps using a list or pregenerating a list of items or material required to complete a task. This included a shift from the use of an external strategy to an internal

(Continued)

CASE EXAMPLE 20.1. Brian, a Client With Multiple Brain Tumors *(Cont.)*

TABLE 20.3. Description of Multicontext Treatment Sessions for Brian

TREATMENT CONSIDERATIONS	VERY SIMILAR → SESSIONS 1–3	SOMEWHAT SIMILAR SESSIONS 4–6	DIFFERENT SESSIONS 7–9	VERY DIFFERENT → SESSIONS 10–12
Focus of sessions	Facilitate error recognition and self-awareness of performance *Strategies* • Preplanning by generating a list of steps or creating self-cues to get started • Self-generating an external reminder strategy to keep track of items	Facilitate self-monitoring, error recognition, and self-awareness of performance *Strategies* • Preplanning by generating a list of steps or creating self-cues to get started • Self-generating an external reminder strategy to keep track of items	Facilitate self-exploration of strategies before activity, self-monitoring during activity, and self-evaluation of performance after activity *Strategies* • Preplanning by organizing and associating items needed to initiate and carry out steps • Self-generating an internal reminder strategy in combination with an external strategy to keep track of items	Facilitate self-exploration of strategies before activity, self-monitoring during activity, and self-evaluation of performance after activity *Strategies* • Preplanning by organizing and associating items needed to initiate and carry out steps • Self-generating an internal reminder strategy in combination with an external strategy to keep track of items
Sample activities	Prepare a morning routine calendar and checklist using a list of 10 essential self-care tasks; organize on the basis of specific sequence and flow Medication management, including self-generating a list of medications and setting up a weekly pill caddy according to pill labels and instructions	Prepare an exercise routine by generating a list of steps needed to initiate signing up for a local program, joining a gym, or subscribing to online workout videos Self-generate smartphone reminders and an external visual reminder (e.g., empty glass out on the countertop) to remind client to drink water when entering the kitchen	Prepare a list of things to do during the week, including medical, social, and personal appointments and errands; then enter them into a weekly calendar by using talk-aloud verbal rehearsal to help keep track Create a list to take to the local grocery store to make a simple lunch, and check kitchen pantry to see what items are missing from the list; self-monitor and keep track of ingredients using talk-aloud verbal rehearsal and associations as a self-generated internal strategy	Generate a list of things to pack when traveling for an overnight stay; preplan and identify the steps needed using internal visual imagery Make a list of local restaurants before searching on the computer for reviews and possible reservation times; find a way to keep track of the restaurants that have 4- or 5-star reviews by using internal verbal rehearsal and note taking

(Continued)

CASE EXAMPLE 20.1. Brian, a Client With Multiple Brain Tumors *(Cont.)*

TABLE 20.3. Description of Multicontext Treatment Sessions for Brian *(Cont.)*

TREATMENT CONSIDERATIONS	VERY SIMILAR → SESSIONS 1–3	SOMEWHAT SIMILAR SESSIONS 4–6	DIFFERENT → SESSIONS 7–9	VERY DIFFERENT → SESSIONS 10–12
Techniques used	Brian practiced detecting errors and correcting them both in and out of treatment. Self-awareness of difficulties was facilitated by the therapist's pretask and posttask questions, aimed at • Bridging and helping Brian see the similarities between situations, and • Reflecting on and exploring performance and comparing actual performance with the estimation of it. The therapist facilitated Brian's awareness of using self-generated lists as a strategy by joined exploration of different ways to approach tasks to optimize how he kept track of details.	Guided questioning was used pretask to facilitate the use of strategies, including self-generated list making in similarly structured tasks (e.g., planning steps to being successful with creating an exercise routine). Guided questioning was also used pre- and posttask to promote self-awareness for anticipation of challenges and for generation of alternative strategies. The therapist facilitated use of an external visual reminder strategy by asking questions that guided Brian in anticipating the need to use a strategy that did not require him writing down steps. Brian's wife facilitated guided questioning outside of therapy during functional performance.	Guided questions encouraged a shift from using a more external strategy to an internal strategy, which required a higher level of self-awareness and monitoring. Brian was encouraged to look for a method that would decrease distraction to promote execution of tasks without interruption. The therapist used post-task guided questioning to facilitate the use of an internal strategy (e.g., talk aloud and associations) to better keep track of items he was searching for.	Brian practiced self-choosing relevant activities and exploring needed strategies to accomplish them before the task and with less-structured guided questioning. As tasks became more complex, guided questioning was aimed to facilitate a shift from simpler strategies to more sophisticated strategies.

(Continued)

CASE EXAMPLE 20.1. Brian, a Client With Multiple Brain Tumors (Cont.)

TABLE 20.3. Description of Multicontext Treatment Sessions for Brian (Cont.)

TREATMENT CONSIDERATIONS	VERY SIMILAR →	SOMEWHAT SIMILAR	DIFFERENT →	VERY DIFFERENT
	SESSIONS 1–3	SESSIONS 4–6	SESSIONS 7–9	SESSIONS 10–12
Outcomes	*Awareness:* During more-structured tasks, Brian began to vaguely bridge previously experienced errors or difficulties. With questioning, he was able to identify difficulties pretask and began to self-monitor by correcting 1–2 errors made. However, he was still making additional unnoticed errors. Self-reflection was emergent: He could identify errors made and think of alternative methods to reduce errors if he tried the task again. *Strategy generation:* Brian required mediation to begin to think about possible strategies to help with preplanning and organizing. After he engaged in multiple similarly structured tasks, he was able to recall use of list making but still required mediation to think of using it. *Strategy initiation and frequency:* Brian was using 1–2 strategies 50% of the time, mostly external strategies that included making lists of items or steps. Strategy frequency increased with practice; it required mediation initially but improved to more self-directed list making with practice.	*Awareness:* With repeated engagement in similarly structured novel tasks, Brian began to master anticipation of challenges, strategy initiation, and self-monitoring and reflection. He still had difficulty with recognizing and managing errors during the task or self-check period, as these periods were not being consistently implemented or used. Posttask, he was able to identify that self-checking was a helpful strategy he should be using more often. He even identified using a self-check worksheet as a visual aid to remind him to do so. *Strategy generation:* Brian could now report previously discussed strategies with minimal questioning. These included • Breaking down a task into smaller steps by generating a list to formulate a plan before jumping in; • Organizing his materials, crossing off or highlighting items on his list as they were completed; and • Using a self-check period to look back to the instruction sheet or to check for errors.	*Awareness:* During less structured and more functional activities, Brian anticipated challenges he had experienced in previous tasks and began to verbalize a pattern of errors he was likely to make. This led to an increased use of self-monitoring; he spontaneously implemented stop-and-check periods without use of a visual aid 75% of the time to assess for any errors. He even used self-talk as a way to self-monitor—for example, when he noticed he was becoming more distracted, he said aloud to himself, "Brian, stay focused and check your list." *Strategy generation:* Brian was identifying at least 3 strategies (both internal and external) in pretask questioning with no additional probing. He did still show some difficulty in generating alternative strategies in posttask guided questioning if a strategy he had tried to use was not an efficient one to use in a specific task.	*Awareness:* Overall, Brian was aware of his strengths, which decreased the burden of care placed on his wife. He could readily anticipate errors and self-correct them in the moment, and he was implementing self-check periods without mediation or use of an external visual cue. Brian was also more aware of when performance was more difficult and could identify why a challenge or error might have occurred. *Strategy generation:* Brian was identifying at least 3 strategies before starting a task, and his strategies had shifted from simple and heavily external to internal and complex. He showed a higher level of adaptability: He was able to generate 1–2 alternative strategies to a given task when engaged in posttask guided questioning. Brian's wife reported that if he was given a new, unfamiliar task outside of therapy sessions, he would even begin each activity by talking aloud and writing down some ideas of strategies he could use to effectively and efficiently compete the task.

(Continued)

CASE EXAMPLE 20.1. Brian, a Client With Multiple Brain Tumors (*Cont.*)

TABLE 20.3. Description of Multicontext Treatment Sessions for Brian (*Cont.*)

TREATMENT CONSIDERATIONS	VERY SIMILAR → SESSIONS 1–3	SOMEWHAT SIMILAR SESSIONS 4–6	DIFFERENT SESSIONS 7–9	→ VERY DIFFERENT SESSIONS 10–12
	Functional performance: Brian was able to execute his daily morning self-care routine using his paper checklist, but with verbal guidance 30% of the time from his wife to initiate. He was able to set up his pill caddy 3 times with supervision using his premade list, and he self-corrected errors made on the 3rd trial without guidance.	Although pretask strategy generation had improved, strategy implementation remained difficult; Brian successfully used 1–2 strategies 75% of the time overall. *Strategy initiation and frequency:* Brian showed improved follow-through of strategy use during tasks. He was more consistent in making a list with multiple-step activities, and 50% of the time he used a self-check period. He spontaneously used a new strategy in Session 6 (visual external reminder) after pretask questioning. This showed a large shift from a more assistive external cue to a less direct external cue that required increased self-awareness. At times, Brian attempted to use strategies in activities for which the strategy might not be helpful or conducive to success.	*Strategy initiation and frequency:* Brian was now using external strategies, such as making lists, using visual aids, and self-checking, 100% of the time without additional prompts or mediation periods during activities. He was beginning to use internal strategies in combination with external strategies; however, he was implementing these only 50% of the time. Brian used talk-aloud self-cueing as a self-monitoring strategy and used rote verbal rehearsal to manage multiple steps or items at once.	*Strategy initiation and frequency:* Brian was independently implementing at least 2 strategies during a given task 100% of the time. He was phasing out the use of a checklist and relying more heavily on visual imagery, internal verbal rehearsal, and even note taking when appropriate.

(Continued)

CASE EXAMPLE 20.1. Brian, a Client With Multiple Brain Tumors *(Cont.)*

TABLE 20.3. Description of Multicontext Treatment Sessions for Brian *(Cont.)*

TREATMENT CONSIDERATIONS	VERY SIMILAR — SESSIONS 1–3	→	SOMEWHAT SIMILAR — SESSIONS 4–6	DIFFERENT — SESSIONS 7–9	→	VERY DIFFERENT — SESSIONS 10–12
			Functional performance: Brian's wife reported she was no longer providing verbal guidance to assist him in initiating his morning routine, because he was using a paper checklist to check off activities as they were completed. He was now able to use his premade list of medications to set up his pill caddy and was self-correcting errors spontaneously. On the last trial, he completed the task without an error. With managing his daily water intake, Brian still required a mediation period to facilitate use of his external reminder (i.e., glass on the counter) approximately 75% of the time.	*Functional performance:* Brian was now independent with his ADL morning routine, reporting he had begun to phase out the use of his checklist. He now skimmed the list before his routine and used talk-aloud verbal rehearsal to keep track of the ADLs he needed to perform. As a way to self-monitor and check himself, he referred back to his checklist only when the entire routine was done. Brian had begun to take responsibility for managing his daily errands and appointments. He was independent in generating a list of errands and activities for the week after discussing with his wife, then used self-talk to manage placing 2–3 tasks at a time into his calendar. He did require mediation 25% of the time to consistently use self-talk and not just refer to his list, which was more costly on time.		*Functional performance:* Brian was managing his daily schedule without assistance from his wife. He checked it daily, made updates to it as needed, and even used it to plan social activities. Brian was also now independently monitoring and managing his daily water intake without requiring a visual cue (i.e., glass on the counter), which optimized his health and recovery during treatments. Brian's wife reported that she no longer felt as though she had to monitor him when he was cooking or running errands, such as grocery shopping or going to the bank. She was confident he could anticipate challenges and use strategies to perform tasks efficiently. Brian also reported an increased sense of self-confidence and autonomy with his day-to-day routines.

(Continued)

strategy. Using internal strategies helped Brian progress in his ability to manage multiple steps and keep a consistent flow and plan without needing to refer back to an external aid or cue. This allowed him to execute a task with more efficiency, not lose track of steps or items, and optimize his overall autonomy.

During Sessions 7–9, Brian began to independently recognize that the strategies he was using could bridge across a continuum of activities. With guided questioning and mediation, he discovered that making lists could maximize his execution of more novel, complex tasks, such as cooking and grocery shopping. Brian reported that when preparing a list and searching the pantry to make a simple lunch, he was able to use check marks to keep track of items he found. However, in a more noisy, crowded environment (e.g., his wife walking around the kitchen, television or music playing in the background), he found himself more distracted and was not 100% compliant with checking off items. This led to additional searches for items he had already found. Nevertheless, Brian needed mediation to identify that noisy environments might be an obstacle.

Once Brian mastered strategy use and generalized it across the horizontal continuum (Sessions 1–6), activities were increased in difficulty (Sessions 7–12), and strategies were expanded and applied to more complex tasks. Progressing along a horizontal continuum, Sessions 1–6

- Began with near transfer, in which activities were very similar in cognitive demands;
- Progressed to somewhat similar demands;
- Further progressed to different and more complex demands; and
- Finally progressed to far transfer, in which activities and cognitive demands were completely different but shared common cognitive challenges.

When Brian was able to spontaneously use strategies and self-monitor his performance across activities at 1 level (Sessions 1–6), activities were increased in difficulty along a vertical continuum. For example, probing with more complex tasks (Session 7–12) focused on facilitating a shift from using lists to taking notes as well as from associations to visual imagery. This demonstrated a higher level of self-regulation and self-monitoring as well as increased ability to use strategies that were more sophisticated.

During Sessions 9–12, Brian experienced more challenges with these complex tasks. However, he was better at anticipating potential difficulties, and he knew what types of performance errors he needed to watch out for. This awareness allowed him to generate and use multiple appropriate strategies to effectively complete the task error free. Brian chose strategies he had previously used successfully or identified as alternatives. For example, when creating a list to pack for an overnight stay, Brian showed some difficulty in bridging previously used strategies (e.g., list making and associations, talk-aloud verbal rehearsal) to a more complex, novel activity. The therapist asked him to look for similarities between preparation for grocery shopping, meal prep, or his daily morning routine as a way to facilitate identifying and generalizing previous strategies to many types of tasks and activities.

In summary, the therapist structured the first 6 treatment sessions horizontally from near to far, using transfer activities to help Brian recognize and self-monitor his tendency to lose track of information across activities and identify the need for strategies. Once Brian was more independently anticipating challenges and the need for specific strategies (i.e., making and generating lists and using verbal rehearsal externally) as well as using strategies with less mediation and pretask questioning during the initial 6 sessions, the therapist increased the activities in difficulty level during Sessions 7–12. These latter sessions focused on Brian's use of more internal strategies (e.g., using internal verbal rehearsal and association vs. external list making).

During all treatment sessions, the therapist asked questions before each activity to promote Brian's overall awareness and anticipation of performance and to assess whether he was preemptively considering strategies for use. During the activities, the therapist used task mediation as needed on the basis of observed task challenges or recognition of errors. The therapist used posttask discussion interviews to assess perceived level of task difficulty

(Continued)

and strategy use (if used at all). Discussion included generating alternative methods or strategies for similar types of tasks and identifying daily activities in which strategies could be helpful.

Assessment Results Postintervention

Brian showed significant increases in self-awareness, strategy use, and performance across the intervention period, as indicated in Table 20.3. By the end of treatment, Brian was able to anticipate at least 1 to 2 potential task challenges and identify strategies to prevent performance errors, such as breaking the task down into more manageable steps or parts. He spontaneously self-corrected errors, either in the moment or after a self-check period. Posttask discussions illustrated that Brian could now verbalize strategies he used; recognize and describe any performance errors; and, when appropriate, identify potential strategies that he could use with similar activities in the future.

These observations were confirmed by significant changes in awareness, strategy use, and performance assessed by objective measures, including the SRSI, CMT, and WCPA. They were also supported by subjective reports from Brian and his wife.

Overall, Brian's functional performance and independence improved after the intervention. He was managing his medications daily, setting up and using a pill caddy to manage his morning and nighttime medications. He also used an alarm to remind him to take his medications; however, once this became rote and routine, the alarm was phased out. Brian was using a water reminder application on his smartphone to initiate drinking and keeping track of his daily water intake.

Brian's wife reported that if she asked him to follow through with a household task, such as washing a dish or taking out the trash, he could do this using self-cueing techniques and a motivational phrase to drive initiation. Brian still had some difficulty initiating steps in novel tasks in a timely fashion. For example, if tasks were complex and included more than 5 to 7 steps or criteria, he required increased time to process and plan how he would approach the task. However, despite these ongoing challenges, he was able to independently self-generate and use strategies to sequence multistep activities without guidance.

Brian and his wife reported an overall improved dynamic in their marriage and felt they were able to resume their social life, going out to dinner with friends and engaging in activities as a couple. The MC strategy approach was instrumental in guiding Brian through self-exploration of performance, strategy generation and use, and self-monitoring, which increased his quality of life and overall autonomy.

Summary

The MC Approach provides the occupational therapist with guidelines for facilitation and training of strategy use, self-awareness, self-monitoring, and self-regulatory skills across everyday activities to treat a wide range of functional–cognitive lapses that interfere with daily life. An MC Approach can be used seamlessly in a variety of settings, including acute, inpatient rehabilitation, and outpatient settings. It also can be suitable for a variety of ages and diagnoses when mild cognitive limitations may impede functional performance.

It is important to use functionally meaningful and relevant activities in MC treatment sessions to optimize a client's participation. This also increases the chance for generalization and transfer of strategies across a continuum of activities spanning from simple, basic ADLs and IADLs to more complex IADLs and work-related tasks. Activities should also remain at the same level of cognitive complexity until evidence of strategy transfer is observed.

Once strategies are applied horizontally across the transfer continuum, activities are increased in difficulty or along a vertical continuum to increase challenge and optimize generalization of strategy in more structurally complex and different tasks. The MC Approach uses techniques, including mediation and guided questioning before, during, and after the activity, to increase self-awareness and self-monitoring and promote strategy use in a wide array of contexts and situations. Direct cueing is avoided, because treatment involves empowering clients to cope with cognitive challenges and identify strategies themselves.

Preparing structured activities, mediation guidelines, pre- and posttask questions, and probes ahead of time can prove helpful in implementing a seamless MC Approach treatment session. Structured activity sets found on www.multicontext. net are available for use and can optimize implementation. A variety of other techniques, including role reversal, video feedback, and goal-attainment scales, can be used to administer an MC Approach and should also be considered when appropriate and deemed useful.

References

American Occupational Therapy Association. (2018). Guidelines for documentation of occupational therapy. *American Journal of Occupational Therapy, 72*(Suppl. 2), 7212410010. https://doi.org/10.5014/ajot.2018.72S203

Birnboim, S., & Miller, A. (2004). Cognitive rehabilitation for multiple sclerosis patients with executive dysfunction. *Journal of Cognitive Rehabilitation, 22,* 11–18.

Cermak, S. A., & Toglia, J. (2018). Cognitive development across the lifespan: Development of cognition and executive functioning in children and adolescents. In N. Katz & J. Toglia (Eds.), *Cognition, occupation, participation across the lifespan: Neuroscience, neurorehabilitation, and models of intervention in occupational therapy* (4th ed., pp. 9–27). Bethesda, MD: AOTA Press.

Fleming, J. M., & Ownsworth, T. (2006). A review of awareness interventions in brain injury rehabilitation. *Neuropsychological Rehabilitation, 16,* 474–500. https://doi.org/10.1080/09602010500505518

Fleming, J. M., Strong, J., & Ashton, R. (1996). Self-awareness of deficits in adults with traumatic brain injury: How best to measure? *Brain Injury, 10,* 1–15.

Foster, E. R., Spence, D., & Toglia, J. (2018). Feasibility of a cognitive strategy training intervention for people with Parkinson's disease. *Disability and Rehabilitation, 40,* 1127–1134. https://doi.org/10.1080/09638288.2017.1288275

Giles, G. M. (2018). Neurofunctional Approach to rehabilitation after brain injury. In N. Katz & J. Toglia (Eds.), *Cognition, occupation, and participation across the lifespan: Neuroscience, neurorehabilitation, and models of intervention in occupational therapy* (4th ed., pp. 419–442). Bethesda, MD: AOTA Press.

Goverover, Y., Johnston, M. V., Toglia, J., & Deluca, J. (2007). Treatment to improve self-awareness in persons with acquired brain injury. *Brain Injury, 21,* 913–923. https://doi.org/10.1080/02699050701553205

Harrison, M. J., Morris, K. A., Horton, R., Toglia, J., Barsky, J., Chait, S., . . . Robbins, L. (2005). Results of intervention for lupus patients with self-perceived cognitive difficulties. *Neurology, 65,* 1325–1327. https://doi.org/10.1212/01.wnl.0000180938.69146.5e

Josman, N., & Regev, S. (2018). Dynamic Interactional Model in severe mental illness: Metacognitive and strategy-based intervention. In N. Katz & J. Toglia (Eds.), *Cognition, occupation, and participation across the lifespan: Neuroscience, neurorehabilitation, and models of intervention in occupational therapy* (4th ed., pp. 387–403). Bethesda, MD: AOTA Press.

Katz, N., Fleming, J., Keren, N., Lightbody, S., & Hartman-Maeir, A. (2002). Unawareness and/or denial of disability: Implications for occupational therapy intervention. *Canadian Journal of Occupational Therapy, 69,* 281–292. https://doi.org/10.1177/000841740206900504

Levine, B., Schweizer, T. A., O'Connor, C., Turner, G., Gillingham, S., Stuss, D. T., . . . Robertson, I. H. (2011). Rehabilitation of executive functioning in patients with frontal lobe brain damage with goal management training. *Frontiers in Human Neuroscience, 5,* 9. https://doi.org/10.3389/fnhum.2011.00009

Nasreddine, Z. S., Phillips, N. A., Bédirian, V., Charbonneau, S., Whitehead, V., Collin, I., . . . Chertkow, H. (2005). The Montreal Cognitive Assessment, MoCA: A brief screening tool for mild cognitive impairment. *Journal of the American Geriatrics Society, 53,* 695–699. https://doi.org/10.1111/j.1532-5415.2005.53221.x

Ownsworth, T. L., McFarland, K. M., & Young, R. M. (2000). Development and standardization of the Self-Regulation Skills Interview (SRSI): A new clinical assessment tool for acquired brain injury. *Clinical Neuropsychologist, 14,* 76–92. https://doi.org/10.1076/1385-4046(200002)14:1;1-8;FT076

Perez, F. M., Tunkel, R. S., Lachmann, E. A., & Nagler, W. (1996). Balint's syndrome arising from bilateral posterior cortical atrophy or infarction: Rehabilitation strategies and their limitation. *Disability and Rehabilitation, 18,* 300–304. https://doi.org/10.3109/09638289609165884

Robnett, R., & Toglia, J. (2015). Evidence-based interventions for older adults with mild cognitive impairment. *OT Practice, 20,* CE-1–CE-8.

Roebers, C. M. (2017). Executive function and metacognition: Towards a unifying framework of cognitive self-regulation. *Developmental Review, 45,* 31–51. https://doi.org/10.1016/j.dr.2017.04.001

Rosenblum, S., Josman, N., & Toglia, J. P. (2017). Development of the Daily Living Questionnaire (DLQ): A factor analysis study. *Open Journal of Occupational Therapy, 5,* 1–17. https://doi.org/10.15453/2168-6408.1326

So, Y. P., Toglia, J., & Donohue, M. V. (1997). A study of memory functioning in chronic schizophrenic patients. *Occupational Therapy in Mental Health, 13*(2), 1–23. https://doi.org/10.1300/J004v13n02_01

Sohlberg, M. M. (2000). Assessing and managing unawareness of self. *Seminars in Speech and Language, 21*(2), 135–152.

Toglia, J. P. (1989). Visual perception of objects: An approach to assessment and intervention. *American Journal of Occupational Therapy, 4,* 587–595. https://doi.org/10.5014/ajot.43.9.587

Toglia, J. P. (1991). Generalization of treatment: A Multicontext Approach to cognitive perceptual impairment in adults with brain injury. *American Journal of Occupational Therapy, 45,* 505–516. https://doi.org/10.5014/ajot.45.6.505

Toglia, J. P. (1992). A Dynamic Interactional Approach to cognitive rehabilitation. In N. Katz (Ed.), *Cognitive rehabilitation: Models of intervention in occupational therapy* (pp. 104–143). Boston: Andover Medical.

Toglia, J. P. (1993). *Contextual Memory Test.* San Antonio: Therapy Skill Builders.

Toglia, J. P. (2011). A Dynamic Interactive Model of cognition in cognitive rehabilitation. In N. Katz (Ed.), *Cognition, occupation, and participation across the lifespan: Neuroscience, neurorehabilitation, and models of intervention in occupational therapy* (3rd ed., pp. 161–202). Bethesda, MD: AOTA Press.

Toglia, J. (2015). *The Weekly Calendar Planning Activity: A performance measure of executive dysfunction.* Bethesda, MD: AOTA Press.

Toglia, J. (2017). *Schedule Activity Module: Functional cognitive rehabilitation activities and strategy-based intervention.* Hastings on Hudson, NY: MC CogRehab Resources.

Toglia, J. (2018). The Dynamic Interactional Model and the Multicontext Approach. In N. Katz & J. Toglia (Eds.), *Cognition, occupation, and participation across the lifespan: Neuroscience, neurorehabilitation, and models for intervention in occupational therapy* (4th ed., pp. 355–383). Bethesda, MD: AOTA Press.

Toglia, J., & Cermak, S. A. (2009). Dynamic assessment and prediction of learning potential in clients with unilateral neglect. *American Journal of Occupational Therapy, 63,* 569–579. https://doi.org/10.5014/ajot.63.5.569

Toglia, J., & Foster, E. (in press). *The Multicontext Approach: A metacognitive strategy based intervention for functional cognition.* Hastings on Hudson, NY: MC CogRehab Resources.

Toglia, J., Goverover, Y., Johnston, M. V., & Dain, B. (2011). Application of the Multicontextual Approach in promoting learning and transfer of strategy use in an individual with TBI and executive dysfunction. *OTJR: Occupation, Participation and Health, 31*(Suppl. 1), S53–S60. https://doi.org/10.3928/15394492-20101108-09

Toglia, J., & Johnston, M. V. (2017). *Cognitive Self Efficacy Questionnaire II (CSEQ).* Hastings on Hudson, NY: MC CogRehab Resources.

Toglia, J., Johnston, M. V., Goverover, Y., & Dain, B. (2010). A Multicontext Approach to promoting transfer of strategy use and self regulation after brain injury: An exploratory study. *Brain Injury, 24,* 664–677. https://doi.org/10.3109/02699051003610474

Toglia, J., & Kirk, U. (2000). Understanding awareness deficits following brain injury. *NeuroRehabilitation, 15,* 57–70.

Toglia, J. P., Rodger, S. A., & Polatajko, H. J. (2012). Anatomy of cognitive strategies: A therapist's primer for enabling occupational performance. *Canadian Journal of Occupational Therapy, 79,* 225–236. https://doi.org/10.2182/cjot.2012.79.4.4

Waldman-Levi, A., & Obermeyer, I. S. (2018). Addressing executive function in schools. In N. Katz & J. Toglia (Eds.), *Cognition, occupation, and participation across the lifespan: Neuroscience, neurorehabilitation, and models of intervention in occupational therapy* (4th ed., pp. 259–271). Bethesda, MD: AOTA Press.

Zlotnik, S., Sachs, D., Rosenblum, S., Shpasser, R., & Josman, N. (2009). Use of the Dynamic Interactional Model in self-care and motor intervention after traumatic brain injury: Explanatory case studies. *American Journal of Occupational Therapy, 63,* 549–558. https://doi.org/10.5014/ajot.63.5.549

21

Cognitive Disabilities Model: Intervention for Clients With Dementia

KARI C. BURCH, OTD, OTR/L, AND PEGGY P. BARCO, OTD, OTR/L, SCDCM, CDRS, FAOTA

LEARNING OBJECTIVES

After completing this chapter, readers should be able to

- Explain the importance of including a care partner in assessment and intervention for selecting and implementing appropriate strategies and techniques,
- Recognize the difference between appropriate and inappropriate interventions at each functional–cognitive level of dementia progression, and
- Apply evidence-based occupational therapy intervention techniques to adapt and modify activities and environments to help care partners manage difficult behavioral and psychological dementia symptoms.

KEY TERMS AND CONCEPTS

- Behavioral and psychological symptoms of dementia • Care partners • Cognitive Disabilities Model

Intervention Introduction

Occupational therapy rehabilitation is a fundamental part of the management of neurodegenerative diseases, such as dementia. Occupational therapy is well suited to dementia care because of its focus on enabling engagement in meaningful and necessary occupations throughout disease duration for both the client and their care partners (American Occupational Therapy Association, 2014). *Care partners* are informal (unpaid) caregivers, usually family members, who provide the vast majority of care to individuals with dementia. Care partners' health is often negatively affected by caregiving (Alzheimer's Association, 2018; Zhu et al., 2015). Occupational therapy intervention focuses on optimizing clients' remaining abilities and modifying activity demands, contexts, and environments (e.g., care partner training in communication and cueing, activity simplification techniques, environmental modifications, strategies emphasizing

care partner problem solving; e.g., Gitlin & Hodgson, 2015; Gitlin et al., 2009, 2010a, 2010b, 2016).

Occupational therapy intervention for persons with irreversible cognitive impairment was first deemed worthwhile and subsequently systematized in the late 1960s by Claudia Allen in the form of the *Cognitive Disabilities Model* (CDM; McCraith et al., 2011; McCraith & Earhart, 2018). The CDM intervention approach focuses on maximizing the function of persons with dementia by adapting activities, contexts, and environments and providing care partner training tailored to the severity of the client's dementia (Levy, 2018; McCraith & Earhart, 2018). This model was developed to support clinical reasoning and appropriate intervention for different levels of cognitive capacity. It has evolved over time to accommodate current neurocognitive research; this chapter focuses specifically on the CDM as applied to neurodegenerative dementia (Levy, 1986).

The CDM now characterizes the typical pattern of dementia progression into 6 hierarchical levels focusing on the global cognition underlying function (Levy, 2018). The determination of the client's current functional level allows the occupational therapist to develop an effective intervention plan to facilitate an optimal person–environment–occupational performance fit. Interventions incorporate appropriate activities, cueing techniques, and environmental modifications to optimize the client's functional performance and to train care partners to provide the support needed for the client to perform desired tasks as independently and safely as possible (Levy, 2018; Levy & Burns, 2011).

This chapter aims to advance occupational therapy practitioners' understanding and effective treatment of individuals with neurodegenerative illness, in particular dementia, using an indirect care model that includes identifying residual abilities, addressing caregiving challenges, and modifying tasks and environments at any functional–cognitive level or setting of intervention. When the indirect approach is used with clients with dementia, transfer of learning on behalf of the client is not the goal. The goals are environmental adaptation, activity simplification, and external assistance from caregivers.

Principal Intervention Tenets

Principal intervention tenets, regardless of the client's functional–cognitive level, include education, care partner training, activity simplification, and environmental barrier modifications. The specific components must be tailored to each functional–cognitive level, each intervention target, and each client–care partner dyad and their priorities and preferences.

Education

Education of care partners and clients always begins at their current level of understanding. Care partners and, potentially, clients, depending on functional–cognitive level, benefit from education about dementia and the disease process. Education about and understanding of dementia are crucial precursors to the care partner's ability and willingness to change their caregiving approach, implement environmental modifications, and use behavior management techniques.

Care partners need to first understand that ***behavioral and psychological symptoms of dementia*** (BPSDs) are unintentional and part of the disease process. BPSDs are neuropsychiatric symptoms of dementia that influence the function of the person with dementia as well as the ability of the care partner to manage care (e.g., resisting care; forgetting to eat, drink, or bathe; withdrawing from meaningful activities). Current evidence supports the use of functional-analysis-based interventions as the first-line management for BPSDs (Dyer et al., 2018).

Occupational therapy intervention using the CDM approach reduces BPSD presentation (e.g., Gitlin et al., 2009). Education and intervention should take into consideration care partners' readiness to learn (Gitlin & Rose, 2014). For example, a care partner who does not agree that the client is cognitively impaired will not appreciate education and training in behavior management, whereas a care partner who acknowledges dementia and expresses willingness to change their own behaviors and trial strategies will be receptive.

Care Partner Training (Caregiving Approach)

Care partners need assistance to learn and implement proper cueing (use of verbal, visual, and tactile cues) and task facilitation (activity setup and communication) techniques. Many care partners also need continued feedback on their communication approach to the client, such as reminders that rationalizing, arguing, and using incentives are not helpful approaches to modify client behavior because the client's functional cognition will not support reasoning, safety awareness, or following through with agreements. Teaching methods such as verbal education, practice-based training (e.g., modeling, role play, reverse demonstration), and written handouts and resources may be helpful for training care partners to use new strategies (see Video 21.1 for examples; e.g., Family Caregiver Alliance, 2011).

Because dementia is a dynamic disease, care partners need intervention not just to solve their current challenges but also to equip them with the ability to problem solve through future challenges as they arise. Formal caregiver training interventions in behavioral management are efficacious in decreasing dementia behaviors and increasing care partner and client outcomes over time (e.g., Gitlin et al., 2009, 2010a, 2010b, 2017).

Activity Simplification

Occupational therapists are proficient in activity analysis to determine components of tasks that clients may be able to perform even if, for safety or quality reasons, they can no longer perform the whole task. Clients often benefit from activity setup (i.e., visual cueing) to perform tasks and are particularly successful if distracters and clutter are removed. For example, care partners could implement the following strategies:

- Set up laundry on a table for folding. The client may be able to fold laundry with activity setup even if they cannot manipulate the washing appliances or sequence the steps of doing laundry.

- Clear the bathroom counter to include only the materials needed for the desired task. The client might still be able to brush their teeth if only a toothbrush, toothpaste, and cup are in sight on the counter.

- Make food available without comment. Many clients may report they are not hungry but will eat when a meal is placed in front of them.

Care partners may believe the client is incapable of or is "refusing" to do these tasks when in fact the greatest barrier is locating and attending to the selected items needed for performing the task safely and effectively. Furthermore, apathy and lack of initiation are common and pervasive dementia symptoms that reduce participation in meaningful tasks, which then exacerbates dementia behaviors (e.g., anxiety, agitation, wandering, sleep disturbance). Providing tailored activities for clients and training the care partner in facilitating these activities can have a significant impact on quality of life for all involved (e.g., Gitlin et al., 2009).

Of greatest importance is that care partners must be taught that the process, not the product, of meaningful leisure activities is what matters. As long as clients are engaged and enjoying themselves, the accuracy of leisure activities is of no concern. Clients at any functional–cognitive level benefit from a consistent day-to-day routine involving not only regular wake–sleep, meal, and medication timing but also times for meaningful leisure activities.

Environmental Modification

Some environmental barriers are physical and biomechanical; however, many barriers are sensory and cognitive in nature. Small changes, such as the addition of color contrast to steps, bathtub, and shower ledges, and setup for grooming and even feeding tasks can increase the client's performance by reducing the visual–perceptual task demands. The removal of excess clutter and choices reduces attentional demands when the client navigates the environment and may decrease anxiety.

Removing access to appliances (e.g., the stove or microwave if the client can no longer use them independently), vehicles (e.g., locking up keys or putting a club on the steering wheel), any weapons (e.g., firearms, knives), and chemicals and cleaners (which can be easily confused with hygiene or food products) is advisable even in the early stages to prevent accidents. Setting up wandering deterrents (e.g., window chimes on doors, laser or remote motion sensors) can increase a care partner's peace of mind and improve sleep.

Target Population

Clients who are a good fit for intervention with the CDM vary greatly, because it is appropriate for clients with dementia at any level of functional–cognitive impairment. However, dementia is a progressive, neurodegenerative condition associated with distinct symptoms and brain abnormalities and a characteristic pattern of decline (regardless of type of dementia; e.g., Alzheimer's disease, vascular dementia, Lewy body dementia, frontotemporal degeneration, Parkinson's dementia). This pattern involves progressive loss of cognitive abilities, including executive dysfunction, impairments in episodic and semantic memory, attentional deficits, and lack of anticipatory or emergent awareness (and eventually lack of intellectual awareness). This pattern also involves gradual loss of occupational performance, beginning with work, IADLs, leisure, and ADLs.

Unfortunately, in the current health care system, individuals with dementia do not typically receive occupational therapy referrals specifically for dementia-related challenges, other than specialty occupational therapy community-based practices (e.g., Memory Care Home Solutions; Gitlin et al., 2017). Research, however, has demonstrated the capacity

of occupational therapy services to effectively intervene to improve occupational performance as well as to address functional deficits caused specifically by dementia-related symptoms and difficult behaviors, through caregiver training and environmental modifications (e.g., Gitlin et al., 2016, 2017; Pimouguet et al., 2017; Struckmeyer & Pickens, 2016).

More typically, occupational therapists encounter individuals with dementia when they are referred for other reasons indirectly related to underlying cognitive impairment, including falls resulting in orthopedic or other injuries; deconditioning; failure to thrive or weight loss; urinary tract infections; exacerbations of chronic conditions, such as congestive heart failure or chronic obstructive pulmonary disease; or frequent unplanned health care use. In fact, according to the Centers for Medicare and Medicaid Services (2017), 80% of people living with dementia have 3 or more additional chronic health conditions and use health care at greater rates than peers without dementia.

Occupational therapists work with clients with cognitive impairment, often secondary to dementia, regardless of referral diagnosis across a spectrum of service settings, including acute care, inpatient or outpatient rehabilitation, long-term care, skilled nursing facilities, independent or assisted living facilities, and home health therapy. Even if the occupational therapy referral was not made because of cognitive impairment, the occupational therapist, when addressing functional cognition, can and must understand the client's functional–cognitive status to assess and intervene appropriately for their level of functioning, to maximize the effectiveness of the intervention.

Furthermore, occupational therapists will encounter individuals with dementia who have not yet been diagnosed and whose medical charts may lack mention of any type of cognitive impairment. Therapists can serve a crucial role in identifying clients with functional–cognitive impairment so that care can be appropriately tailored by all involved professions and to improve overall health outcomes.

Lesser identified but significant deficits important to a functional–cognitive approach are typically present in the following areas:

- Sensory factor deficits (olfactory, somatosensory, auditory, visual–perceptual processing) and motor factor deficits are typically present and may begin prior to onset of memory changes or other dementia symptoms (Albers et al., 2015).

- Gait and balance tend to be affected early in the disease, and persons with dementia have a higher rate of frailty and risk of falling (Kojima et al., 2017).

- Mood disturbances (including depression and/or anxiety) are common in persons with dementia (Ryu et al., 2017).

Care partners will likely report frustration with managing BPSDs that interfere with daily activities, particularly resistance to ADL care, IADL errors (e.g., medication, finances, driving, meal preparation), sleep disturbance, wandering, withdrawal from meaningful activities, and apathetic or agitated mood (Choi et al., 2017; Fauth et al., 2016; Gitlin et al., 2017; Mukherjee et al., 2017). Administering a BPSD assessment to the care partner can be revealing and necessary to assist in determining intervention priorities; examples include the Neuropsychiatric Inventory (Cummings, 1997) or the Revised Memory and Behavior Problems Checklist (Teri et al., 1992).

Care partners should be included in both initial assessment and intervention planning. Lack of metacognitive awareness is common among individuals for whom the CDM is most appropriate. This is particularly troublesome for clients who have a high level of social comportment, whose functional–cognitive abilities may be easily overestimated. Furthermore, occupational therapists must compare their own appraisal of the client's functional–cognitive abilities (objective, performance-based assessments) with that of the care partner, who may be over- or underestimating the client's abilities (e.g., not aware that the client is not managing IADLs correctly or is not bathing regularly, because they are taking the client's report at face value and are unaware of the client's level of anosognosia).

It is important for the occupational therapist to be aware of the care partner's potential need for education about dementia and implications functionally. The occupational therapist considers the results of the multifaceted evaluation process and uses clinical judgment in interpreting the results to begin the intervention planning.

In the CDM, the occupational therapist uses all of the evaluation information, including the additional caregiver assessment information, to determine the client's functional–cognitive level (see Table 21.1; Levy, 2018; Levy & Burns, 2011). Determining the client's functional–cognitive level is crucial to knowing where to begin the intervention. In some cases, nonstandardized approaches that use skilled and experienced clinical reasoning of functional observations, medical background, and care partner reports may be sufficient.

For a standardized and rigorous method, there are several lines of thought and preferences in the literature for determining a client's functional–cognitive level (see Table 21.1). The client's functional–cognitive level gives insight into their ability to learn and apply techniques, as opposed to what is necessary to modify the task or environment. That is, it helps

the occupational therapist determine to what extent external cues are needed on a day-to-day basis to maintain optional functioning, to identify potential safety concerns, and to educate the care partner on the client's function and how to best assist for occupational performance and safety.

The occupational therapist might consider administering the following measures:

- Scoring for the Cognitive Performance Test (Burns, 2006, 2011) is tied to the 6 functional–cognitive profiles associated with CDM, along with half-levels at 3.5 and 4.5 (Levy & Burns, 2011; Schaber et al., 2013, 2016).

- The Global Deterioration Stages (Reisberg et al., 1982, 1999, 2002) and corresponding Functional Assessment Staging Instrument stages (Sclan & Reisberg, 1992) scores are inversely related to the functional–cognitive level and also follow the progression of the disease (Levy, 2018; Levy & Burns, 2011).

- The Allen Cognitive Level (Allen et al., 1995; McCraith & Earhart, 2018), as determined by the Allen Cognitive Level Screen (Allen et al., 2007) and confirmed by the Allen Diagnostic Module (Earhart, 2006), may be used to determine the client's functional–cognitive level directly (Levy, 2018).

- The Functional Capacity Card Sort can be used to compare care partners' appraisal of function with standardized assessment results (Piersol et al., 2016).

Administration

Specific foci of intervention with the CDM vary by functional-cognitive levels, which have been described in detail in various textbooks and resources (highlights are presented in this chapter, along with practical intervention examples). For more information, reference the original works (e.g., Levy, 2018; Levy & Burns, 2011; McCraith & Earhart, 2018; McCraith et al., 2011; Reisberg et al., 1982; Sclan & Reisberg, 1992). Each of the

TABLE 21.1. Methods to Ascertain Functional–Cognitive Level

CDM FUNCTIONAL–COGNITIVE LEVEL	CORRESPONDING ASSESSMENT SCORES		
	ACL	GDS/FAST	CPT
6: Absence of functional–cognitive disability	6	1–2	5.6
5: Mild functional decline	5	3	5
4: Moderate to moderately severe functional decline	4	4–5	4
3: Severe functional decline	3	6	3
2: Very severe functional decline	2	7	2
1: Very severe functional decline	1	7	1

Note. ACL = Allen Cognitive Level; CDM = Cognitive Disabilities Model; CPT = Cognitive Performance Test; FAST = Functional Assessment Staging Instrument; GDS = Global Deterioration Stages.

principal intervention tenets is considered uniquely by the determined functional–cognitive level. Additionally, each level provides specific information on functional–cognitive abilities that are common at the level, safety recommendations, and caregiver approaches best suited for intervention (Levy, 2018; Levy & Burns, 2011; McCraith & Earhart, 2018; McCraith et al., 2011).

Any specific intervention target must be tailored and taught to the client or care partner in a manner appropriate to the client's functional–cognitive level (e.g., see Table 21.2). This chapter focuses on practical intervention principles in the CDM and commonly used techniques and strategies in occupational therapy practice for persons with dementia (e.g., Gitlin et al., 2017).

TABLE 21.2. Examples of Interventions for Medication Management at Each Functional–Cognitive Level

FUNCTIONAL–COGNITIVE LEVEL	ENVIRONMENTAL MODIFICATIONS	ACTIVITY SIMPLIFICATION	CAREGIVING APPROACH
6: Absence of functional–cognitive disability	None needed	None needed	None needed
5: Mild functional decline	• Use a pillbox. • Write a medication list to be used as a checklist.	Remove extra medication bottles and throw away expired medications.	• Teach care partner to give reminders or set timers. • Teach care partner how to double-check that medications have been filled in pillbox correctly and taken appropriately.
4: Moderate to moderately severe functional decline	• Use pillbox. • Lock extra medications out of sight and reach.	• Remove extra medication bottles. • Choose a medication box where each day can be removed so that client does not have to identify correct day of the week. • Use an automatic pill dispenser that locks away untaken medication to prevent overdosing.	• Teach care partner how to set up and cue to help the client initiate the activity safely and correctly. • Retrieve pills and place in a separate cup or show the client which pills to take; deliver to the client with a glass of water. • Watch to make sure the client swallows the pills and does not place them somewhere else and then forget about the task. • Care partner can take their pills at the same time if the client feels agitated; change the language to "We will take these pills together" or "I forgot to give you these earlier—I'm sorry!" to shift the focus to themselves for clients whose performance suffers when they feel they are being criticized or told what to do.
3: Severe functional decline	• Remove access to all medications. • Lock medications out of sight and reach.	• All medications must be organized and administered by care partner. • Fewer pills can be given at a time if the client is resistant (wait 5–10 minutes or until the client has forgotten, and then resume the task).	• Teach the care partner how to set up and cue throughout the task. • Give the pills to the client in a small cup, and provide a glass of water at the same time. • Give the client only a few pills at a time if a large number of pills results in the client feeling anxious or perturbed. • Watch the client swallow the pills (otherwise the pills may end up elsewhere, e.g., in pockets or fed to the pet). • Ask the doctor if pills can be crushed or ground and put into applesauce or pudding.
2: Very severe functional decline	Client should have no access to medications.	Medications must be administered by care partner.	• Ask the doctor if pills can be crushed or ground. • Administer the medications to the client's mouth, or assist the client in hand to mouth using hand-under-hand technique.
1: Very severe functional decline	The client should have no access to medications.	Medications must be administered by care partner.	• Ask the doctor if pills can be crushed or ground. • Administer the medications to the client's mouth, or assist the client in hand to mouth. • If the client qualifies for hospice, this service can help reduce care partner burden for organizing and monitoring medications.

Functional–Cognitive Levels

Level 6: Absence of Functional–Cognitive Disability

At this level, no intervention is needed to address functional–cognitive abilities because they are within typical limits. Clients can learn through traditional teaching methods, including verbal instruction, hands-on training, and written handouts and instructions, and they do not need care partner training (Levy, 2018; Levy & Burns, 2011; McCraith & Earhart, 2018; McCraith et al., 2011).

Level 5: Mild Functional Decline

Functional cognition impairments are often secondary to attentional control, disinhibition, and working-memory impairments, leading to difficulties with IADLs, especially if they are complex or new (e.g., driving, meal preparation, medication management, financial management). This level may include subjective or diagnosed mild cognitive impairment or very early-stage dementia (Levy, 2018; Levy & Burns, 2011; McCraith & Earhart, 2018; McCraith et al., 2011; Reisberg et al., 1982; Sclan & Reisberg, 1992).

Safety Recommendations

Clients need someone to check on them at least daily to ensure their safety. Some families choose to use in-home cameras to monitor the client or to help determine the level of assistance they need, because the family cannot take the client's report for granted.

Caregiving Approach

IADLs and other complex tasks requiring the client to make good decisions, keep track of details, use multitasking and simultaneous attention, and exercise judgment must be monitored because of safety concerns. Care partners need training in how to monitor and provide assistance for IADLs. Thoughtful communication techniques can reduce the client's agitation; clients might resist help because of lack of insight (e.g., fixing the pill organizer without the client being present to avoid making them feel defensive, monitoring their driving without necessarily telling them they are being monitored).

Activity Simplification

If any tasks are assessed to be unsafe and the client needs more support, care partners need training in how to take over components without necessarily taking over the entire task. Conducting activity analysis and practicing with the care partner are helpful techniques (e.g., modeling, role play, and reverse demonstration).

Environmental Modification

Environmental safeguards should also be put in place surrounding IADLs. Examples include the following:

- *Medication management:* Pillboxes or automatic pill dispensers can be useful to prevent medication over- or underdosing.

- *Financial management:* Reducing access to credit cards and checks can prevent scams or poor judgment during purchases; having mail and bills forwarded to the care partner if they do not live with the client can ensure that bills are paid on time.

- *Meal preparation:* Smoke detectors should be in working order, and automatic fire extinguishers should be placed above stove if possible. Expired or spoiled foods should be regularly removed from the refrigerator.

- *Driving:* Monitoring or removing vehicle access is advised to avoid any unsafe events. If unsafe driving behaviors have occurred, recommending driving cessation to the physician is advisable. If no unsafe behaviors have occurred, care partners and clients still need education and empowerment on conversing with the physician or scheduling a driving evaluation if appropriate.

- *Other environmental modifications:* External memory aids and cues may be helpful for orienting the client to locations of items or to the day and date of planned activities (see Figure 21.1).

Level 4: Moderate to Moderately Severe Functional Decline

Functional cognition is often impaired secondary to attentional deficits (difficulty inhibiting irrelevant cues) and significant working memory and executive functioning impairments, which can result in impaired IADLs (need partial or full assistance) and ADLs (requiring task reminders or setup). In particular, the client may now need assistance for ADLs for adequate frequency or quality of bathing, hygiene, dressing, and eating.

The client may have BPSDs such as wandering; rummaging; losing or misplacing items; asking repetitive questions; shadowing the caregiver; or experiencing delusions, hallucinations, or paranoia. Because clients may resist bathing and changing and may forget to eat or drink, urinary tract infections, malnutrition, or failure to thrive may be the reason for occupational therapy referral. This functional–cognitive level may include early to moderate dementia (Levy, 2018; Levy & Burns, 2011; McCraith & Earhart, 2018; McCraith et al., 2011; Reisberg et al., 1982; Sclan & Reisberg, 1992).

Safety Recommendations

The client is no longer safe to perform IADLs without assistance (see information for Level 5). Recommendations for IADL safety include the following:

- Medications should be monitored or administered by care partners.

- Driving should be removed or further assessed.

- Money management should be restricted.

- Meal preparation should be supervised or simplified.

FIGURE 21.1. Visual cues for orientation to time and locations of items.

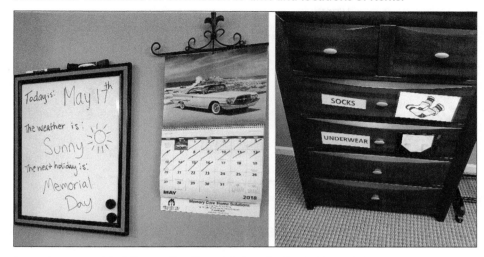

Source. Image copyright © Memory Care Home Solutions. Reprinted with permission.

Furthermore, care partners must provide safety and structure and monitor all health needs. Twenty-four-hour supervision is recommended; if the client lives alone, an assisted living environment should be considered. Clients at this level benefit from a consistent day-to-day routine and schedule incorporating physical, mental, and social activities. In-home care, adult day care, or both are recommended. Care partners benefit from other, more formal supports, such as support groups.

Caregiving Approach

Care partners need training in how to assist with IADLs and ADLs in a way that is most appropriate for the individual client, with an emphasis on safety as well as communication and cueing approaches to reduce agitation caused by resistance to care. Clients may no longer initiate activities without assistance, and this should not be mistaken for lack of interest or motivation. The client no longer performs familiar tasks, including ADLs, regularly or without activity setup (see Figure 21.2) from a care partner, and they may require additional prompting during tasks to perform with quality (e.g., clients may say they are bathing, and care partners may believe they are bathing, but performance-based assessment might reveal that the client is not washing thoroughly, only attending to visible areas and ignoring less visible areas or not using soap).

Finding the "just-right" approach for each client that also matches the care partner's abilities and willingness requires creativity and a trial-and-error approach. Use of single-step cueing can be helpful, with an emphasis on caregiver reverse demonstration to refine their approach (see Video 21.1).

FIGURE 21.2. Activity setup to decrease attentional and problem-solving demands.

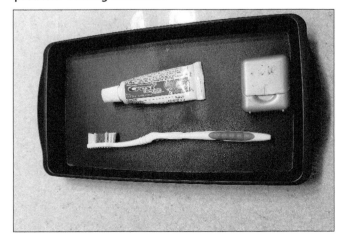

Source. Image copyright © Memory Care Home Solutions. Reprinted with permission.

Activity Simplification

Clients take very concrete actions focused on cause and effect, and they can do familiar tasks only when the activity is set up for them in advance. Clients pay attention to what is in sight and are distracted by clutter or excess choices and options. Care partners need education on activity setup, simplification, and cueing needs throughout tasks. They need training in communication techniques that rely more on step-by-step instructions and timed prompting for ADLs.

Examples are as follows:

- Care partners should be taught to give single-step cues, such as saying, "Come with me" to the bathroom, then cueing the client to get in the shower, rather than giving a multistep instruction (e.g., "Go take a shower"). Additionally, use of a shower calendar with "shower" written on certain days of the week may allow the caregiver to shift the blame to a schedule when providing cueing, and reduce client agitation over "being told what to do."

- Care partners should use set schedules and calendars (e.g., "It's time to eat this delicious lunch," with presentation of food) rather than questions or choices (e.g., "Are you hungry?" or "Do you want to eat lunch?").

- Simplifying enjoyed leisure activities and training the care partner to help the client initiate activities is essential at this stage for increased mood, improved quality of life, and reduced BPSDs. Clients respond better to single-step directives with activity setup (e.g., "Look at this") rather than questions or choices (e.g., "Do you want to do this?" or "What do you want to do?").

Activities that are familiar and repetitive (i.e., 1 step) may be most successful. Simplified household management tasks (e.g., folding towels, sorting items or silverware, wiping down surfaces) or leisure tasks (e.g., simple color-blocked 24-piece puzzles, word searches or simplified letter searches [e.g., "Find all the *A*'s"], or craft activities) may be appropriate, with consideration of the client's previously enjoyed activities and occupational profile.

Environmental Modification
Environmental simplification, removal of fall hazards, and reduction of clutter will decrease attentional demands for the client. Adding visual color contrast to indicate changes in floor thresholds, in bathrooms (e.g., shower, toilets, grab bars), and on other key task supplies will increase the client's ability to perceive what is needed during tasks (see Figure 21.3). The client will attend to what is in sight; thus, all medications, chemicals and cleaners, weapons, and knives should be removed and locked in a closet or in a cabinet with safety locks (unobtrusive magnetized locks may be preferable if the client is irritated by visible locks).

Removing access to cooking appliances, such as the stove (removing knobs) and microwave (adding a lock or covering up buttons), as well as the thermostat (with a locked box), will prevent safety concerns. Wandering deterrents should be implemented before any incidents occur. External orientation aids (e.g., whiteboard with day, date, planned activities) may help the client understand and give the care partner options for communicating about the plan for the day and managing repetitive questions.

Visual cues and labels may improve function. For example, labeling "hot" or "cold" on faucets or labeling drawers with a word and visual of interior contents (such as "underwear") may increase the client's ability to locate and perform tasks with fewer verbal cues.

Level 3: Severe Functional Decline
Clients at this level have functional cognition impaired secondary to attentional and working-memory impairments that are severe enough to prevent the client from following through with goal-directed actions. This level designates moderately severe dementia, as indicated by assistance needed for all

FIGURE 21.3. Color contrast to decrease visual–perceptual demands.

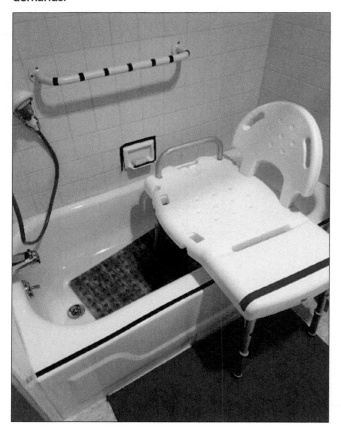

Source. Image copyright © Memory Care Home Solutions. Reprinted with permission.

ADLs, including step-by-step instructions and provision of items needed for tasks. The client's actions are more exploratory in interacting with the environment.

Orientation to time, place, and sometimes people is impaired. The client needs assistance for all ADLs and is dependent for IADLs. They will make some contribution when presented with the proper activity supplies and setup. Pacing, searching for something, and "wanting to go home" are common at this level (Levy, 2018; Levy & Burns, 2011; McCraith & Earhart, 2018; McCraith et al., 2011; Reisberg et al., 1982; Sclan & Reisberg, 1992).

Safety Recommendations
The client needs 24-hour supervision. Close monitoring and prevention of access to potential hazards as well as step-by-step assistance for all ADLs will ensure safety and quality of performance.

Caregiving Approach
The client needs step-by-step cues and assistance for all tasks. Some care partners at this level might have taken over ADL

tasks completely, but learning strategies to involve the client as much as possible can reduce stress for both the client and the care partner. BPSDs contribute to care partners' difficulty in assisting the client. Care partners (both family and professional) need education in strategies for interpreting and responding to behaviors. Behavioral management training and performance-based problem solving will increase caregivers' skills and abilities to manage difficult BPSDs (e.g., to analyze the antecedents or triggers for behavior and ways to modify for a better outcome). Because care partners at this level tend to be exhausted mentally, emotionally, and physically, they need education and encouragement to use self-care and stress-reduction strategies, including practicing deep breathing, taking breaks from caregiving, and engaging more formal supports.

Activity Simplification

Whereas activity setup might have been sufficient for Level 4, at this level, clients need step-by-step instructions to sequence all ADLs (including eating) and other activities. Removal of clutter or excess materials is crucial, as is task setup (only the items needed for the given activity should be in sight or reach). Leisure activities that are rote, repetitive, and 1 step will be most successful (e.g., folding towels or napkins instead of clothing).

The provision of meaningful activities is crucial at this stage, because ability to initiate meaningful tasks is lost, and napping during the day leads to risk of sleep disturbance at night. Activity engagement (e.g., listening to music through headphones, folding towels, performing simple 2-item sorting tasks, looking at photo albums and reminiscing) should be selected and attempted with consideration for the client's prior interests and occupational profile. Care partners need training in how to set up and cue the client during leisure activities.

Environmental Modification

See Level 4 (all material and fall hazards should be removed, wandering deterrents enacted, color contrast added to select or troublesome thresholds or activity supplies). Some clients may not recognize their own reflection; removing or covering mirrors or windows with fabric or paper may relieve fear or distraction. Signs incorporating visuals on doors may help the client with wayfinding in their home (see Figure 21.4).

Level 2: Very Severe Functional Decline

At this level, the client's functional cognition is impaired secondary to extremely impaired attention and memory abilities, and the client is more internally focused (e.g., proprioceptive cues). Most behavior and movement seems to be purposeless or in direct response to touch, sounds, or other sensory stimulation. The client may not be able to ambulate (either with or without assistance).

Restlessness and agitation are common, particularly when the client is overstimulated by the environment. The client is

FIGURE 21.4. Visual cue for location of bathroom.

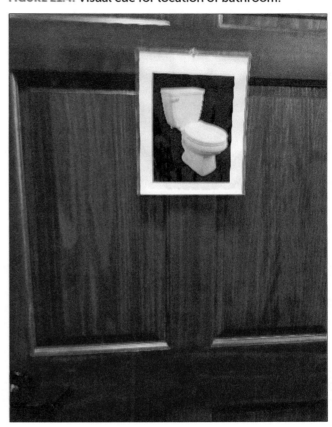

Source. Image copyright © Memory Care Home Solutions. Reprinted with permission.

unable to take care of any basic needs and requires maximal if not complete assistance for all ADLs and IADLs. This level designates severe dementia (Levy, 2018; Levy & Burns, 2011; McCraith & Earhart, 2018; McCraith et al., 2011; Reisberg et al., 1982; Sclan & Reisberg, 1992).

Safety Recommendations

The client needs 24-hour supervision and assistance and requires total care. The client is at risk for falls, improper use of objects, and other safety concerns as a result of apraxia and inability to notice or respond to safety hazards. Feeding programs (reduced nutrition and hydration or changes with swallowing can occur), fall prevention, and movement and positioning programs are key for the client's safety and can help care partners manage day-to-day care (e.g., Levy, 2018). The client is on the verge of qualifying for hospice services for dementia diagnosis (see Level 1 for more information).

Caregiving Approach

Care partners must be taught total-care techniques. Behavior management training (as in Level 3) can help care partners to learn to problem solve through difficult tasks and behaviors.

Clients respond best to 1 direction at a time (1-step cues) for all ADLs. For example, at mealtime, the caregiver should use a series of 1-step directives (e.g., "Come with me," "Sit down," place a piece of food in the client's hand, "Taste") rather than multi-step suggestions (e.g., "Let's go to the dining room to eat"). For toileting, single-step directives such as, "Come with me," "Push down your pants," and "Sit down" work better than "Go to the bathroom."

Care partners need education and hands-on training in cueing and comfort-care techniques. Resistance to care for ADLs is common when too many verbal directions are given, unanticipated touch occurs, or the client is overstimulated. This stage can be exhausting for care partners, particularly if the client is still very mobile and needs constant monitoring, such as in the case example of John and his wife Holly (see Case Example 21.1 at the end of this chapter). Care partners need encouragement to use community resources, ask family members for help, and take breaks.

Activity Simplification

The care partner now may need to do activities for the client rather than just giving verbal and visual directives. The client may no longer be able to perform purposeful leisure activities. The care partner should try activities incorporating sensory stimulation (e.g., music, dancing, simple exercises, colorful and textured objects, lotion and massages) to help calm the client and reduce BPSDs.

Environmental Modification

The environment needs to be completely safety proofed at this stage because of the client's complete unawareness of safety hazards. Ensuring that any hazardous objects are out of sight and inaccessible is ideal.

Level 1: Very Severe Functional Decline

At this level, functional cognition is impaired secondary to attention limited completely to internal cues; the client may seem unaware of external stimuli. The client is dependent for all ADLs and IADLs. This level designates very severe or end-stage dementia (Levy, 2018; Levy & Burns, 2011; McCraith & Earhart, 2018; McCraith et al., 2011; Reisberg et al., 1982; Sclan & Reisberg, 1992).

Safety Recommendations

Twenty-four-hour care is needed. Complications such as aspiration, pneumonia, pressure ulcers, malnutrition, sepsis, and urinary tract infections are common at this stage. Because this is the final stage of the disease, the client may benefit from hospice services. If the care partner has not heard of hospice, it is important to facilitate a conversation about it, given that physicians might not bring up the subject with the family. Hospice services can help greatly with managing pain, preventing pressure ulcers, observing swallowing deficits, keeping an eye on the client's comfort, managing medications, and providing supplies at no out-of-pocket cost for the family.

Caregiving Approach

Negative behaviors, such as agitation, pushing away, or hitting, may occur with overstimulation (e.g., excess noise, unanticipated touch). Care partners should speak calmly and give short, basic cues. Any behaviors or actions are automatic and may be elicited by 1-step cues (e.g., "Turn," "Open mouth," "Swallow"; e.g., Levy, 2018). Care partners need training in ADLs and total-care techniques, behavioral management, and sensory stimulation programs (as in Level 2).

Activity Simplification

Care providers may note that the client has a short attention span for items in sight in the environment or in response to perceiving movement (e.g., washcloth, gentle touching or massage, stuffed animals, meaningful music from the person's late teens and early 20s). Familiar activities or stimulation with meaningful items can help the person to feel safe and calm.

Environmental Modification

Care partners benefit from training in use of durable medical equipment (e.g., hospital bed, bedside commode or bedpan) as well as care techniques (e.g., how to change incontinence supplies or clothing in bed). Placing enjoyed items in the client's line of sight may help the client to notice and engage. Keep environmental stimulation low, with 1 stimulus at a time (e.g., turn television or radio off, gently notify before touch, keep conversation and speech calm and at a level that does not irritate the client).

Goals and Documentation

All intervention provided with the CDM should be documented thoroughly, including but not limited to the following:

- Performance-based training in ADLs and IADLs;

- Task-oriented therapeutic activity, including leisure tasks for increased activity and reduced BPSDs; and

- Recommendations and communications provided to the client, the caregiver, or both (e.g., cueing training during ADLs and IADLs, activity facilitation techniques, environmental adaptations, behavioral management, and training in use of durable medical or adaptive equipment).

It is important to document that all interventions should be specifically stated in relationship to improving ADL and IADL performance, safety, and management of BPSDs. The level of cueing required (whether verbal, visual, or tactile) and amount of time needed for processing should be documented for the client. Furthermore, it is important to specify the reason for any adaptations made, whether for cognitive, visual–perceptual, sensory, motor, or other reasons (e.g., adding color contrast in the shower to help with visual–perceptual impairment and explaining the difference between a transfer before and after adding the color contrast).

Occupational therapists should document care partner training by including statements about education provided and for what topic (e.g., dementia, progression of disease, communication and cueing training, benefits and purpose of equipment or environmental modifications). Moreover, documentation should include care partner training components (e.g., caregiver performance and the level of assistance the care partner needs from the therapist to implement proper cueing, transfer, or ADL and IADL technique) as well as what other types of care partner training were provided (e.g., role play, brainstorming, training in problem solving). In summary, the therapist should document the caregiver's ability to implement and perform tasks with use of recommended strategies and what type of training was needed to facilitate this.

Goals for work with this population may include both client and care partner involvement. Goal documentation should strategically specify desired performance of the task, with a specified level of cueing and physical assistance from the caregiver, rather than in general or just from the therapist. To help facilitate a continual focus on care partner training, when documenting goals, occupational therapists should specify the particular care partner who will be performing the challenging task in question after occupational therapy is over.

Example goals are as follows:

- Bathing
  - *Short-term goal:* Client will perform tub or shower transfer with supervision and minimal verbal cues from the caregiver, with appropriate environmental modifications.
  - *Short-term goal:* Client will bathe with moderate physical assistance and moderate verbal cues from the caregiver.
  - *Long-term goal:* Client will bathe 3 times a week, with minimal assistance and appropriate environmental setup and equipment for safety.

- Medication management
  - *Short-term goal:* Client will take medications with minimal physical assistance and moderate verbal cues from the caregiver.
  - *Long-term goal:* Client will take medications with minimal verbal cues from the caregiver and appropriate environmental setup.

- Leisure activity performance for BPSD management
  - *Short-term goal:* Caregiver will return-demonstrate the home activity program with the client (to reduce behavioral symptoms and improve participation in meaningful activity) with minimal assistance.
  - *Long-term goal:* Client and caregiver will be independent in the home activity program.

Intervention Considerations

The CDM is an adaptive and compensatory approach designed for persons with an irreversible cognitive impairment. The premise of occupational therapy interventions using the CDM with persons with dementia differs from a traditional occupational therapy model in that rather than attempting to remediate cognitive abilities or discharging the client from occupational therapy because of their inability to learn, the occupational therapist determines the residual abilities of the person and focuses on improving their engagement in meaningful activity as well as making environmental modifications to support their remaining capabilities and improve their quality of life.

Even very brief or time-limited occupational therapy interventions focused on simplifying tasks, modifying environments, and bolstering caregiver skills have been shown to improve health outcomes for persons with dementia and their caregivers (Gitlin et al., 2017). Occupational therapy interventions have been shown to improve the function of persons with dementia despite a progressive prognosis (Jensen & Padilla, 2011; Pimouguet et al., 2017). Furthermore, randomized controlled trials have shown that occupational therapy interventions for persons with dementia that heavily incorporate care partner training can reduce BPSDs, improve ADL function, and increase caregiver skills and well-being (e.g., Gitlin et al., 2009, 2010a, 2010b).

A systematic review of effective interventions for Alzheimer's and dementia identified the following priorities for intervention across the duration of the disease:

- Occupation-based ADL training

- Physical exercise for improved sleep, ADLs, and physical function

- Social activity for improved sleep

- Errorless learning and prompting for the performance of ADLs and IADLs

- Cognitive stimulation for improved quality of life and socialization (Smallfield & Heckenlaible, 2017).

Key components of effective occupational therapy interventions include focusing on the care partner and their readiness to learn (Gitlin & Rose, 2014), brainstorming and problem solving with the care partner, and providing tools to help them continue to manage dementia symptoms as the disease progresses and changes (Gitlin et al., 2010a, 2010b).

Use of the CDM is optimal and most advantageous when a care partner is able to participate. If no care partner is identified, such as when the client lives alone and has no supports, no one will be able to implement the intervention in the client's day-to-day life. The CDM is helpful in this situation to further inform the occupational therapist's recommendation for appropriate level of assistance needed for safe day-to-day living. It also can justify recommendations for more support or for determining appropriate living arrangements or home and environmental modifications.

Other approaches may be complementary and appropriate for clients, depending on their functional–cognitive level. The Neurofunctional Approach may be used complementarily with this model (e.g., Crowe & Gabriel, 2013). Strategy and learning approaches may be applicable if the client is in the early stages of dementia (e.g., Level 5 or above) but, given the progressive nature of dementia, is not usually a main focus of intervention. The CDM must be used with caution in the event of reversible cognitive impairment, such as a change in cognitive status resulting from urinary tract infections or delirium, and should be revised as any related acute health problems resolve.

Perhaps the most important consideration of use of the CDM is that the client with dementia might not have been referred to occupational therapy because of dementia or cognitive impairment. Nonetheless, no matter the setting or reason for referral, determining the functional–cognitive level

of the client is essential for effective intervention. Identification of the functional–cognitive level enables the occupational therapist to focus on the client's residual abilities and techniques to

- Support their current capacities,

- Use an appropriate environmental and task adaptation approach, and

- Engage the caregiver in a practical and helpful manner to ensure that the intervention carries over into the client's day-to-day life.

A focus on intervention tailored to the client's current abilities and the care partners' priorities will help support current abilities, maintain ADL function, bolster participation in meaningful activities, and maintain the highest possible quality of life for both the client and their family or care staff throughout the progression of the disease.

CASE EXAMPLE 21.1. Interventions for John and His Wife Holly

John is 59 years old and was diagnosed with early-onset Alzheimer's disease 5 years ago. John was referred to occupational therapy because of frequent falls and deconditioning.

Results of Assessment

The occupational therapist observed that John was unable to perform goal-directed actions and was minimally responsive to environmental stimuli, other than seeking out and being intent on interacting with objects in view or that he could touch with his hands, including keys, cards, magnets on the kitchen counters, and his own pants zipper. John required maximal assistance for all ADLs and full assistance for IADLs. The **occupational therapist** used the Functional Assessment Staging Instrument and Global Deterioration Stages to determine that John was currently at functional–cognitive Level 2 and confirmed this with the Allen Cognitive Assessment Battery.

John's wife, **Holly,** was most concerned about the following problem areas:

1. Preventing John from wandering
2. Preventing him from falling
3. Preventing him from rummaging in drawers and putting items in the toilet
4. Keeping him from urinating in the trash can or on the carpeted floor.

The occupational therapist referenced the CDM and appropriate task and environmental interventions for John and collaborated with Holly to determine appropriate approaches that matched her preferences.

Intervention

Goal 1: Wandering Prevention
Environmental Modification. The occupational therapist suggested environmental modifications to prevent wandering that coincided with functional–cognitive Level 2 for each of the goals Holly identified. For wandering, the therapist helped implement and train Holly in the use of the following modifications:

- Motion sensors were added to detect John's movements at night. If he were to get up, an alarm in Holly's room would notify her that he had moved his legs over the edge of the bed.

(Continued)

- Door chimes were installed on exterior doors of the house so that everyone would hear if John opened a door to leave.

Activity Simplification and Caregiving Approach. The occupational therapist taught Holly that different cueing techniques and environmental approaches would be more successful than reasoning and trying to make agreements with John.

- Trying to convince John not to leave the house would not work, because John was now "living in the moment." Trying to tell him to do or not to do things in advance no longer worked.
- Focusing on monitoring technology and preventing access to unsafe doors and items was the best technique to use, because John could no longer adapt his own behavior.

Goal 2: Fall Prevention
Environmental Modification. The occupational therapist helped Holly to implement fall prevention environmental modifications, including the following:

- They added color contrast using black electrical tape to the changes in thresholds of floors where John had fallen, because he was no longer able to perceive differences between the tan carpet and the tan kitchen floor and between the white tub and the white tile in the bathroom.
- They installed brighter lightbulbs and motion-sensor lights to activate when John walked in darker areas.

Caregiving Approach. The occupational therapist taught Holly new ways to reduce the chances of John falling, including the following:

- A change in cueing technique was needed. Telling John not to go to certain areas of the house was no longer helpful, because he could not comprehend or retain this instruction, and thus could not follow it later.
- Instead, the occupational therapist encouraged Holly to focus on limiting John's access to those areas of the house by keeping him engaged in activity and by implementing the environmental safeguards described previously.

Goal 3: Activity Engagement
Environmental Modification. The occupational therapist taught Holly how to keep John safe and engaged in meaningful activity, including by

- Removing unsafe or important items from countertops to which John had access and placing them in a locked drawer with magnetic childproof locks, and
- Providing an effective sensory "vest" that the occupational therapist created over many sessions using trial and error. This vest served to engage John but also moved with him as he ambulated throughout the household (see Figure 21.5).

Activity Simplification. The occupational therapist trained Holly in activity simplification ideas, including for the goal of engaging John in more (safe) activities.

- The occupational therapist taught Holly that other activities they had been trying were too complex for John now because they had too many steps. John now needed single-step activities (repetitive, rote) or just exploratory activities rather than goal-directed tasks.
- Removing excess supplies from activity areas was crucial to prevent confusion and distraction.
- John needed activities set up for him in full (e.g., putting toothpaste on the toothbrush rather than just handing John a toothbrush and toothpaste separately) to perform tasks as accurately as possible.

(Continued)

CASE EXAMPLE 21.1 Interventions for John and His Wife Holly *(Cont.)*

FIGURE 21.5. Sensory stimulation solution.

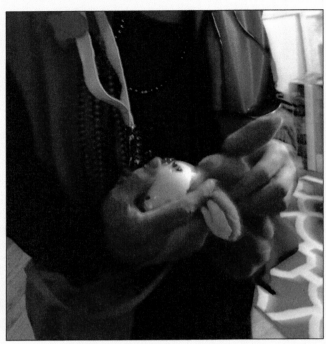

Source. Image copyright © Memory Care Home Solutions. Reprinted with permission.

Caregiving Approach. The occupational therapist helped Holly problem solve ways to make engaging John in activities less stressful for everyone.

- Trying to constantly engage John in conversation and activities was causing Holly to feel exhausted and discouraged.
- The occupational therapist told Holly that it is a full-time job to be a caregiver and helped her to brainstorm about other people who could come over to give her a break and whom she could ask to try different activities with John.

Goal 4: Limiting Urination in Inappropriate Places
Environmental Modification. The occupational therapist helped Holly change the environmental layout of the home to limit John's urination in inappropriate locations, including the following:

- The trash can was removed and placed inside a closet so that it would be out of John's sight.
- A picture of a toilet was also added to the bathroom door in case it would trigger John to use the restroom on his own. The occupational therapist cautioned that it might not help, but Holly was open to a visual, saying, "It can't hurt, and it might help."

Activity Simplification. The occupational therapist trained Holly in activity simplification for toileting tasks to prevent inappropriate urination.

- The occupational therapist taught Holly that use of the sensory vest was reducing excess urination not only by keeping John busy but also seemingly by reducing John's likelihood of touching his zipper, which was a sensory cue that he should unzip his pants to urinate. Thus, preventing John from seeing, touching, or feeling

(Continued)

sensations that reminded him of automatic bodily needs kept those undesired tasks from happening. Conversely, providing reminders of or "similar feelings" to a desired task can help to facilitate it.

- When the sensory vest was being washed or not in use, the occupational therapist taught Holly to dress John in pants without a zipper so that he was less likely to be cued to unzip and pull down his pants to urinate in inappropriate locations.

Caregiving Approach. The occupational therapist taught Holly that John was no longer able to rationally decide when and where to use the bathroom.

- John could not be "convinced" to use the bathroom and also could not find the bathroom even if he wanted to, given his impaired memory and problem solving.
- Holly should focus on noticing John's body cues and anticipating when he would try to go to the bathroom (e.g., reaching for his pants). She should try to redirect him in that moment rather than telling him in advance what to do.
- Holly should try to preemptively take John to the bathroom at key times during the day or every few hours to empty his bladder intentionally rather than waiting for an accident to happen, by using single-step cues (e.g., "Come with me") to get him to go into the bathroom.

Results of Intervention

After the occupational therapy intervention, Holly reported great relief with the behaviors that had caused her so much stress (see Exhibit 21.1 for John's progress documented in a SOAP [Subjective, Objective, Assessment, Plan] note). She reported that she was able to sleep much better not having to be "on alert" all night, and she felt confident that John had a higher level of safety with use of the motion sensors and color contrast. In addition, Holly reported that John seemed less agitated and had a better mood now that he was more stimulated by the sensory vest.

EXHIBIT 21.1. John's Progress SOAP Note

S: Care partner reports client has had fewer instances of urinating in inappropriate locations since last visit with addition of sensory vest and after moving the trash can. Care partner is still concerned about client getting up at night.

O: Provided caregiver training in use of environmental modifications to reduce instances of dementia behaviors (wandering and pacing at night). Trialed adaptive equipment, including motion sensor and door chimes, to alert care partner of client's movement. Care partner verbalizes and demonstrates understanding of use of equipment with 3 repetitions to trial and gain proficiency. Client performed bed transfers with moderate visual cues, with care partner responding to and using motion sensor correctly and safely after practice. Assisted in installation of door chimes and provided education in benefits and purpose of use; care partner verbalizes understanding.

A: Client's performance of ADLs, IADLs, leisure tasks, functional mobility, and transfers is limited by intrinsic impairments (including cognitive, motor, sensory, and mobility concerns) but is improving with implementation of environmental modifications (visual cues and visual contrast in the environment) as well as caregiver training (in dementia education, cueing and behavioral management skills, and activity facilitation skills). Client and care partner will benefit from continued training in task performance, addition of visual cues for tasks and other environmental modifications, and gradual progression in daily activity program with care partner use of recommended behavioral management skills.

P: Client and care partner are progressing toward all goals.

Note. SOAP = Subjective, Objective, Assessment, Plan.

Conclusion

Occupational therapists have an integral role in the treatment of individuals with neurodegenerative illnesses such as dementia. By using an indirect approach to cognitive intervention, occupational therapists are uniquely able to address the dynamic challenges caregivers face throughout the disease. They creatively assist in solutions involving task and environmental modifications to enable engagement in meaningful and necessary occupations for both the client and their care partners.

References

Albers, M. W., Gilmore, G. C., Kaye, J., Murphy, C., Wingfield, A., Bennett, D. A., . . . Zhang, L. I. (2015). At the interface of sensory and motor dysfunctions and Alzheimer's disease. *Alzheimer's and Dementia, 11*, 70–98. https://doi.org/10.1016/j.jalz.2014.04.514

Allen, C. K., Austin, S. L., David, S. K., Earhart, C. A., McCraith, D. B., & Riska-Williams, L. (2007). *Manual for the Allen Cognitive Level Screen–5 (ACL–5) and Large Allen Cognitive Level Screen (LACLS–5).* Camarillo, CA: ACLS and LACLS Committee.

Allen, C. K., Blue, T., & Earhart, C. A. (1995). *Understanding the modes of performance.* Ormond Beach, CA: Allen Conferences.

Alzheimer's Association. (2018). 2018 Alzheimer's disease facts and figures. *Alzheimer's and Dementia, 14*, 367–429. https://doi.org/10.1016/j.jalz.2018.02.001

American Occupational Therapy Association. (2014). Occupational therapy practice framework: Domain and process (3rd ed.). *American Journal of Occupational Therapy, 68*(Suppl. 1), S1–S48. https://doi.org/10.5014/ajot.2014.682006

Burns, T. (2006). *Cognitive Performance Test* (rev. ed.). Pequannock, NJ: Maddak.

Burns, T. (2011). *Cognitive Performance Test Revised draft manual.* Pequannock, NJ: Maddak.

Centers for Medicare & Medicaid Services. (2017). *State level chronic conditions table: Prevalence, Medicare utilization and spending, 2015.* Retrieved from https://www.cms.gov/Research-Statistics-Data-and-Systems/Statistics-Trends-and-Reports/Chronic-Conditions/CC_Main.html

Choi, S. S. W., Budhathoki, C., & Gitlin, L. N. (2017). Co-occurrence and predictors of three commonly occurring behavioral symptoms in dementia: Agitation, aggression, and rejection of care. *American Journal of Geriatric Psychiatry, 25*, 459–468. https://doi.org/10.1016/j.jagp.2016.10.013

Crowe, J., & Gabriel, L. (2013). Errorless learning and spaced retrieval training for clients with Alzheimer's dementia. *Physical and Occupational Therapy in Geriatrics, 31*, 254–267. https://doi.org/10.3109/02703181.2013.796037

Cummings, J. L. (1997). The Neuropsychiatric Inventory: Assessing psychopathology in dementia patients. *Neurology, 48*(Suppl. 6), S10–S16. https://doi.org/10.1212/WNL.48.5_Suppl_6.10S

Dyer, S. M., Harrison, S. L., Laver, K., Whitehead, C., & Crotty, M. (2018). An overview of systematic reviews of pharmacological and non-pharmacological interventions for the treatment of behavioral and psychological symptoms of dementia. *International Psychogeriatrics, 30*, 295–309. https://doi.org/10.1017/S1041610217002344

Earhart, C. A. (2006). *Allen Diagnostic Module: Manual* (2nd ed.). Colchester, CT: S&S Worldwide.

Family Caregiver Alliance. (2011). *Ten real-life strategies for dementia caregiving.* Retrieved from https://www.caregiver.org/ten-real-life-strategies-dementia-caregiving

Fauth, E. B., Femia, E. E., & Zarit, S. H. (2016). Resistiveness to care during assistance with activities of daily living in non-institutionalized persons with dementia: Associations with informal caregivers'

stress and well-being. *Aging and Mental Health, 20*, 888–898. https://doi.org/10.1080/13607863.2015.1049114

Gitlin, L. N., Cigliana, J., Cigliana, K., & Pappa, K. (2017). Supporting family caregivers of persons with dementia in the community: Description of the "Memory Care Home Solutions" Program and its impacts. *Innovation in Aging, 1*, igx013. https://doi.org/10.1093/geroni/igx013

Gitlin, L. N., & Hodgson, N. (2015). Caregivers as therapeutic agents in dementia care: The evidence base for interventions supporting their role. In J. Gaugler & R. Kane (Eds.), *Family caregiving in the new normal* (pp. 305–353). Philadelphia: Elsevier. https://doi.org/10.1016/B978-0-12-417046-9.00017-9

Gitlin, L. N., Hodgson, N. A., & Choi, S. S. W. (2016). Home-based interventions targeting persons with dementia: What is the evidence and where do we go from here? In M. Boltz & J. Galvin (Eds.), *Dementia care: An evidence-based approach* (pp. 167–188). New York: Springer. https://doi.org/10.1007/978-3-319-18377-0_11

Gitlin, L. N., & Rose, K. (2014). Factors associated with caregiver readiness to use nonpharmacologic strategies to manage dementia-related behavioral symptoms. *International Journal of Geriatric Psychiatry, 29*, 93–102. https://doi.org/10.1002/gps.3979

Gitlin, L. N., Winter, L., Dennis, M. P., Hodgson, N., & Hauck, W. W. (2010a). A biobehavioral home-based intervention and the well-being of patients with dementia and their caregivers: The COPE randomized trial. *JAMA, 304*, 983–991. https://doi.org/10.1001/jama.2010.1253

Gitlin, L. N., Winter, L., Dennis, M. P., Hodgson, N., & Hauck, W. W. (2010b). Targeting and managing behavioral symptoms in individuals with dementia: A randomized trial of a nonpharmacological intervention. *Journal of the American Geriatrics Society, 58*, 1465–1474. https://doi.org/10.1111/j.1532-5415.2010.02971.x

Gitlin, L. N., Winter, L., Earland, T. V., Herge, A., Chernett, N. L., Piersol, C. V., & Burke, J. P. (2009). The Tailored Activity Program to reduce behavioral symptoms in individuals with dementia: Feasibility, acceptability, and replication potential. *Gerontologist, 49*(3), 428–439. https://doi.org/10.1093/geront/gnp087

Jensen, L., & Padilla, R. (2011). Effectiveness of interventions to prevent falls in people with Alzheimer's disease and related disorders. *American Journal of Occupational Therapy, 65*, 532–540. https://doi.org/10.5014/ajot.2011.002626

Kojima, G., Liljas, A., Iliffe, S., & Walters, K. (2017). Prevalence of frailty in mild to moderate Alzheimer's disease: A systematic review and meta-analysis. *Current Alzheimer Research, 14*, 1256–1263. https://doi.org/10.2174/1567205014666170417104236

Levy, L. L. (1986). A practical guide to the care of the Alzheimer's disease victim: The cognitive disability perspective. *Topics in Geriatric Rehabilitation, 1*, 16–26. https://doi.org/10.1097/00013614-198601000-00006

Levy, L. L. (2018). Neurocognition and function: Intervention in dementia based on the Cognitive Disabilities Model. In N. Katz & J. Toglia (Eds.), *Cognition, occupation, and participation across the lifespan: Neuroscience, neurorehabilitation, and models of intervention in occupational therapy* (4th ed., pp. 499–522). Bethesda, MD: AOTA Press.

Levy, L. L., & Burns, T. (2011). The Cognitive Disabilities Reconsidered Model: Rehabilitation of adults with dementia. In N. Katz (Ed.), *Cognition, occupation, and participation across the life span: Neuroscience, neurorehabilitation, and models of intervention in occupational therapy* (3rd ed., pp. 407–441). Bethesda, MD: AOTA Press.

McCraith, D. B., Austin, S. L., & Earhart, C. A. (2011). The Cognitive Disabilities Model in 2011. In N. Katz (Ed.), *Cognition, occupation, and participation across the life span: Neuroscience, neurorehabilitation, and models of intervention in occupational therapy* (3rd ed., pp. 383–406). Bethesda, MD: AOTA Press.

McCraith, D. B., & Earhart, C. A. (2018). Cognitive Disabilities Model: Creating fit between functional cognitive abilities and cognitive activity demands. In N. Katz & J. Toglia (Eds.), *Cognition, occupation, and participation across the lifespan: Neuroscience, neurorehabilitation, and models of intervention in occupational therapy* (4th ed., pp. 469–497). Bethesda, MD: AOTA Press.

Mukherjee, A., Biswas, A., Roy, A., Biswas, S., Gangopadhyay, G., & Das, S. K. (2017). Behavioural and psychological symptoms of dementia: Correlates and impact on caregiver distress. *Dementia and Geriatric Cognitive Disorders, 7,* 354–365. https://doi.org/10.1159/000481568

Piersol, C. V., Herge, E. A., Copolillo, A. E., Leiby, B. E., & Gitlin, L. N. (2016). Psychometric properties of the Functional Capacity Card Sort for caregivers of people with dementia. *OTJR: Occupation, Participation and Health, 36,* 126–133. https://doi.org/10.1177/1539449216666063

Pimouguet, C., Le Goff, M., Wittwer, J., Dartigues, J. F., & Helmer, C. (2017). Benefits of occupational therapy in dementia patients: Findings from a real-world observational study. *Journal of Alzheimer's Disease, 56,* 509–517. https://doi.org/10.3233/JAD-160820

Reisberg, B., Ferris, S. H., De Leon, M. J., & Crook, T. (1982). The Global Deterioration Scale for assessment of primary degenerative dementia. *American Journal of Psychiatry, 139,* 1136–1139. https://doi.org/10.1176/ajp.139.9.1136

Reisberg, B., Franssen, E. H., Souren, L. E., Auer, S. R., Akram, I., & Kenowsky, S. (2002). Evidence and mechanisms of retrogenesis in Alzheimer's and other dementias: Management and treatment import. *American Journal of Alzheimer's Disease and Other Dementias, 17,* 202–212. https://doi.org/10.1177/153331750201700411

Reisberg, B., Kenowsky, S., Franssen, E. H., Auer, S. R., & Souren, L. E. (1999). Towards a science of Alzheimer's disease management: A model based upon current knowledge of retrogenesis. *International Psychogeriatrics, 11,* 7–23. https://doi.org/10.1017/S1041610299005554

Ryu, S. H., Jung, H. Y., Lee, K. J., Moon, S. W., Lee, D. W., Hong, N., . . . Lee, C. U. (2017). Incidence and course of depression in patients with Alzheimer's disease. *Psychiatry Investigation, 14,* 271–280. https://doi.org/10.4306/pi.2017.14.3.271

Sclan, S. G., & Reisberg, B. (1992). Functional Assessment Staging (FAST) in Alzheimer's disease: Reliability, validity, and ordinality. *International Psychogeriatrics, 4*(Suppl. 1), 55–69. https://doi.org/10.1017/S1041610292001157

Schaber, P., Klein, T., Hanrahan, E., Vencil, P., Afatika, K., & Burns, T. (2013). Using cognitive–functional assessment to predict self-care performance of memory care tenants. *American Journal of Alzheimer's Disease and Other Dementias, 28,* 171–178. https://doi.org/10.1177/1533317512470206

Schaber, P., Stallings, E., Brogan, C., & Ali, F. (2016). Interrater reliability of the revised Cognitive Performance Test (CPT): Assessing cognition in people with neurocognitive disorders. *American Journal of Occupational Therapy, 70,* 70052900110. http://doi.org/10.5014/ajot.2016.019166

Smallfield, S., & Heckenlaible, C. (2017). Effectiveness of occupational therapy interventions to enhance occupational performance for adults with Alzheimer's disease and related major neurocognitive disorders: A systematic review. *American Journal of Occupational Therapy, 71,* 7105180010. https://doi.org/10.5014/ajot.2017.024752

Struckmeyer, L. R. & Pickens, N. D. (2016). Home modifications for people with Alzheimer's disease: A scoping review. *American Journal of Occupational Therapy, 70,* 7001270020. https://doi.org/10.5014/ajot.2015.016089

Teri, L., Truax, P., Logsdon, R., Uomoto, J., Zarit, S., & Vitaliano, P. P. (1992). Assessment of behavioral problems in dementia: The Revised Memory and Behavior Problems Checklist. *Psychology and Aging, 7,* 622–631. https://doi.org/10.1037/0882-7974.7.4.622

Zhu, C. W., Scarmeas, N., Ornstein, K., Albert, M., Brandt, J., Blacker, D., . . . Stern, Y. (2015). Health-care use and cost in dementia caregivers: Longitudinal results from the Predictors Caregiver Study. *Alzheimer's and Dementia, 11,* 444–454. https://doi.org/10.1016/j.jalz.2013.12.018

Appendix: Case Examples

Case examples are adapted from "Cognition, Cognitive Rehabilitation, and Occupational Performance," by the American Occupational Therapy Association, 2019, *American Journal of Occupational Therapy*. Copyright © 2019 by the American Occupational Therapy Association. Adapted with permission.

Introduction

This appendix presents 2 case examples that were developed to help illustrate the entire process of using a functional–cognitive approach with clients as outlined in this text. The case examples were adapted from the American Occupational Therapy Association's (2019) official statement on cognition and are also consistent with the content of that statement. The two case examples involve

1. A client with a mild stroke, and

2. A client with major neurocognitive disorder related to Alzheimer's disease.

These cases were selected to illustrate how the general approach to addressing functional cognition discussed in this text can be applied to individuals with very different neurological impairments. Each case is approached from the perspective of functional cognition. However, because of the unique circumstances of each case (e.g., different types of neurological injury, varying prognoses and occupational history), the occupational therapist in each case selected different assessments and used different intervention approaches to help maximize functional–cognitive ability for each client.

CASE EXAMPLE A.1. Client With Mild Stroke: Combined Problem-Solving and Task-Specific Approach

Background

Martha is a 65-year-old woman and an experienced circuit court judge. She lives in a suburban community with her husband. She has 3 children and 3 grandchildren younger than 5 years old. One month ago, Martha fell down a flight of stairs in her home and has not been able to resume work. Before the fall, Martha provided care for her grandchildren and traveled frequently for both work and pleasure.

Symptoms and Complaints

Since her fall, Martha has felt dizzy and fatigued and has reported physical, cognitive, and emotional challenges. She says that it takes her more effort to smile and make facial expressions and that her speech is less clear, especially when she is tired. She reports difficulty picking up and not dropping items, such as her hairbrush, during functional tasks. She states that she used to enjoy spending time with her grandchildren, but now she feels impatient and intolerant with them. During a recent work trip, Martha lost track of time while having a meal at the airport and missed her flight.

Medical Evaluation and Referral to Occupational Therapy

The consulting neurologist working with Martha informed her that her magnetic resonance imaging scan showed that she had a mild stroke, due to a clot in her right anterior cerebral artery, which damaged the middle region of her right frontal lobe. This accounted for her mild facial weakness, dysarthria, and mild weakness in her left hand.

(Continued)

The neurologist recommended that Martha take more time to rest before returning to work. He also referred her to outpatient occupational therapy, which is where her assessment took place and her treatment plan was developed.

Occupational Profile and Screening

The **occupational therapist** conducted an informal interview with Martha and her husband and concluded that Martha was aware of her deficits. Martha revealed that she found situations that were out of her control to be the most difficult: "I don't like not knowing what is going to happen. I lose my cool, and that is when I make mistakes." According to Martha and her family, these errors were new and seemed to be a consequence of her stroke.

The occupational therapist used the Canadian Occupational Performance Measure (COPM; Law et al., 2014) to identify Martha's priorities for treatment. The Activity Card Sort (Baum & Edwards, 2008) revealed that Martha retained only 80% of her usual activities since her stroke. Among the activities she had given up were eating in restaurants, playing golf, dancing, going to parties and picnics, playing with her grandchildren, and doing laundry and yard work. Table A.1 gives an overview of Martha's COPM scores. COPM scores range from 1 to 10, with a score of 1 indicating least or worst, and 10 indicating highest or best.

The occupational therapist completed the Montreal Cognitive Assessment (MoCA; Nasreddine et al., 2005) with Martha, and she scored a 30 out of 30. This would be expected given her current functional status as well as her level of education. The results of the MoCA, in conjunction with the results from the occupational profile, do not indicate any concern with performance-based testing for Martha.

Performance-Based Testing

On the basis of Martha's occupational profile, the occupational therapist chose the Complex Task Performance Assessment (CTPA; Wolf et al., 2008; see Chapter 10), a multitasking work-related assessment, as a performance-based test for administration. Two of Martha's goals involved a high level of multitasking, and work was also 1 of her highest rated activities on the COPM. The CTPA requires high-level multitasking and overlaps with Martha's goals.

On the CTPA, Martha did not complete 2 of the prospective memory tasks. She also had multiple inefficiencies (e.g., not sorting the cards before starting the calculations) as well as rule breaks (e.g., she continued to talk to the examiner and ask questions throughout the assessment). Martha also had some difficulty with some of the fine-motor tasks (e.g., filling in the inventory control sheet while completing the assessment). Martha was, however, aware of her deficits and was able to articulate clearly to the occupational therapist what her difficulties were after she completed the assessment.

The occupational therapist also assessed Martha with the Performance Assessment of Self-Care Skills (PASS; Rogers et al., 2016; see Chapter 12), a performance-based test of IADLs. Two of Martha's goals focused on taking

TABLE A.1. Martha's COPM Results

ACTIVITY	IMPORTANCE SCORE	PERFORMANCE SCORE	SATISFACTION SCORE
Taking care of grandkids	10	6	2
Multitasking activities (e.g., cooking)	9	6	2
Returning to work as a judge	10	7	3
Taking care of house	8	7	4

Note. COPM scores range from 1 to 10, with a score of 1 indicating *least or worst*, and 10 indicating *highest or best*. COPM = Canadian Occupational Performance Measure.

(Continued)

care of her house and completing multitasking activities, such as cooking. The occupational therapist assessed Martha using the changing bed linens (heavy housework), sweeping (home maintenance), and meal preparation (oven use, stovetop use, use of sharp utensils) tasks of the PASS. All the selected tasks focused on physical (changing bed linens, sweeping) and cognitive (meal preparation) IADLs.

Martha was able to perform both the changing bed linens and the sweeping tasks of the PASS with verbal support (both nondirective and directive), and she had 1 safety concern while completing the sweeping task. She demonstrated decreased quality while performing both tasks, mostly because of decreased upper extremity strength, coordination, and fine-motor skills and frustration with her inability to complete the tasks without mistakes.

Martha was able to perform the meal preparation tasks with verbal assistance (both nondirective and directive) and needed gestures as well as task-rearrangement assistance to perform some of the subtasks of the task. She also had a couple of safety concerns that the occupational therapist noted: Martha reached inside the oven without an oven mitt and left the towel on the stove while cooking soup on the stovetop. Martha had adequacy problems, mainly because of her left-hand weakness and her frustration with the demands of the tasks at different times during the performance of the tasks.

Goal Setting

On the basis of Martha's occupational therapy evaluation, the occupational therapist determined that a direct-intervention, strategy-based approach would be the most appropriate to help Martha improve her functional–cognitive ability during complex IADL tasks. The therapist selected the Cognitive Orientation to daily Occupational Performance Approach (CO–OP; Polatajko & Mandich, 2004; see Chapter 19) to address Martha's long-term (1-month) goals, which were to

- Be proficient at applying a global Goal–Plan–Do–Check (GPDC) strategy to complex IADL tasks,
- Use GPDC to identify 3 strategies to improve her ability to complete cooking activities independently, and
- Use GPDC to identify 3 strategies to improve her ability to complete work and scheduling activities independently.

Intervention Approach

The goal-setting and problem-solving approach (i.e., CO–OP) aimed to empower Martha to use a specific problem-solving framework to develop, with the occupational therapy practitioner's guidance, her own self-training program. Appropriate steps for problem-solving training include

- Problem orientation, definition, and formulation;
- Generation of alternatives;
- Decision making; and
- Solution verification.

Task-specific training requires task analysis and a graded approach as the client accomplishes sequential tasks.

Using both training methods, Martha accomplished her goal to improve her cooking ability by identifying specific aspects of cooking that caused her to feel stressed and frustrated. Martha was encouraged to define the problem (e.g., "When I leave 1 task and forget to come back, I feel anxious and frustrated."). She then identified strategies she could try to help her remember where she left off (e.g., use timers, limit how many things she is cooking at 1 time, prepare portions of meals in stages).

With practice, Martha improved at self-monitoring and needed her husband's assistance less. With the encouragement and guidance of the occupational therapy practitioner, Martha used GPDC to help her identify the use of timers as the primary strategy she would use when cooking. Martha also developed plans using GPDC to address work-related tasks, such as different ways to keep her schedule for work or new ways to take notes to help her remember things discussed at work.

CASE EXAMPLE A.2. Client With Alzheimer's Disease: Task- and Environmental-Modification Approach

Background

Raymond is a 79-year-old man who lives with his wife, **Dorothy,** in a rural community. Raymond and Dorothy have lived in the same house for 42 years, where they raised 5 children. They have made few upgrades to the home, so all the bedrooms and the only full bath are on the 2nd floor (clawfoot tub only).

Medical Evaluation and Referral to Occupational Therapy

The event that first led to medical evaluation occurred 1 year ago, when Raymond became lost when driving to a neighboring town and ended up 150 miles beyond his intended destination. A state trooper helped him when his car ran out of gas, and Raymond was returned home to a worried Dorothy. Subsequently, Raymond was diagnosed with Alzheimer's disease (AD), and over the following year his symptoms progressed, triggering a referral to occupational therapy by Raymond's internist.

Occupational Profile and Screening

Dorothy responded to most of the questions at the initial interview, with Raymond responding only when questioned directly. She reported that Raymond required assistance for self-care tasks, although he remained independent with feeding and toileting. Dorothy completed the Functional Behavior Profile (Baum et al., 1993), which provides caregivers with a method of describing the impaired person's capabilities in performing tasks, engaging in social interactions, and solving problems. It was developed to guide practitioners in planning treatment, documenting change, and identifying helpful community resources. Dorothy reported that Raymond could follow 1-step commands and that he positively engaged in social activities in quiet settings with small groups of family or friends. Dorothy also completed the informant version of the Activity Card Sort (Baum & Edwards, 2008). Although Raymond had given up many instrumental and high-demand leisure activities, this assessment helped Dorothy identify leisure and social activities they could do together, such as going for walks, playing card games, and going to church (Baum, 1995).

The Revised Memory and Behavior Problems Checklist (RMBPC; Teri et al., 1992) allowed Dorothy to identify which of Raymond's behaviors were most frustrating to her. This 27-item scale provides a total score as well as scores for 3 subscales: Memory-Related Problems, Affective Distress, and Disruptive Behaviors. Scores are computed first for the presence or absence of each problem and then for caregivers' "reaction" or the extent to which caregivers were "bothered" or "distressed" by each behavior.

On the RMBPC, Dorothy indicated that Raymond was often agitated at night and that she was getting very little sleep. She was also frustrated by his repetitive questions. The RMBPC results provided an opportunity for the occupational therapist to help Dorothy gain a better understanding of how AD affects behavior and the importance of seeking support for herself as well as the types of respite services available in their community.

Raymond owned his own furniture repair business before retiring, and until about 3 months ago he was able to make simple repairs around the house or in his workshop. Dorothy did not feel it was currently safe for him to work unsupervised. Raymond no longer drove or did home chores and was angry about these losses. Dorothy said he was easily angered and bored. She was concerned that he "sits around the house all day and does nothing." Dorothy wanted to help her husband, so she had given up activities she enjoyed. The occupational therapist was concerned about role overload for Dorothy.

Performance-Based Testing

Direct observation of Raymond in his workshop and assessment with the Cognitive Performance Test (Burns, 2018; see Chapter 14) provided findings for symptoms consistent with the moderate stage of AD and difficulties

(Continued)

CASE EXAMPLE A.2. Client With Alzheimer's Disease: Task- and Environmental-Modification Approach *(Cont.)*

completing detailed tasks, consistent with Raymond's need for assistance with most IADLs and supervision and setup for ADLs (Burns, 2018). The occupational therapist also administered the following:

- *Geriatric Depression Scale (Yesavage & Sheikh, 1986):* Raymond's score indicated that he should visit his physician for diagnostic testing for possible major depressive disorder.
- *Safety Assessment of Function and the Environment for Rehabilitation–Health Outcome Measurement and Evaluation (Chiu et al., 2006):* Safety issues were moderate and were isolated primarily to lighting and bathroom issues.

Goal Setting

Dorothy and the occupational therapist, with input from Raymond, agreed on the following goals:

- Through use of environmental and verbal cueing, Raymond would
  - Dress and bathe independently on 5 of 7 days,
  - Complete simple home chores with distant supervision, and
  - Assemble simple wooden kits with distant supervision.
- Raymond would engage in desired activities, with no more than 1 agitated outburst per week.

Intervention Approach

The intervention used environmental modification and task simplification during self-care, leisure, and work activities. The occupational therapist helped the couple set a daily routine and instructed Dorothy about how to interact with Raymond to provide a calming atmosphere.

The occupational therapist proposed 6 visits per month (twice weekly for 2 weeks, once weekly for 2 weeks), followed by a reevaluation. In collaboration with Dorothy, the therapist worked with Raymond to determine the types of cueing that worked best to support his occupational performance. The overall approach was to support his retained procedural memory with cues (e.g., lists or other types of instructions, placement of objects, verbal instruction).

Interventions included the following:

- *Daily routine:* The development of a daily routine with activities occurring at specific times provided both Dorothy and Raymond with a structure for the day.
- *Verbal cueing:* To avoid conflict, the occupational therapist taught Dorothy to use implicit guiding by setting up the environment and making appropriate activity choices. When explicit guidance was needed, Dorothy was taught to provide instructions 1 step at a time in a neutral voice.
- *Task simplification:* Dorothy and Raymond learned to choose simple activities or to modify existing activities so they involved few steps and reduced opportunities for errors.

References

American Occupational Therapy Association. (2019). Cognition, cognitive rehabilitation, and occupational performance. *American Journal of Occupational Therapy.*

Baum, C. (1995). The contribution of occupation to function in persons with Alzheimer's disease. *Journal of Occupational Science, 2*(2), 59–67. https://doi.org/10.1080/14427591.1995.9686396

Baum, C., & Edwards, D. F. (2008). *Activity Card Sort* (2nd ed.). Bethesda, MD: AOTA Press.

Baum, C., Edwards, D. F., & Morrow-Howell, N. (1993). Identification and measurement of productive behaviors in senile dementia of the Alzheimer type. *Gerontologist, 33,* 403–408.

Burns, T. (2018). *Cognitive Performance Test Revised manual.* Pequannock, NJ: Maddak.

Chiu, T., Oliver, R., Ascott, P., Choo, L., Davis, T., Gaya, A., & Letts, L. (2006). *Safety Assessment of Function and the Environment for Rehabilitation–Health Outcome Measurement and Evaluation (SAFER–HOME), Version 3.* Toronto: COTA Health.

Law, M., Baptiste, S., Carswell, A., McColl, M. A., Polatajko, H., & Pollock, N. (2014). *Canadian Occupational Performance Measure* (5th ed.). Ottawa: CAOT Publications.

Nasreddine, Z. S., Phillips, N. A., Bédirian, V., Charbonneau, S., Whitehead, V., Collin, I., . . . Chertkow, H. (2005). The Montreal Cognitive Assessment, MoCA: A brief screening tool for mild cognitive impairment. *Journal of the American Geriatrics Society, 53,* 695–699. https://doi.org/10.1111/j.1532-5415.2005.53221.x

Polatajko, H., & Mandich, A. (2004). *Enabling occupation in children: The Cognitive Orientation to daily Occupational Performance (CO–OP) Approach.* Ottawa: CAOT Publications.

Rogers, J. C., Holm, M. B., & Chisholm, D. (2016). *Performance Assessment of Self-Care Skills—Version 4.1.* Pittsburgh: University of Pittsburgh.

Teri, L., Truax, P., Logsdon, R., Uomoto, J., Zarit, S., & Vitaliano, P. P. (1992). Assessment of behavioral problems in dementia: The Revised Memory and Behavior Problems Checklist. *Psychology and Aging, 7,* 622–631.

Wolf, T. J., Morrison, T., & Matheson, L. (2008). Initial development of a work-related assessment of dysexecutive syndrome: The Complex Task Performance Assessment. *Work, 31,* 221–228.

Yesavage, J. A., & Sheikh, J. I. (1986). Geriatric Depression Scale (GDS): Recent evidence and development of a shorter version. *Clinical Gerontologist: Journal of Aging and Mental Health, 5,* 165–173. https://doi.org/10.1300/J018v05n01_09

Index

Note. Page numbers in *italic* indicate exhibits, figures, tables, and boxed material.